I0043919

THE WHY BEHIND

WILDERNESS MEDICINE

ESSENTIAL KNOWLEDGE FOR GUIDES & WILDERNESS RESPONDERS

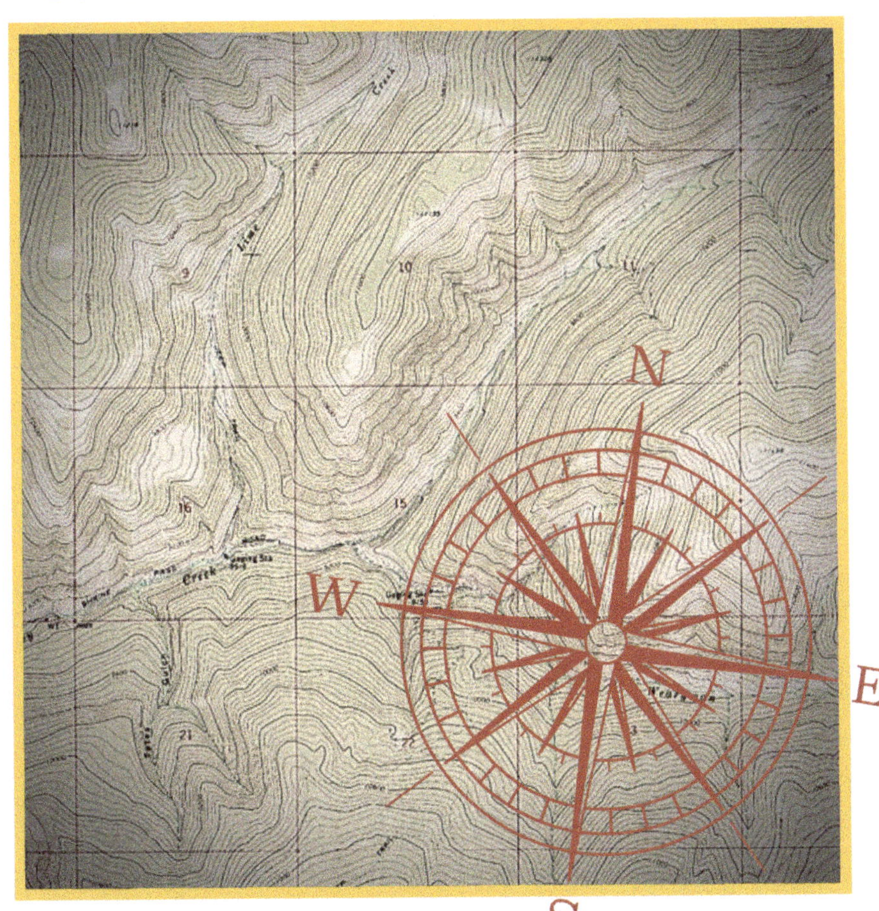

CAPT. JASON MOORE, PhD, PA.

The Why Behind Wilderness Medicine

MILTON & HUGO L.L.C.
4407 Park Ave., Suite 5
Union City, NJ 07087, USA

Website: *www. miltonandhugo.com*
Hotline: *1- 888-778-0033*
Email: *info@miltonandhugo.com*

Ordering Information:
Quantity sales. Special discounts are granted to corporations, associations, and other organizations. For more information on these discounts, please reach out to the publisher using the contact information provided above.

Library of Congress Control Number:		2025919113
ISBN-13:	979-8-89285-438-2	[Paperback Edition]
	979-8-89285-439-9	[Hardback Edition]
	979-8-89285-440-5	[Digital Edition]

Rev. date: 09/12/2025

Wilderness is not a luxury but a necessity of the human spirit.

—Edward Abbey (*Desert Solitaire*, 1968)

Contents

Acknowledgments

This project reflects decades of learning, collaboration, and the support of countless individuals who have profoundly influenced my career, my passion for guiding, and my understanding of medicine. To each of you, I owe my deepest gratitude.

To my mentors, colleagues, and collaborators—thank you for the expertise, the lessons, and the laughs. Drs. Franciose, Lawrence, Downey, Hammaker, E.E. Moore, Johnson, Hearne, Wenzel, Podgorney, Kamper, Gaul, Hackett, Dent, McNeill, Heick, Dowdy, Bernard, Coleman, Pavlick, Knudson, and Fischione are just a few of the many who shaped my training in surgery, medicine, and research—and who taught me what it truly means to care for patients.

To the nurses, respiratory therapists, pharmacists, physical and occupational therapists, EMTs, paramedics, SAR teams, ski patrollers, firefighters, and law enforcement officers—who have quite literally saved my ass, and likely that of my patients, more than once—thank you for always having my back.

Special thanks to Sean, Eric, Freddie, Gary, Chip, Caretto, and to the tribe of guides who share a passion for wilderness and adventure. Your wisdom, camaraderie, and commitment to connecting people with the natural world have shaped this work—and my life—in more ways than I can count. I'm deeply grateful.

To Zoe and Jezzy—always ready for the next adventure, always by my side, always in my heart.

To my wonderful family and friends, who have stood by me through every challenge and triumph—thanks and love.

To Guzman Martinez and Marie Parker—thank you for your support throughout the editing and publication process.

Ashley—your support, encouragement, and partnership are everything. This book would not exist without you.

Why This Book

Welcome to the book I've long wanted to write. Over the past 25 years, I've worked as a guide, educator, researcher, and clinician. My path has taken me across all four hemispheres—through mountains, deserts, jungles, rivers, and oceans. I've rowed a raft through the Himalaya, slept in the sand of the Sahara, and built Island Fly to guide serious anglers in some of the best fisheries on the planet. These experiences have shaped how I think, teach, lead—and how I move through the world.

This book is for guides, wilderness responders, expedition leaders, and anyone working in remote settings. It won't focus much on complex techniques or equipment—there are already excellent resources that do, and in true wilderness settings far from care, advanced procedures rarely change outcomes.

While I have deep respect for herbalists, naturopaths, survivalists, and indigenous healers, this isn't a survivalist manual or a guide to traditional remedies. Where treatments are discussed, I've focused on what's commonly taught in wilderness responder courses or found in base camps, fishing lodges, or the kitchen box on a multi-day river trip. The book focuses on the principles and science that shape decision-making in the field—the "why" behind adventure medicine: why certain calls are made; why some risks aren't worth taking; and why real improvisation relies on a deep understanding of how the body responds to stress, illness, and injury.

This book assumes a baseline familiarity with core medical concepts on the part of the reader and is meant to supplement that knowledge, not replace it. The structure is based on questions I've asked over the years; and the ones that have come from students, colleagues, guests, and fellow guides. It covers topics often left out of standard training, including the guiding philosophy, women's health, psychiatric emergencies, and the medical realities of remote care. Scattered throughout are real cases from my own experiences—situations that pushed past protocol and forced improvisation in places far from help.

Wilderness medicine isn't just a guiding skillset—it's a foundation built on knowledge, experience, and judgment that gives guides the confidence to lead with clarity—even in the face of uncertainty.

What follows is my gift to you—lessons learned through experience; some mistakes; and the wisdom of mentors, colleagues, and clients. I hope it gives you the tools and perspective to lead not only with competence—but with intention, clarity, and respect for the places and people you meet along the way.

Enjoy.

sjm

Disclaimer

This book is not a substitute for formal medical training, clinical supervision, or professional judgment. Wilderness medicine is inherently situational, and no single resource can account for the variables present in remote environments. What works in one setting may be unsafe in another.

Medical practices evolve. As Samuel Arbesman notes in *The Half-Life of Facts*, "Many medical schools inform their students that within several years *half* of what they've been taught will be wrong, and the teachers just don't know which half." While this book aims to provide accurate and current information, readers are responsible for verifying details through appropriate medical direction and current clinical guidelines. All medical decisions, including the use of medications or interventions, must be guided by proper education, training, experience, and professional oversight.

Medication discussions are provided for educational purposes only and do not constitute medical advice or authorization for unsupervised use. Understanding indications, contraindications, and limitations is essential. When uncertain, seek qualified medical guidance.

All care provided in wilderness settings must fall within the responder's scope of training and available resources. This book is intended to inform—not to prescribe or direct care. Readers must use their own judgment, prepare appropriately, and recognize their limits.

A Guide's Perspective

The Realities of Connection, Responsibility, and Risk

Who is this book written for?

The *Why Behind Wilderness Medicine* is written for guides, trip leaders, wilderness responders, healthcare professionals, or anyone who finds themselves leading or safeguarding others in remote environments. It speaks to those who shoulder responsibility when medical resources are distant, delayed, or unavailable. This project assumes a working understanding of basic medical concepts on the part of the reader and aims to deepen both knowledge and judgment—skills that matter when conditions are far from ideal.

In full transparency, I recognize that this book can't be truly comprehensive or universally applicable. Some topics are too complex to cover entirely, and others may require additional study to fully grasp. Oversimplifying them would sacrifice scientific accuracy and nuance. That focus on depth over simplicity is intentional. Medical knowledge is always evolving, and so is the ability to apply it in the field. Some sections may challenge you, push you to revisit unfamiliar material, or reframe how you approach problems you've seen before. That's the point. Wilderness medicine demands critical thinking, adaptability, and a working grasp of physiology, pathology, and improvisation.

What makes a guide great?

True greatness in guiding goes beyond technical skill, logistics, or even leadership. It lies in the deeper appreciation for what guiding really is: a responsibility not just for the trip, but for the experience itself. A great guide understands that they are entrusted with something much bigger than logistics—they are building connection, trust, and meaning in wild places where comfort and certainty do not exist.

Not to wax poetic, but guiding isn't just about where you take guests or what you do—it's just as much about what they take away from the experience. It's more than technical skill and safety checks—it's connection and responsibility. Guiding means building relationships—with the landscape you move through, the people you lead, and, ultimately, yourself. The discipline runs deeper than logistics; it sits at the intersection of safety, challenge, and growth.

A great guide understands both the physical and psychological needs of the group. It's not just about getting people from point A to point B, climbing a mountain, catching a fish, or skiing a ridge—it's about reading their strengths and limitations, adjusting the experience to match their abilities, and creating something that's not just safe but deeply fulfilling. Equally important is self-awareness—knowing your own limits, recognizing when to push and when to pull back, and staying grounded in the purpose that brought you here in the first place.

Guiding is also about respect—for the environment, for local cultures, and for the individuals who put their trust in you. A guide is both a steward and a bridge—connecting people to the wild, to each other, and to something bigger than themselves.

How much of guiding is about mindset?

More than most people realize, a guide is the stabilizing force in any emergency. That doesn't just mean providing care—it means controlling the environment, setting the tone, and leading with clarity even when things feel uncertain.

Fear, doubt, and hesitation are normal; but they don't change what needs to be done. What defines a guide is how they act.

Mindset starts long before a crisis—with preparation that is as much mental as it is physical. It begins with how you approach the trip, how you plan, and how you think about risk. Medical readiness means tailoring your kit to the group, the environment, and the duration of the trip. It also means knowing your clients. Anticipation is a core skill of effective leadership. The guides who think ahead are the ones who prevent problems before they happen.

In an emergency, people follow your lead. Your mannerisms, tone of voice, and behavior shape the group's response. Panic spreads—so does calm. If you project confidence and control, your group will respond in kind. Your job isn't just treating the patient; it's keeping the group steady, occupied, informed—or simply out of the way. Your ability to assess, prioritize, and lead under pressure determines how the story ends. No one knows what you were feeling. They remember what you did.

Does any of this *really* matter for a guide?

Nope. Until it does—and then it matters more than anything else. Most days, even full seasons, it won't. But when it happens, it sticks—with you, and with your patient—for life. Trust me. Properly handled emergencies build reputations for excellence—for guides, outfitters, and lodges alike. The flipside of this conversation is never good, and if you're lucky, it only ends with a bad review or a damaged reputation. Sometimes it doesn't. Sometimes it follows you, and leads to hard conversations with outfitters, owners, and even lawyers. Remember, when things go sideways, guests rarely remember the hunting, fishing, or skiing—they remember how you handled their worst moments.

That's why I encourage you to go further—further than you think you need to. Read more. Take classes. Learn from others. There are more tools than ever—courses, podcasts, social media. Embrace them. Treat guiding as a profession, not just a job. A medical emergency can define your career—one way or the other. Preparation, planning, and training matter. These moments aren't scheduled—but your preparation certainly can be.

You can't predict everything—so how do you prepare?

You won't always have the answers. Wilderness medicine lives in the gray—between what you were taught and what's actually in front of you. Things go wrong. Conditions shift. Patients rarely follow the script. In that space, improvisation becomes essential—but not in the way most people think. It's not about cleverness or quick fixes. It's about understanding. "The eyes can only see what the mind knows." Most people see a pile of rocks; a paleontologist sees a fossil. You can't improvise a solution if you don't recognize the problem—and you won't recognize the problem if you've never learned it exists.

This book isn't about expanding your kit. It's about building the kind of understanding that makes gear secondary. When you know how the body works, how it breaks down, and how the environment affects both—you're adapting with intent. That's what real improvisation looks like: drawing on core knowledge when it matters most.

Perception vs. Reality: Understanding Risk

Is the wilderness riskier than daily life?

Risk is unavoidable—whether crossing a street, driving to work, or stepping into the wilderness. The difference is in how we perceive it. Familiar risks—like walking through a city—feel routine, even though they carry real danger. Meanwhile, the unpredictability of the wilderness often feels more hazardous, even when the actual risk is no greater than daily life.

This disconnect between perception and reality is where guides must lead with knowledge and preparation. A shifting weather system, a medical emergency, or a navigation error can create a heightened sense of danger, even if the actual risk is manageable with proper preparation. Understanding this gap in perception allows guides to make better decisions, educate their clients, and maintain control in difficult situations.

How do guides manage risk?

A competent guide minimizes risk before the trip even begins. Proper training, preparation, and adaptability ensure that challenges become manageable obstacles rather than emergencies.

- *Mindset and Mental Readiness* - Your ability to stay calm, think clearly, and manage stress before it manages you determines how effectively you lead. Panic is contagious—so is confidence.
- *Training and Knowledge* - Wilderness medicine, navigation, rescue techniques, and activity-specific skills aren't just useful—they're essential. Personality and a certain degree of leadership skill may be natural; but true expertise is built through education, training, and experience.
- *Preparation and Planning* - Risk is reduced before stepping into the field. Thorough gear checks, contingency planning, and understanding the environment allow for flexibility when conditions change. A prepared guide anticipates problems before they arise.
- *Physical Readiness* - Strength, stamina, and mental resilience are just as important as technical skill. A guide must assist clients, navigate difficult terrain, and remain sharp under stress. The ability to function in extreme conditions and make critical decisions after long hours is critical.
- *Equipment Familiarity* - Reliable gear prevents minor issues from escalating. Well-maintained, field-tested equipment—including medical supplies, navigation tools, and protective clothing—must match the environment and the demands of the trip. A guide

should be intimately familiar with their gear, knowing its limitations and how to adapt when things break, or supplies run low.

- *Client Awareness and Management* - Your group is part of the risk equation. Understanding their experience levels, medical concerns, and expectations allows you to adapt your approach and keep them engaged rather than overwhelmed. Clear communication builds trust and turns clients into assets rather than liabilities.
- *Adaptability and Decision-Making* – No plan survives first contact with the wilderness. Weather shifts, injuries happen, and conditions change without warning. The ability to think clearly, adjust strategies, and make sound decisions in real time is what separates competent guides from exceptional ones.

Can risk ever be eliminated?

Nope. Wilderness guiding isn't about eliminating risk—it's about preparing for it. The more you refine your skills, anticipate challenges, and control what you can, the better you'll handle what you can't. Uncertainty becomes something you manage, not something you fear. Preparation doesn't remove risk—but it lines up your bullets for when it matters.

What does it mean to "line up your bullets"?

One of my early guide trainers, Gary—affectionally known as "G5"—had a saying: "Line up your bullets." The idea was simple: Control what you can—so when the uncontrollable shows up, you're ready. Just like bullets lined up on a cartridge belt in the Old West, preparedness means having your mindset, physical conditioning, gear, environmental awareness, client understanding, and team readiness all in order. When the unexpected hits—and it always does—you're reaching for a solution that's probably already in place.

How should a guide approach an emergency?

In a medical emergency, a guide's responsibility is to assess the situation, prioritize actions, and lead decisively. This means managing not just the patient but the entire group, ensuring everyone remains safe and focused. A guide who stays calm and organized sets the tone for the response, preventing panic and fostering trust. Adaptability and clear decision-making under pressure transform a potentially chaotic situation into a manageable one.

Next, a wilderness medical mindset hinges on calm, clarity, and adaptability. Guides work in environments where resources are limited, conditions are unpredictable, and evacuation may be far off. Success isn't about having every tool—it's about making the most of what's available. An effective response means addressing immediate needs, anticipating complications, and staying focused on what can be controlled.

Skill matters but so does how it's applied under pressure. A guide who hesitates or second-guesses in a crisis risks losing the group's trust. Emergencies evolve quickly, and even the best-laid plans drift and shift. The ability to adapt, stay focused, and lead with purpose is what keeps people safe and situations under control.

How can guides avoid becoming a patient?

Rescuing others in the wilderness carries significant risks. Guides and responders must balance patient care with personal safety, ensuring they do not become casualties themselves.

- *Scene safety always comes first.* Before approaching a patient, assess for immediate hazards—unstable terrain, falling debris, rising water, or dangerous wildlife. A secondary injury to the rescuer compromises the entire team. If conditions are unsafe, do not proceed until risks are mitigated.
- *Use personal protective equipment (PPE).* Gloves should be worn to reduce exposure to blood-borne pathogens,

and eye protection is ideal if there is a risk of splashes. If body fluids are involved, consider improvised barriers like a buff or rain jacket sleeve if medical gloves are unavailable.

- *Be mindful of physical exhaustion*. Wilderness rescues often involve prolonged exertion—lifting, carrying, and navigating rough terrain while assisting an injured person. Pacing, hydration, and shared workload among team members prevent overexertion and injury.
- *Avoid unnecessary risks*. Swift-water rescues, steep terrain extractions, wildlife concerns, and hazardous weather conditions require specific skills and equipment. If untrained or unequipped, wait for more experienced help or reassess the approach. The best intentions can't trump physics.
- *Maintain situational awareness*. Conditions can change rapidly. A safe rescue environment can deteriorate due to weather shifts, nightfall, or worsening terrain. Constant reassessment of safety is essential throughout an incident.

The priority is stabilizing the patient while ensuring safety for everyone involved. The best rescue is the one where all responders walk away.

Communication During Emergencies

Why is communication so important?

Clear communication is one of a guide's most powerful tools in an emergency. Calm, direct instructions keep people focused, reduce confusion, and help maintain control of the situation. The way you speak—your tone, clarity, and composure—does more than relay information; it reassures your group that you know what needs to be done and that you can be trusted to lead.

Good communication isn't just about speaking—it's about listening. Engaging the group, gathering input, and encouraging teamwork improves response efforts and helps ensure everyone understands their role. A frantic or uncertain guide breeds panic; a calm, composed one fosters confidence. Your preparation, knowledge, and expertise should come through in both your words and demeanor. Clear, steady communication doesn't just manage the situation—it sets the tone for how others respond. And yes, it's okay to project calm until you find your footing.

How should a guide communicate during an emergency?

Effective communication is a guide's most powerful tool in an emergency. It keeps the group focused, prevents confusion, and ensures that necessary actions are taken efficiently. The way a guide speaks, listens, and presents themselves directly influences how the group responds. Remember, under stress, the body activates the sympathetic nervous system—the "fight or flight" response. This causes a surge of adrenaline (among other stress hormones), narrowing attention, speeding up heart rate, and prioritizing survival over complex thinking. In this state, people process information differently: Reaction time decreases but decision-making, memory recall, and fine motor skills often suffer. Clear, simple communication becomes critical—because when stress rises, the brain favors familiar patterns and direct commands over nuance or abstraction. Here are the things to keep in mind when communicating during an emergency:

1. *Assess Before You Speak* - Before giving instructions, take a moment to evaluate the situation. Identify immediate threats, determine priorities, and decide what information needs to be communicated first. Rushing into commands without a clear plan will add to the chaos.
2. *Be Direct* - As described above, in high-stress situations, people process information differently. Keep instructions short, specific, and calm. Avoid

unnecessary details—actionable, to-the-point communication is most effective.

3. *Ensure Understanding* – Don't assume instructions were heard or interpreted correctly. Have group members repeat back critical steps to confirm clarity. Miscommunication in a high-pressure scenario can lead to mistakes that worsen the situation.
4. *Use Nonverbal Cues* – Your body language, facial expressions, and tone can either instill confidence or create uncertainty. Standing tall, making eye contact, and speaking with authority reassures the group, while hesitation or uncertainty can trigger anxiety and doubt.
5. *Adapt as the Situation Changes* – Emergencies are fluid. Plans may shift, and new priorities may emerge. A guide must continuously reassess conditions, update the group, and modify communication strategies as needed. Staying flexible and responsive ensures the group remains informed and engaged.

A guide who communicates clearly, confidently, and decisively fosters trust, maintains order, and keeps the team moving in the right direction—even under pressure.

What if communication breaks down?

It happens. Stress, fear, and fatigue can cause miscommunication and confusion. If a team member panics, resists evacuation, or misunderstands directions, it's up to the guide to reset the situation.

- Stay calm and reset expectations. Lower your voice, slow your speech, and bring the focus back to what needs to happen next.
- Delegate roles and responsibilities. Assign tasks to capable team members to prevent chaos and give structure to the response.

- Use physical demonstrations. If words fail, show what needs to be done.
- Avoid information overload. Stick to essential instructions, reinforcing them as needed.

When technology is available, use it to enhance clarity and coordination, but remember, verbal leadership and clear messaging remain the most important skills in guiding a team through an emergency.

What role does technology play in wilderness communication?

While verbal communication and leadership skills are critical, technology provides an essential lifeline in wilderness emergencies. Traditional means of communication, such as whistles and signal mirrors, still have their place, but modern satellite devices and emergency beacons dramatically improve a guide's ability to call for help and coordinate rescues.

- Satellite messengers and Personal Locator Beacons (PLBs)—allow guides to send alerts with GPS coordinates, providing emergency responders with real-time location data. Unlike cell phones, which can be unreliable in remote areas, these devices bypass standard cell networks and communicate via satellite, ensuring that distress signals reach help even in the most isolated environments.
- Two-way satellite communicators offer another advantage: the ability to send and receive custom messages. This allows for more detailed updates to emergency responders and helps coordinate evacuation logistics before rescuers arrive. Some devices even provide weather updates, which can influence decision-making during prolonged incidents.
- Handheld radios are valuable for group communication and coordination *within* an expedition, especially in rugged terrain or when members are spread out. In

areas with ranger stations or emergency services, a VHF or UHF radio may also provide a direct line to help.

While these tools enhance safety, they should never replace fundamental emergency response skills, leadership, and decision-making. A guide must still rely on clear, confident verbal communication; active listening; and a well-structured response plan—because technology is only useful if it's available, functional, and used correctly.

Pre-Trip Planning

What are the foundational questions for trip planning?

The questions; Where are you going? Who are you taking? What will you be doing? are more than planning prompts—they form the blueprint for every aspect of guiding. These three questions shape preparation, influence decision-making, and ultimately determine the safety and success of a trip or an expedition. Guides who approach trips with these in mind lead with intention rather than reaction, ensuring preparedness rather than scrambling when conditions slip.

A trip can unravel before it even begins if these questions aren't fully considered. A well-planned expedition is not just about logistics—it's about anticipating variables, mitigating risks, and ensuring a seamless experience for both guides and clients.

Why does where you're going matter?

Understanding the environment is the cornerstone of preparation. Each setting—whether a remote tropical flat, a dense forest, a high-altitude ridge, or an arid desert canyon—presents distinct challenges that demand a tailored approach. Terrain, climate, and potential hazards shape every aspect of planning, from gear selection to medical preparedness to emergency response plans.

Weather patterns, wildlife encounters, water sources, and terrain difficulty all impact a trip's logistics. Knowing what's normal for the environment helps identify when something isn't. A tropical storm rolling in, an unexpected cold snap, or a changing tide can turn an average day into a serious problem. The more you understand about the location before stepping into it, the less you leave to chance.

Maps, local knowledge, and firsthand scouting provide a baseline for decision-making in the field. Preparation transforms information into actionable readiness, ensuring that the trip is both safe and successful.

Why is it essential to understand who you're guiding?

The group defines the scope, rhythm, and safety of the trip. Their physical abilities, medical needs, experience levels, and personalities directly impact planning, risk management, and how the trip plays out. A seasoned team moves differently-decisions come faster, and adversity is met with resilience. Newer clients may need more structure, slower pacing, and clearer boundaries. Tailoring your pace, itinerary, and communication style to match the group prevents unnecessary risk and makes for a better experience across the board.

Not all experience levels are equal—and not all clients are here for the same reasons. Some come to travel. Others come for vacation. *Travel* is about exploration, adaptation, and uncertainty. *Vacation* is about comfort, control, and predictability. Both can be accommodated, but the guide must be clear about what kind of experience is being offered. Misaligned expectations lead to frustration, resentment, and poor decisions in the field. A traveler rolls with the unexpected; a vacationer might see it as failure. If someone expecting comfort finds themselves in an unpredictable wilderness scenario, it can quickly escalate into a problem—for them, for the guide, and for the group.

Understanding medical needs is just as important as gauging experience. Chronic conditions, medications, and prior medical history all shape contingency planning. Does a guest have asthma, diabetes, or a history of heart issues? Recent surgeries? Severe allergies? This information isn't just helpful—it's essential. Participants should always bring their own medications, but guides should carry backups when possible and have a clear action plan. A forgotten inhaler or missing EpiPen can turn a minor issue into a medical emergency.

Psychology matters just as much as physiology. A group that trusts each other, listens, and stays calm under pressure is easier to manage than one prone to panic, silence, or conflict. Some people step into leadership. Others need reassurance. Early in the trip, watch how the group reacts under stress. Do they communicate and help each other—or do they fracture when things go wrong? Groups that function well make your job easier—groups that don't become another variable to manage.

As a last consideration, alcohol and substance use add another, not insignificant layer of complexity. A few drinks around the fire may seem harmless; but alcohol impairs judgment, balance, and reaction time—none of which mix well with wilderness settings. The culture of the group matters. Are they expecting a relaxed, responsible social drink at camp—or are they treating the trip like a party? If alcohol is involved, you need to consider interactions with medications, dehydration, and altitude. And if someone's impaired, you have the final say on whether they continue.

A well-planned trip isn't just about terrain, weather, or tides—it's about who you're taking into it. Experience, medical background, group dynamics, and individual risk profiles shape every decision you make. A guide who understands their group leads from the front. One who doesn't, ends up reacting to problems that should've been spotted before the trip ever began. The best trips don't happen by luck.

How does what you're doing affect planning?

Activities dictate the risks, equipment, and skill demands of a trip. Fly fishing, mountaineering, rafting, hiking, and diving all present unique hazards, gear requirements, and technical skills that must be factored into planning. Preparation means more than packing the right equipment—it requires anticipating how participants will engage with the activity and where potential pitfalls lie.

A guide's ability to think ahead, predict challenges, and work through each day before it happens is critical to both mental and logistical preparedness. What happens if a boat motor fails? If the group gets delayed on a hike and loses daylight? If a client panics during a dive? Thinking through possible failures in advance allows for better decision-making in real time. Guides who prepare for the what-ifs are far less likely to be caught off guard when that something inevitably goes wrong.

Risk tolerance varies widely, and not all participants fully grasp the demands of an activity before stepping into it. Some overestimate their abilities, while others have no frame of reference for the challenges ahead. A guide must read the group; adjust plans in real time; and ensure that the trip remains within safe, manageable limits.

A successful trip isn't about pushing limits—it's about knowing when to adjust them. There's a fine line between challenge and recklessness; and guides must recognize when an activity should be slowed down, modified, or even abandoned for safety. The best guides don't just react to problems—they anticipate them, ensuring that risk remains controlled while still delivering an experience that feels both rewarding and adventurous.

Why do these questions matter?

These questions separate reactive guiding from intentional leadership. Trips rarely fall apart due to bad luck—they usually unravel because of poor preparation. Guides who *ask and answer* these questions aren't just leading—they're building experiences that balance risk, adventure, and safety with purpose.

Ultimately, a well-planned trip turns uncertainty into preparation and keeps risks from spiraling. Traditional training focuses on how to *respond* when things go wrong—and that's what makes a good guide. Great guides are defined by something else: the ability to shape their preparation around the risks and *anticipate* problems before they derail a trip.

Let's dig in.

Things to Know

Water & Hygiene

Why is clean water such a big deal?

Contaminated water is one of the most common causes of illness in remote settings. Globally, the combination of unsafe drinking *water*, poor *sanitation*, and inadequate *hygiene*—collectively known as WASH—contributes to an estimated 830,000 deaths each year. While most wilderness travelers won't face risks on that level, the threat is real. One case of waterborne illness can derail an entire trip. In the absence of clean water and basic hygiene, even the strongest can become a liability.

What is the most reliable way to disinfect water in the wilderness?

There's no perfect answer, but if we need to pick one, boiling is the most reliable method. It kills bacteria, viruses, and parasites, making it the gold—or at least silver—standard for disinfection. Water should be brought to a rolling boil for at least one minute at sea level, and for three minutes at higher elevations, where lower boiling temperatures reduce effectiveness and require longer boil times.

While foolproof, boiling requires fuel and time, making it impractical for large volumes or when resources are limited.

In most backcountry settings, a high-quality filter is the most practical option, as bacteria and protozoa are the primary threats. If viral contamination is a concern—especially in water exposed to human or animal waste—chemical treatment with chlorine dioxide is a lightweight, effective backup. UV purifiers work well for clear water but rely on batteries, which can fail when needed most. Stagnant pools or agricultural runoff require more aggressive treatment. Understanding the risks associated with different water sources allows for better decision-making in the field.

Do water filters make water safe?

Not always. Filters are highly effective at removing sediment, bacteria, and protozoa, including threats like *Giardia* and *Cryptosporidium*, which are the primary concerns in most wilderness environments. However, viruses—such as norovirus, hepatitis A, and rotavirus—are much smaller and can pass through standard filters. These viruses are more common in water sources contaminated by human or animal waste, making filtration alone insufficient in those settings.

To ensure full protection, filtration should be combined with chemical treatment or UV purification, both of which effectively neutralize viruses. Filters also require regular maintenance, as clogged or damaged units will fail to remove contaminants. Understanding the microbial risks in different water sources is fundamental to wilderness medicine, as waterborne illness can rapidly lead to dehydration, impaired judgment, and increased medical risk in remote environments.

How effective are chemical treatments for water disinfection?

Chemical treatments like chlorine dioxide and iodine are lightweight, easy to use, and effective against bacteria, viruses, and most protozoa. However, their effectiveness depends on water temperature, clarity, and contact time. In cold or cloudy water, chemical agents work more slowly, making prefiltering a good idea. Chlorine dioxide is preferred for its broad-spectrum action and lack of taste, while iodine is less effective against *Cryptosporidium* and has some restrictions, particularly for pregnant individuals or those with thyroid conditions. Following the correct dosage and waiting period is essential, as cutting corners reduces effectiveness.

How do UV purifiers work?

UV purifiers effectively disinfect water by neutralizing bacteria, protozoa, and viruses by exposing the bugs to ultraviolet light, which disrupts the DNA of microorganisms, preventing them from replicating and causing infection. Unlike chemical treatments, UV purification does not alter the taste or odor of water, making it an attractive option for water disinfection. However, UV purifiers require *clear water* to function properly. Sediment or turbidity can block the light, significantly reducing its effectiveness. Prefiltration is necessary if the water is cloudy. Additionally, UV purifiers rely on batteries or electricity, making them less reliable for extended trips or cold environments where electronics can fail.

A simpler, low-tech alternative in extreme cases is solar water disinfection (SODIS). This method involves placing clear plastic bottles (found worldwide) in direct sunlight, where exposure to UVA radiation and a bit of heat neutralizes pathogens. On a sunny day, at least 6 hours of direct sunlight is required. On a partly cloudy day, exposure should be extended to at least 12 hours. If the sky is heavily overcast, the process can take up to two full days. SODIS is ineffective at night or in conditions where sunlight is too weak to penetrate the water.

Determining when the water is safe to drink after SODIS depends on proper exposure and, of course, is a bit of a gamble. The bottles should remain in direct sunlight for the full recommended time based on weather conditions. The bottle itself must be clear as any cloudiness or tinting of the plastic can reduce effectiveness. The water should also be free of turbidity—clear enough to read text through the bottle. If the water is warm after exposure, it is a good sign (not a guarantee) that enough solar energy has been absorbed. Best to drink within 24 hours.

Both SODIS and UV purifiers *are* effective in clear water but will *not* remove chemical contaminants, heavy metals, or toxins. A backup treatment method, such as filtration or chemical disinfection, is essential for ensuring safe drinking water in all conditions.

Can you find clean water by digging a hole?

In some environments, digging a "seep well" near a known water source can provide filtered groundwater. This works because sand and soil act as natural filters, reducing sediment and some contaminants. However, this method does not remove bacteria, viruses, or chemical pollutants; so further treatment is still required. In arid regions, digging in dry riverbeds or low-lying areas with signs of groundwater, such as green vegetation or damp sand, may yield water; but it will likely accumulate slowly. Even when water is found, it must be treated before drinking.

Can water be strained to make it safe?

Straining water through sand or cloth only removes sediment and improves clarity—it does not disinfect the water. Some pathogens, particularly bacteria and viruses, are too small to be removed this way. However, prefiltering through sand, gravel, or even a shirt before chemical or UV treatment can improve effectiveness. This is especially useful for murky or turbid water that would otherwise reduce the efficiency of chemical disinfectants or UV purifiers.

What are the biggest mistakes people make with water treatment?

The most common mistakes include failing to treat water at all, rushing the treatment process, using a clogged or damaged filter, failing to prefilter cloudy water before chemical or UV treatment, and assuming one method is always enough. Many people also fail to clean and maintain their filters, reducing their effectiveness. Another critical error is recontamination of water—touching clean water with dirty hands, cups, or containers can undo proper treatment.

Which matters more in the field—staying hydrated or having clean water?

In extreme conditions, dehydration can be a more immediate threat than contaminated water. While drinking untreated water carries risks, severe dehydration can be life-threatening in a matter of hours. In survival situations, drinking untreated water may be necessary to prevent heat stroke or other complications. However, in non-emergency settings, proper treatment should always be used to prevent illness.

What is the best backup method for water treatment?

It depends. Always carry a secondary purification option. If using a filter, pack chemical tablets as a backup. If relying on UV purifiers, bring extra batteries and an alternative method like chlorine dioxide. Boiling is always an option if fuel is available. Having multiple ways to treat water ensures safe drinking water, regardless of the conditions.

Water security in the wilderness is about balancing safety, practicality, and available resources. Knowing the limitations of different treatment methods and adapting to the specific environment ensures access to clean water while minimizing risks.

Is handwashing really that big of a deal?

More than I can put into words. The simple act of handwashing has an extraordinary history and profound impact on public health. Ignaz Semmelweis, a 19th-century Hungarian physician, is credited with championing hand hygiene after he observed that handwashing drastically reduced maternal deaths from puerperal fever in obstetrics wards. Despite his findings, Semmelweis faced significant resistance from the medical community of his time. Today, however, hand hygiene is universally recognized as *the* most effective methods to prevent the spread of infection. Handwashing becomes even more critical in wilderness settings where medical care is limited, and the consequences of infection can be severe.

Wait, what's puerperal fever?

Puerperal fever, also known as "childbed" fever, is a bacterial infection of the female reproductive system that can occur after childbirth, often caused by the bacteria *Streptococcus pyogenes*. It was historically a leading cause of maternal death due to unsanitary birthing practices. In the 1840s, Dr. Semmelweis revolutionized its management by demonstrating that handwashing with chlorinated lime significantly reduced its incidence and saved lives, laying the foundation for modern infection control practices—namely handwashing.

How does soap work?

Soap molecules have two parts: a hydrophilic head and a hydrophobic tail. Hydrophilic means "water-loving"—from the Greek *philos*, meaning fondness. Hydrophobic means "water-fearing"—from the Greek *phobos*, meaning fear. When lathered with water, the hydrophobic tails embed into oils, grease, and other fats on the skin, while the hydrophilic heads remain in the water. This forms micelles—tiny spheres that trap dirt, oils, and microbes—which are then rinsed away. Many microbes cling to the skin by becoming embedded in natural skin oils, which water alone cannot remove. Soap disrupts that oil barrier and allows contaminants to be physically washed off the skin.

Is "antibacterial" soap better?

No. Antibacterial soap offers no real advantage over plain soap. All soap is effectively antimicrobial because it disrupts microbial membranes and removes pathogens from the skin. The outer layers of many bacteria and viruses—like influenza and coronaviruses—are made of lipids. Soap molecules break through these lipid structures—destroying bacterial cell walls and inactivating viruses.

Antibacterial soaps often contain added agents like triclosan or triclocarban. These ingredients are marketed as superior, but studies show they offer no additional health benefit over regular soap and water. In fact, the U.S. Food and Drug Administration banned several of these additives from over-the-counter soaps due to lack of proven efficacy and concerns over long-term safety.

In the field, what's more important is the mechanical removal—scrubbing, rinsing, and removing—dirt, organic material, and microbes. Not to sound like a marketing ploy, but unscented dish soap—formulated to break down grease—is often more effective than so-called "antibacterial" options. It performs well in cold-water, cuts through grime, and does exactly what's needed to eliminate pathogens from skin and surfaces.

When to Pull the Plug

What factors should be considered when deciding to evacuate a patient?

This is one of the tougher calls a guide will make. Evacuation decisions hinge primarily on three factors: (1) the patient's medical condition, (2) logistical feasibility, and (3) the broader impact on both the patient and the group. Medical urgency dictates whether immediate evacuation is required, while logistics determine *how* evacuation can be executed safely. The emotional and psychological effects—such as the patient's reluctance to leave or the group's response—also influence the decision. Balancing these factors ensures the best outcome for all involved. These decisions can be defining moments—not only for the patient's outcome but for a guide's career. Wilderness emergencies push guides into high-stakes decisions where uncertainty, pressure, and responsibility converge. I've watched great guides—friends—walk away from the career they loved, not because they lacked skill but because a difficult moment in the field left them questioning themselves. That confidence—the ability to stand by the decision made under pressure—is what keeps great guides guiding.

What *medical* factors determine the need for evacuation?

The first step is assessing whether the patient's condition can be managed in the field or requires advanced care. Life-threatening conditions—such as uncontrolled bleeding, neurological abnormalities, respiratory distress, severe pain, or shock—require immediate evacuation.

For less severe cases, the key question is whether the condition is stable or likely to worsen. A guide's ability to anticipate complications and recognize when a stable patient may soon become unstable is often the difference between a controlled evacuation and an emergency. Minor injuries or illnesses can sometimes be managed in the field, but if there is any doubt about the patient's ability to continue safely, early evacuation is always the better option

What *logistical* challenges affect evacuation decisions?

Even when evacuation is medically necessary, logistics dictate how and when it can happen. Terrain, weather, and available resources all influence the plan. In some cases, these constraints may require adjusting the urgency or method of evacuation—whether by land, water, or air.

Guides must work backward from definitive care, identifying the safest and most feasible route to get the patient to medical treatment. The first question isn't how to move the patient—it's where they need to go. A clinic, hospital, or emergency transport hub should be the endpoint; and every decision should be made in reverse from *that* destination.

If an air evacuation is possible, the focus shifts to finding an extraction point rather than moving the patient unnecessarily. If the only option is a prolonged ground evacuation, guides must factor in terrain, weather, available manpower, and medical stability. A seemingly straightforward extraction can be derailed by environmental surprises or exhaustion, forcing an alternative route or even sheltering in place.

These situations demand patience, adaptability, and a clear head under pressure. A guide must be comfortable being uncomfortable, making tough decisions that balance medical urgency with real-world constraints. The best evacuation is not the fastest—it's the one that ensures the highest chance of survival with the least risk to everyone involved.

What are the *emotional* considerations when deciding to evacuate a patient?

Evacuation isn't just a medical decision—it's often tangled in personal investment, cost, and group dynamics. In critical cases, the decision is clear, but when the urgency is less obvious, emotions cloud judgment, and guides must navigate both medical needs and client resistance.

Patients may feel guilt, embarrassment, or reluctance, especially if their condition isn't immediately life-threatening. The thought of leaving a trip they've planned and paid for—or feeling like they're inconveniencing others—can be overwhelming. Many hesitate to speak up, fearing they'll ruin the experience for the group or waste money on what was meant to be a once-in-a-lifetime trip.

Common emotional barriers include:

- Guilt and Embarrassment - Patients may downplay symptoms to avoid being seen as a burden.
- Financial Impact - The high cost of wilderness trips makes some reluctant to leave, especially if refunds aren't an option.

- Group Pressure – Some worry about disappointing others and may try to push through rather than disrupt the trip.

Guides must recognize these emotions and communicate clearly. The conversation isn't about whether the patient wants to evacuate—it's about what's in their best interest. Framing the decision around long-term health and safety rather than short-term disappointment helps ease resistance. Patients should feel heard, but they also need to understand that their well-being comes first. A firm, confident, and empathetic approach helps guide them toward the right decision while maintaining group cohesion.

What should guides know about helicopters?

Helicopter evacuation in the wilderness requires deliberate preparation and strict attention to safety. The landing zone (LZ) should be at least 100 feet by 100 feet; flat; open; and clear of overhead obstructions, large rocks, or loose debris. All gear must be secured. Nothing should be used to mark the LZ unless it is heavy and immobile. If the aircraft requires a visual reference, body positioning or arm signals may be used, but only when coordinated and safe.

As the aircraft approaches, rotor wash creates hurricane-force winds capable of lifting unsecured items and blasting sand, snow, and debris across the area. Any airborne material—especially fine debris, sand, or snow—can cause eye injuries. All individuals should be positioned on one knee, facing the aircraft, with sunglasses or other eye protection in place. When material is blowing around, eyes should be closed and the head kept low. One knee down, head low, and body stable is the safest position near rapidly turning blades.

The patient should be positioned flat on the ground with eyes and ears covered. A jacket or shirt can be pulled over the face, and soft gear wrapped around the head for protection. Blankets must be tightly secured to prevent them from becoming airborne. Patients have sustained injuries from debris or disorientation during rotor wash, making early shielding essential.

Direction from the flight crew must be followed without hesitation. The crew is in charge once the aircraft is on scene. Approach should only occur when clearly signaled. Movement should remain *forward* of the main cabin and within the pilot's line of sight. The tail rotor is silent, low, and deadly—crossing behind the aircraft is *never* acceptable.

When the aircraft begins to shut down, the main rotor blades lose lift and begin to droop under their own weight. These blades, which appear high overhead during operation, can swing low enough to strike anyone standing upright. Fatal injuries have occurred during this phase. Low posture must be maintained until directed otherwise by the flight crew.

Once the patient is in the care of the flight crew, guides, guests, and wilderness responders should back away and maintain distance. The safest place at that point is away from the aircraft. When the blades begin spinning again for departure, rotor wash will intensify, and debris will fly—everyone should already be clear.

The Red Flag Framework: Defined

Is there an easy-to-use framework for deciding who should be evacuated?

Glad you asked. The Red Flag Framework is a simple, yet effective decision-making tool designed for wilderness trauma, medical, and environmental emergencies. It removes the burden of diagnosing in situations where definitive diagnostic tools are unavailable, focusing instead on clinical symptoms and patterns. This approach doesn't limit a responder—it provides clarity—helping guides make decisive, informed choices based on the patients signs and symptoms rather than working through a list of possible diagnoses.

The Red Flag Framework is woven throughout this book, providing specific Red Flags for different medical conditions and environmental hazards. These sections highlight key warning signs and include mnemonics to make critical symptoms easier to recognize.

The Red Flag Framework is not about having every answer every time—it was created to help responders make the best possible decision with imperfect information when it matters most.

The Signs: What's Vital?

What are vital signs, and why are they essential in wilderness medicine?

Vital signs—pulse rate, respiratory rate, temperature, and blood pressure—are called vital for a reason. They provide critical insight into a patient's condition and serve as a guide's most reliable tool for assessing severity, making informed decisions, and prioritizing evacuation needs in remote settings.

Observing vital signs offers a wealth of information. A rapid pulse with pale or clammy skin often signals shock, while abnormal respiratory patterns can indicate respiratory failure, lung injury, or metabolic distress. Temperature, whether measured with a thermometer or assessed through touch, helps identify systemic infections, hypothermia, or heat-related illness.

While some tools, like thermometers, are practical to carry in the field, others, like blood pressure cuffs, are often unreliable due to operator technique and environmental challenges. Much of the information a blood pressure cuff provides can be inferred from skin signs, capillary refill, and mucous membrane assessment. In the wilderness, the ability to assess and interpret vital signs through observation and palpation is often more practical than relying on devices.

Vital signs are more than just numbers; they guide medical decision-making. Tracking trends over time helps assess a patient's status and determine whether their condition is improving, stable, or worsening—key factors in deciding if evacuation is necessary.

What's the best way to assess pulse rate in the wilderness?

Pulse rate provides valuable insight into cardiovascular status and blood volume. To measure it, use the pads of your first two fingers (not your thumb) to palpate a pulse, count beats for 15 seconds, and multiply by four to determine beats per minute (bpm).

The radial pulse, located at the wrist near the base of the thumb, is most useful for assessing circulation. A strong radial pulse generally indicates a systolic blood pressure above 80 mmHg, suggesting adequate perfusion. If the radial pulse is weak or absent, check the carotid pulse, located in the neck beside the trachea. The carotid pulse is stronger and more reliable, correlating with a systolic blood pressure of roughly 60 mmHg, and should be used when the radial pulse is difficult to detect.

Normal resting pulse rates by age:

- Adults: 60-100 bpm
- Children: 80-120 bpm
- Infants: 120-130 bpm

A rapid pulse (tachycardia) may indicate dehydration, blood loss, infection, pain, or shock, while a slow pulse (bradycardia) may suggest hypothermia, head injury, or metabolic dysfunction. Persistent abnormalities should not be ignored, as they often signal worsening illness or injury.

How about respiratory rate?

Respiratory rate reflects both respiratory function and metabolic status. A stethoscope isn't required, but it can help identify abnormal breath sounds—like wheezing, crackles, or diminished airflow—that might not be obvious on visual exam. To measure the rate, observe chest or abdominal movement, count breaths for 30 seconds, and multiply by two.

Normal respiratory rates by age:

- Adults: 12-20 breaths per minute

- Children: 20-30 breaths per minute
- Infants: 30 breaths per minute

A rapid breathing rate (tachypnea) may indicate pain, anxiety, dehydration, lung infection, or metabolic acidosis (such as in diabetic ketoacidosis). Slow breathing (bradypnea) can signal head injury, opioid overdose, or late-stage shock. Any irregular, labored, or shallow breathing should raise concern, especially if paired with cyanosis (bluish lips or nail beds), confusion, or worsening fatigue, which are all signs of impending respiratory failure.

Is measuring blood pressure practical in the wilderness?

Rarely. Blood pressure cuffs are often unreliable and impracticable in remote settings. They require consistent use and familiarity—something that's uncommon in the wilderness setting. Intraoperator variability is high, and even minor errors in placement, technique, or interpretation can throw off results. The equipment itself is prone to failure without preventative maintenance and the components doesn't tolerate rough handling, dust, wet, cold, or dry conditions well.

In reality, blood pressure readings rarely change field management. What really matters is whether the body is perfusing—getting oxygen to where it's needed. That can be assessed more reliably through physical signs:

- Skin signs: Cool, pale, or clammy skin suggests peripheral vasoconstriction and possible hypovolemia or shock.
- Capillary refill: Refill over two seconds, especially in warm conditions, points to poor peripheral circulation.
- Mucous membranes: Dry, sticky, or pale mucosa reflects significant fluid loss.
- Radial pulse: A weak or absent radial pulse usually means a systolic pressure is below 80 mmHg and, in the right setting, demands immediate attention. A strong,

regular radial pulse *generally* indicates adequate perfusion.

Blood pressure readings give you numbers. *Perfusion* signs tell you if the body is delivering oxygen where it needs to go. In the wilderness, where treatment decisions must be made quickly and gear is limited, physiology matters more than numbers.

Is the capillary refill time a reliable tool to assess perfusion in the field?

It's reliable anywhere—whether in the field or the ICU. Capillary refill time (CRT) measures how long it takes blood to return to the skin after briefly pressing on the nail bed. Normal CRT is less than 2 seconds. This response depends on blood volume and vascular tone—both of which are impaired in bad disease—shock, dehydration, low-volume states, and critical illness

CRT is fast, repeatable, and gear-free. Its real value is in trending: It may look normal early, then delay, as perfusion drops. Paired with mental status and heart rate, it's a solid tool—just interpret it cautiously in the cold or in poor lighting.

Why do trends in vital signs matter?

Vital signs should be monitored over time to detect trends. A patient whose pulse, breathing, or skin signs progressively worsen—especially in the setting of dehydration, shock, or traumatic injury—requires evacuation.

Minor deviations can sometimes be monitored, but worsening abnormalities signal the need for intervention. Recognizing when a stable patient is becoming unstable is often the difference between a controlled evacuation and a much bigger emergency.

A Little Air Goes a Long Way

Why is airway management critical?

Airway management is critical because it directly protects ventilation, oxygenation, and survival. Without an open and functional airway, oxygen cannot reach the lungs, blood oxygen levels fall, carbon dioxide accumulates, and the body rapidly enters respiratory failure. In the wilderness, where evacuation may be delayed, a compromised airway can quickly become fatal. Early recognition and simple interventions can prevent deterioration and keep a patient stable until definitive care is available.

How do you open the airway in an unconscious patient?

In an unconscious patient without suspected spinal trauma, the airway is opened using the head-tilt, chin-lift maneuver. Tilting the head backward and lifting the chin moves the tongue and soft tissues away from the back of the throat, restoring a clear path for air to enter the lungs. This simple technique corrects the most common cause of airway obstruction in unconscious patients: the tongue falling back against the posterior pharynx. If there is any suspicion of cervical spine injury, use a jaw-thrust maneuver instead—grasping the angles of the lower jaw and lifting it forward without moving the head or neck. This protects the cervical spine while still attempting to clear the airway. In either case, restoring airflow is the first priority, as airway obstruction leads quickly to hypoxia, hypercapnia, and worsening brain injury.

What should you do if the airway is obstructed?

Clear it—carefully. If the airway is obstructed, immediate action is required to restore airflow. First, reposition the patient using a head-tilt, chin-lift or jaw-thrust maneuver, as soft tissue collapse is the most common cause. If repositioning fails, look inside the mouth for visible obstructions such as vomit, blood, or foreign objects, and remove them manually if safe to do so. Blind finger sweeps should be avoided, as they can push obstructions deeper. If the obstruction persists, use abdominal thrusts (Heimlich maneuver) to attempt expulsion. In an unconscious patient with a persistent airway obstruction that cannot be relieved, consider transitioning to rescue breathing with careful repositioning between attempts. If basic maneuvers fail and no air movement is possible, advanced interventions like supraglottic airway placement or emergency cricothyrotomy may be required—depending on the responder's training and available equipment.

How do you keep the airway open after clearing it?

In an unconscious or semiconscious patient, airway adjuncts help maintain patency:

- Oropharyngeal airway (OPA): Use in unconscious patients with no gag reflex. Insert upside-down, then rotate 180° to keep the tongue from falling back.
- Nasopharyngeal airway (NPA): Use in semiconscious patients or those with a gag reflex, unless there is facial trauma. NPAs can be lubricated with saliva or water in an emergency.

If available, supraglottic devices like a laryngeal mask airway (LMA) provide better airway protection without requiring advanced training. In an unconscious patient with a persistent airway obstruction, the tongue can be manually pulled forward, but this is difficult to maintain. In an extreme survival scenario, a safety pin can be used to pierce the tongue and secure it to the lower lip to prevent it from falling back and obstructing the airway. This may seem like a desperate measure but can be lifesaving if no airway adjuncts are available. If the patient is breathing but unconscious, rolling them into the recovery position prevents the tongue from falling back and blocking the airway.

When should you consider an emergency airway procedure?

If airway obstruction cannot be relieved with standard techniques and the patient is unable to breathe, an emergency cricothyrotomy may be the only option. This is a last-resort, high-risk procedure requiring proper training and significant management if successful. In the wilderness, where prolonged care is needed, even a successful cricothyrotomy may not be survivable without rapid evacuation.

What are the evacuation considerations for airway-compromised patients?

Airway-compromised patients require immediate evacuation. If maintaining an airway demands constant intervention, every minute drains team resources and increases risk. In rugged terrain, managing a patient who needs continuous airway support for hours or days is rarely survivable. Guides and responders must assess the feasibility of transport early—and act without delay.

In wilderness medicine, airway management is about rapid assessment, decisive action, and understanding that evacuation decisions are often made within minutes—not hours. The best intervention is the one that protects both the patient and the team while offering the highest realistic chance of survival.

Is CPR useful in the wilderness?

Everyone should know CPR and stay current on how to perform it. That said, its utility in the wilderness is limited. Cardiac arrest in adults is usually caused by an underlying cardiac event or severe metabolic disturbance—problems that are rarely reversible without advanced medical intervention. In pediatric patients, arrest is more often the result of respiratory failure, which means early resuscitation may actually correct—or at least temporize—the underlying issue.

Regardless of the cause, the goals of CPR are the same: to prime the heart, circulate blood, and maintain perfusion to the coronary arteries and vital organs. That requires compressions at a rate of 100 to 120 per minute, deep enough to generate flow, and allowing full chest recoil between compressions. Rescue breaths should be delivered with visible chest rise and fall, demonstrating that full ventilations are being achieved.

In wilderness settings, CPR has a low success rate. Without defibrillation, medications, or airway control, prolonged efforts are rarely effective. CPR after traumatic arrest—whether blunt or penetrating—is essentially futile. That said, there are exceptions. Hypothermic patients, especially those pulled from cold water, may survive if CPR is started promptly. Cold temperatures can slow metabolism and preserve brain and organ function longer than expected. Lightning strike victims may also respond if CPR is initiated quickly, particularly as respiratory arrest often occurs before cardiac collapse in these patients.

Generally speaking, CPR should be continued for as long as it's sustainable and doesn't compromise the team. Once it drains resources or puts others at risk, it's reasonable to stop. In the wilderness, unfortunately, extended efforts without advanced cardiac support rarely change outcomes.

With all of that said, performing CPR is often meaningful—for the patient's friends and family, and the team members alike—as a final effort to save a life and an act that carries both emotional and ethical weight.

Environmental Emergencies

Overview

How common are environmental emergencies in the wilderness?

Environmental emergencies—including heat illness, hypothermia, lightning strikes, and altitude-related conditions—are among the most common causes of illness and injury in remote settings. While global incidence is difficult to quantify, mostly due to underreporting, consistent patterns still emerge across regions and activities.

In the U.S., heat illness is the leading cause of weather-related death. Between 1999 and 2023, annual deaths more than doubled, rising from 1,069 to over 2,300. When contributing factors such as medical comorbidities, heat-triggered cardiac events, or delays in care are included, the true number is likely much higher. Globally, heat is responsible for an estimated 489,000 deaths annually, with the highest burdens noted in Asia and Europe.

Lightning injuries are less common but carry high-consequence risk, especially in exposed terrain. Worldwide, lightning strikes cause approximately 24,000 deaths and ten times as many injuries each year. In the U.S., 20–30 fatalities occur annually, with hundreds more injured—many with lasting neurologic effects.

High-altitude illness is a significant risk in expedition settings. Acute mountain sickness (AMS) affects 40–50% of individuals ascending above 3,000 meters. High-altitude pulmonary edema (HAPE) occurs in 0.5–15%, depending on ascent profile and elevation. High-altitude cerebral edema (HACE), while less common, can be fatal and affects up to 2% of travelers without proper acclimatization.

Cold exposure remains a persistent threat in alpine and high-latitude environments. Hypothermia and frostbite are well documented in both recreational and occupational contexts.

Across all these conditions, the primary danger isn't the environment itself—it's the speed at which it degrades decision-making, delays movement, and complicates evacuation. For guides and responders, success often depends less on the diagnosis and more on awareness, early recognition, and timely action.

Lightning

What causes lightning and why is it dangerous?

Lightning forms when electrical charges in the atmosphere discharge—either between clouds or from clouds to the ground. As warm, moist air rises and forms clouds, strong updrafts carry water vapor upward where it cools and condenses. Inside the cloud, ice crystals, graupel (soft hail), and supercooled water droplets collide with each other. These collisions transfer electric charge: Typically, the smaller, lighter ice crystals gain a positive charge and get carried to the top of the cloud by updrafts, while the heavier graupel picks up a negative charge and falls toward the base. This creates charge separation—a strong difference in electrical charge between the top and bottom of the cloud. When the difference becomes large enough, the atmosphere can no longer insulate the charges, and a discharge occurs—lightning. Strikes tend to hit tall, pointed, or isolated objects, making open ridges, lone trees, and exposed terrain especially hazardous in wilderness settings.

The danger goes beyond direct strikes. Ground current—electricity radiating from a nearby strike—can travel through soil, water, or the human body, causing serious injury. Side flashes occur when lightning jumps from one object to another, often striking those near trees or rock faces. These mechanisms underscore the need for a strong situational awareness and proper precautions during storms.

Does swimming in a pool or at the beach really increase the risk of being struck by lightning?

Not in any meaningful way—and not because of the water itself. Water doesn't attract lightning. The real risk comes from exposure in wide, open, relatively featureless environments—like beaches, lakes, and open water. In those settings, anything that stands out—like a person, a tree, or a lifeguard tower—is more likely to be struck. A swimmer's risk has more to do with location and surroundings than the act of being in water. Available data support this: Swimming accounts for only a small fraction of documented lightning injuries, and even those are often poorly classified or lack detail about whether the person was actually *in* the water when they were struck. Most lightning-related water deaths occur during boating or fishing, where exposure is far greater.

Being on a boat in the middle of a lake or out at sea carries significantly higher risk. In these settings, the boat is often the tallest object for miles, leaving those aboard far more exposed. Unlike swimmers near shore, they're isolated and lack surrounding structures to deflect or absorb a strike. Lightning near water poses an added danger as current can spread across the surface, affecting anyone in or near the strike zone—even without a direct hit.

The point is, water doesn't attract lightning. Elevation and exposure are what increase the risk of a lightning strike.

How do guides keep guests safe in a lightning storm?

Avoid being exposed and elevated. The safest place during a lightning storm is a fully enclosed structure or vehicle. If no shelter is available, take immediate steps to reduce risk:

- Move to lower terrain, away from ridgelines, peaks, and open ground.
- Avoid tall, isolated objects such as lone trees or metal structures.
- Minimize ground contact by crouching low, feet together, balanced on the balls of the feet.
- If in a group, spread out—maintain at least 50 feet (15 meters) between individuals to reduce the risk of multiple casualties.

What injuries can lightning strikes cause?

Lightning can cause severe—and often unusual—injuries. Burns may appear as Lichtenberg figures, branching patterns on the skin from the electrical discharge. Strikes can disrupt the heart's rhythm, causing cardiac arrest, or paralyze the brain's respiratory center, leading to respiratory arrest. Neurologic injury is common, ranging from temporary Charcot's paralysis to long-term cognitive deficits.

Barotrauma may result from the rapid pressure wave, causing ruptured eardrums, collapsed lung, or other internal injuries. The force of the strike can also throw victims, resulting in secondary blunt or penetrating trauma.

Immediate response is critical. Prioritize resuscitation—initiate CPR if needed—and assess for additional injuries. Any direct strike victim requires evacuation due to the high risk of hidden injury and delayed complications.

How should I manage multiple victims of a lightning strike?

In mass casualty lightning events, the concept of "reverse triage" applies: Unresponsive patients are treated *first*. Lightning-induced cardiac or respiratory arrest has a higher survival rate than other causes of arrest. Begin with those who appear lifeless. If a victim has no pulse or isn't breathing, initiate CPR immediately. Once critical interventions are underway, assess and triage secondary injuries, including burns, blunt traumatic injuries, and musculoskeletal damage. Even patients who regain consciousness after initial unresponsiveness require close monitoring and evacuation due to the risk of delayed complications.

Should all lightning strike victims be evacuated?

Anyone directly struck by lightning requires evacuation due to the risk of delayed complications, including cardiac rhythm disturbances(arrythmias), neurological damage, and internal injuries. Even if the patient appears stable, these risks warrant advanced evaluation.

For indirect lightning injuries, such as ground current or side flashes, evacuation depends on symptom severity. Patients with persistent confusion, paralysis, abnormal vital signs, or even difficulty walking should be evacuated immediately. If a patient appears stable but has been exposed to significant electrical discharge, close monitoring is required in the field.

When in doubt, err on the side of evacuation as injuries can be unpredictable, and the patient's clinical condition may worsen over time.

Altitude Illness

What are high-altitude emergencies?

High-altitude emergencies occur when the body fails to adapt to reduced oxygen availability, typically above 8,000 feet (2,500 meters). Although oxygen still makes up about 21% of the atmosphere at any elevation, the lower *pressure* at altitude means fewer oxygen molecules are delivered with each breath. This drop in *pressure*—not a change in the amount of oxygen—is what makes it harder to breathe and what leads to altitude illness.

To compensate, the body increases the respiratory and heart rate to maintain oxygen delivery to vital organs. Over time, other systems contribute as well—kidneys help regulate acid-base balance, and the bone marrow gradually produces more red blood cells to carry oxygen more efficiently. This acclimatization process takes days to weeks. For some individuals, especially those ascending too quickly, these adjustments fall short. The result may be acute mountain sickness (AMS), high-altitude pulmonary edema (HAPE), or high-altitude cerebral edema (HACE)—conditions that range from uncomfortable to life-threatening.

If symptoms worsen, *descent is the only definitive treatment*. Supplemental oxygen and medications may buy time but cannot substitute for the increased oxygen pressure at lower altitude.

What is acute mountain sickness, and how is it managed?

Acute mountain sickness (AMS) is the most common altitude-related illness. It occurs when the body fails to adapt quickly to reduced oxygen levels. Symptoms include headache, nausea, dizziness, fatigue, and difficulty sleeping—early signs that acclimatization is failing.

The most effective treatment is descent, and even a moderate drop in elevation can relieve symptoms. Rest, hydration, and over-the-counter medications like ibuprofen or acetaminophen may help with discomfort; but if symptoms persist or worsen, assume progression and descend immediately. If descent is delayed, acetazolamide (Diamox) can support acclimatization by stimulating ventilation, but it is not a treatment for severe illness and must never replace evacuation in a symptomatic or deteriorating patient.

What is high-altitude pulmonary edema, and how is it treated?

High-altitude pulmonary edema (HAPE) is a life-threatening condition triggered by low oxygen levels at elevation. In response to hypoxia, small blood vessels in the lungs *constrict*, raising pressure in the pulmonary circulation. This forces fluid into the air sacs (alveoli), impairing gas exchange and worsening oxygenation—a cycle that can quickly spiral without intervention.

Early signs include shortness of breath with exertion (dyspnea), fatigue, and a dry cough. As it worsens, breathing becomes difficult even at rest. Symptoms may include chest tightness, frothy pink sputum, and severe weakness. Blue lips or fingertips (cyanosis) and confusion are signs of dangerously low oxygen and require immediate intervention.

HAPE can affect anyone; but risk increases with rapid ascent, intense physical exertion, a personal history of HAPE, or a family history of the condition. Individuals who have had HAPE before are significantly more likely to experience it again.

Descent is the most effective treatment for HAPE, as even a modest drop in elevation can help relieve symptoms. Supplemental oxygen is highly beneficial. Medications like nifedipine may reduce pressure in the lungs but should never delay evacuation. If descent isn't immediately possible, a portable hyperbaric chamber can offer temporary improvement, but it is not a substitute for descent.

At altitude, any unexplained breathing difficulty should be treated as HAPE until proven otherwise, as delayed treatment can be rapidly fatal.

What is high-altitude cerebral edema (HACE), and how should it be managed?

High-altitude cerebral edema (HACE) is a life-threatening condition caused by fluid leakage into the brain, leading to swelling and increased intracranial pressure (ICP). At high elevations, hypoxia triggers cerebral *vasodilation*, increasing blood flow and pressure within the brain. As pressure rises, fluid leaks into brain tissue increasing the ICP, further reducing oxygen delivery and causing progressive neurologic decline. Without intervention, the cycle worsens—often ending in coma and death.

Symptoms typically begin with worsening acute mountain sickness (AMS), then progress rapidly. Early signs include confusion, poor coordination, and fatigue. As the condition advances, slurred speech, altered mental status, and loss of consciousness may develop.

As with HAPE, descent is the only definitive treatment. Even a moderate drop in elevation can relieve pressure and improve symptoms. Dexamethasone may slow progression by reducing brain swelling, but it is not curative and must not delay evacuation. Supplemental oxygen and portable hyperbaric chambers can provide short-term relief but do not replace descent.

At altitude, any neurologic symptoms—confusion, imbalance, or altered behavior—should be assumed to be HACE until proven otherwise and immediate evacuation is the priority.

What are the evacuation considerations for high-altitude emergencies?

Descent is the first and most critical step in treating all altitude-related conditions. AMS may improve with rest and monitoring, but HAPE and HACE require immediate evacuation. If symptoms worsen or fail to improve with descent, further evacuation to a lower elevation or medical facility is essential.

Guides should always have a plan for rapid evacuation—by foot, stretcher, or air—especially in high-risk environments. Advanced care may be necessary, particularly for patients with HAPE or HACE, who face the risk of sudden deterioration or lasting complications. Never wait to see if symptoms improve at altitude—they won't—and delays in evacuation can be fatal.

Hot & Cold

Hyperthermia

What is hyperthermia, and how is it treated?

Hyperthermia occurs when the body produces more heat than it can eliminate, driving core temperature above 40°C (104°F). Under normal conditions, heat is dissipated through sweating and increased blood flow to the skin. In extreme heat, high humidity, or during prolonged exertion, these cooling mechanisms can get overwhelmed. Humidity is especially dangerous because it limits evaporative cooling—the body's primary method of heat loss through sweat evaporation.

As core temperature rises, proteins denature, enzymes lose function, and electrolyte imbalances disrupt nerve and muscle activity. The clotting system becomes unstable, increasing the risk of both hemorrhage and clotting. High-demand organs—especially the brain, liver, and kidneys—are most vulnerable to excessive heat and without correction, multi-organ failure can occur.

Early symptoms include headache, dizziness, fatigue, nausea, a rapid pulse, and confusion. As the condition worsens, neurologic function deteriorates—seizures, coma, and death may follow.

Hyperthermia is a true medical emergency. The most effective treatment is cold-water immersion (CWI), submerging the patient up to the neck in water between 1.5-15°C (35-60°F). If CWI is not available, move the patient to shade; remove excess clothing; and apply wet sheets or ice packs to the neck, armpits, and groin. Cooling should continue until core temperature stabilizes.

Heat-related illness kills more people annually in the U.S. than hurricanes, tornadoes, and floods combined. Those at highest risk include infants, older adults, and individuals with chronic medical conditions. Risk increases further in humid environments, where evaporative cooling is impaired.

Can't patients just drink water?

Hydration is important, but excessive water intake won't correct hyperthermia—and can even cause harm. Drinking large volumes of plain water without sodium replacement can lead to hyponatremia—a dilutional drop in blood sodium that disrupts nerve conduction, muscle contraction, and fluid regulation.

Early symptoms include headache, nausea, and muscle cramps. As sodium drops further, confusion, vomiting, seizures, and coma may follow.

During heat illness or prolonged exertion, the goal isn't just fluid—it's electrolyte replacement. Use small, frequent sips of cool fluids that contain both sodium and glucose, such as oral rehydration solutions (ORS) or sports drinks. Avoid large volumes of plain water, especially in extreme heat.

Hyperthermia and dehydration require coordinated management: cooling, electrolyte replacement, and rest. (See "Dehydration" for more.)

Is it important to differentiate between heat exhaustion and heat stroke?

Yes, but treatment comes first. These conditions fall on the same spectrum, and in the field, cooling takes priority over classification.

Heat *exhaustion* involves heavy sweating, fatigue, nausea, and a rapid pulse. Core temperature is usually *under* 104°F, and *mental status stays normal.*

Heat *stroke* crosses that threshold—core temperature *exceeds* 104°F, and *mental status deteriorates*, from confusion to coma.

Both require rapid cooling and rehydration. But heat stroke is a dire medical emergency. Signs like confusion, vomiting, inability to take fluids, or seizures signal the need for immediate evacuation to advanced care.

Hypothermia

What is hypothermia, and how does it affect the body?

Hypothermia occurs when the body's core temperature drops below 95°F (35°C), impairing normal function and leading to potentially life-threatening complications. While often associated with cold climates, it can also occur in wet, windy, or even tropical environments where prolonged exposure causes excessive heat loss. Wet clothing, immersion in cool water, wind, or inadequate shelter can all accelerate the process.

To understand how hypothermia develops, it helps to know how the body loses heat. There are five primary mechanisms:

- Radiation – Heat radiates from the body into cooler surrounding air or space.
  Example: Standing still under a clear night sky, you lose body heat even without wind or contact.
- Conduction – Heat transfers directly to colder surfaces or water the body touches.
  Example: Lying on cold ground or sitting on wet rocks rapidly draws heat from your body.
- Convection – Moving air or water carries heat away from the skin.
  Example: Wind strips warmth from exposed skin, even when air temperature isn't cold.
- Evaporation – Sweat or moisture pulls heat from the body as it dries.
  Example: Damp clothing in dry air cools you quickly as moisture evaporates from the fabric.
- Respiration – Warm air is lost on exhale and replaced with cooler air on inhale.
  Example: Breathing heavily in cold weather steadily reduces core temperature, especially at rest.

Once core temperature starts to fall, reversing hypothermia becomes progressively more difficult. Recognizing these mechanisms is essential for hypothermia prevention and management in the wilderness.

What are the signs and symptoms of hypothermia?

Hypothermia presents in stages, with symptoms becoming progressively more severe as core temperature drops. Early signs include shivering, pale or bluish skin, cold extremities, and difficulty performing fine motor tasks.

As hypothermia progresses, shivering may slow or stop. Slurred speech, confusion, clumsiness, and poor coordination signal that the body's ability to regulate temperature is overwhelmed.

In severe cases, patients may develop slowed thinking, bradycardia, shallow or irregular breathing, and loss of consciousness. Left untreated, this leads to arrhythmias, organ failure, and death.

How do I treat hypothermia?

Early intervention is critical in hypothermia. Shivering, fatigue, and coordination problems typically mark the initial stages. Hypothermia can develop even in mild or tropical climates when prolonged exposure to wind, moisture, or cold surfaces results in steady heat loss. The progression from manageable cold stress to life-threatening hypothermia is gradual and thankfully, predictable.

Treatment focuses on limiting further heat loss and supporting gradual rewarming. Wet clothing contributes significantly to conductive and evaporative heat loss and should be replaced with dry, insulated layers. Wind, moisture, and contact with cold ground or surfaces accelerate heat transfer away from the body. Passive rewarming methods—such as insulated wraps, warm fluids for those able to swallow, and shared body heat—can help stabilize and increase core body temperature.

In moderate to severe hypothermia, mental status deteriorates, and the body's protective reflexes diminish.

The heart becomes more prone to irregular rhythms, and even minor movement can trigger dangerous arrhythmias. Rewarming must be gradual, as sudden warming of the extremities can cause afterdrop—recirculating cold blood to the core. Direct heat sources can cause burns due to poor circulation and reduced sensation.

Persistent hypothermia-altered mental status or clinical decline despite rewarming efforts indicate the need for advanced medical care.

How does drinking alcohol contribute to hypothermia?

Alcohol accelerates heat loss by dilating blood vessels near the skin's surface, creating a false sense of warmth while increasing heat loss to the surrounding environment. The sensation may feel comforting, but it speeds core cooling and raises the risk of hypothermia. Alcohol also suppresses natural defenses like shivering and thermoregulation, reducing the body's ability to generate and conserve heat. Impaired judgment adds further risk, as intoxicated individuals may fail to recognize symptoms, seek shelter, or dress appropriately—making prolonged cold exposure more likely.

Frostbite

What is frostbite?

Frostbite occurs when tissues freeze from prolonged exposure to extreme cold. Ice crystals form within cells, disrupting structure and causing cellular injury. It typically affects exposed or poorly insulated body areas—fingers, toes, ears, and the nose.

Frostbite progresses in distinct stages. Frostnip, the mildest form, causes redness, tingling, and numbness and is fully reversible with rewarming. Superficial frostbite follows, marked by pale, waxy skin and possible blistering—this damage is still *mostly* reversible. Deep frostbite involves hard, cold tissue; significant numbness; and discoloration, indicating full-thickness injury and often permanent damage.

How is frostbite treated?

Initial management focuses on protecting the tissue from further injury and preventing thaw-refreeze cycles, which cause the most severe damage. Frozen tissue should not be rewarmed if there is any chance it will refreeze before evacuation—this worsens outcomes.

Once the risk of refreezing is eliminated, rewarming should be done using body heat or warm water immersion (ideally 98–102°F/37–39°C). Do not use hot water, fires, or stoves as numb tissue burns easily. Thawing is often painful and may cause swelling or blistering.

The affected area should be kept clean, dry, and protected from pressure or friction. Blisters should not be ruptured in the field. If walking is necessary, avoid thawing frozen feet or toes. Frozen tissue tolerates mechanical use better than thawed, fragile tissue.

Oral anti-inflammatories (e.g., ibuprofen) may reduce further damage by limiting inflammation and microvascular clotting.

Evacuation is indicated for any deep frostbite, blistering, persistent numbness, or if the patient is unable to keep the area protected and dry.

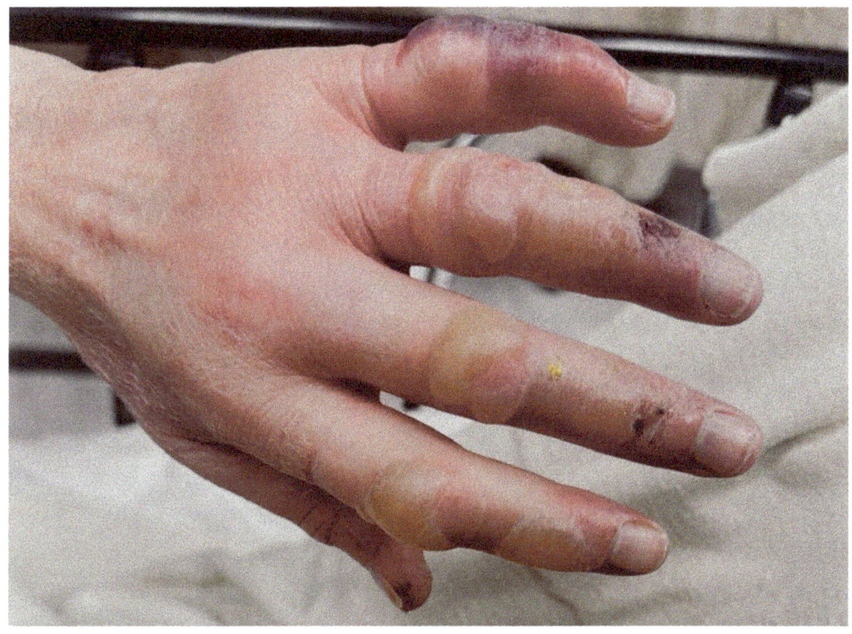

Frostbite sustained while cold camping in the central Rockies. The patient presented with a combination of second-degree (superficial) and third-degree (deep) frostbite, with hemorrhagic blisters and moderate tissue damage involving multiple digits. Image courtesy of the author.

Avalanches

What is an avalanche?

An avalanche is a rapid release of snow down a slope, triggered when weak layers in the snowpack collapse under added weight, temperature shifts, or disturbances from people or animals. Snow can accelerate to 60–80 mph within seconds, carrying enough force to shear trees and cause significant trauma.

As it moves, avalanche snow behaves like a fluid driven by gravity and friction, allowing it to flow freely and wrap around and fill terrain features. When the movement stops, friction also stops, and the snow sets up—transitioning from near-liquid to solid. Victims are immobilized. Chest expansion is restricted, and even the smallest movement becomes impossible. If snow enters the airway, survival is unlikely.

What are the first steps after an avalanche?

Scene safety comes first as secondary slides are a major risk. Once the slope is stable, begin a structured search using transceivers, visual clues, and probe strikes. Shoveling begins as soon as a strike is confirmed.

How long is the window for survival?

The first 15 minutes is the critical window. Most live recoveries occur within that timeframe. Beyond that, oxygen deprivation often becomes fatal unless the victim has an air pocket. By 30 minutes, survival without an airway is rare while trauma deaths often occur immediately or soon after impact.

What types of injuries are expected and how should survivors be managed?

Asphyxiation is the most common cause of death. Blunt trauma to the head, chest, and spine is common. Survivors may have extremity injuries, crush-related complications, and varying degrees of hypothermia.

As with all traumatic events, the airway should be cleared and managed first. Protect the cervical spine and treat based on primary and secondary survey findings. If hypothermic, rewarming should be initiated aggressively in the field with available resources. In cases of cardiac arrest—especially if the core body temperature is below 85°F (30°C)—prolonged resuscitative efforts may be appropriate unless traumatic injuries are incompatible with life. Evacuate all survivors of a complete avalanche burial—regardless of injury, mental status, or exposure time.

What gear improves outcomes?

No piece of gear guarantees survival. While transceivers, probes, and shovels are essential for companion rescue, and airbag systems can reduce burial depth—no gear replaces training.

The most reliable protection is prevention—accurate snowpack assessment, terrain discipline, and group travel protocols.

This one hits close to home, so please live to ski and ride another day.

Dive Medicine

What are "the bends"?

Decompression sickness (DCS), often called "the bends," occurs when dissolved nitrogen forms gas bubbles in the body during ascent from a dive. Standard dive tanks contain compressed air, which—like atmospheric air—is about 78% nitrogen. At depth, increased pressure causes this nitrogen to dissolve into body tissues, particularly fat, joints, and the central nervous system.

If ascent is too rapid, the pressure drops faster than the nitrogen can safely leave solution. Bubbles form—first in the bloodstream and tissues, disrupting circulation, stretching tissue, and triggering inflammatory responses. The effects vary widely—from joint pain and skin rashes to neurologic injury, paralysis, and death.

The name "the bends" comes from a classic presentation: deep joint and muscle pain that forces divers into a bent, stooped posture, first observed in 19th-century caisson workers building underwater tunnels and bridge foundations, who developed these symptoms after surfacing too quickly.

Risk factors include greater depth, longer dive time, repetitive dives, cold water, dehydration, physical exertion, and rapid ascents—especially when decompression stops are missed.

What are the symptoms of DCS, and what is the management in remote settings?

Symptoms of decompression sickness (DCS) can be subtle in onset and are often mistaken for fatigue, soreness, or even a viral illness. Most cases develop within one to six hours of surfacing, but delayed presentations beyond 24 hours are documented.

DCS is categorized into two clinical types. Type I DCS typically presents with localized musculoskeletal symptoms—most commonly a deep, aching pain in joints or limbs. Skin manifestations such as *cutis marmorata* (a mottled, marbled rash) may also occur due to inert gas bubbles in the dermis.

Type II DCS involves neurologic or cardiopulmonary compromise. Symptoms may include dizziness, weakness, bladder dysfunction, confusion, or altered consciousness. In severe presentations, gas emboli to the lungs may cause severe shortness of breath, coughing, or sudden collapse—a condition referred to "the chokes." Any neurological involvement is potentially catastrophic and should be treated as a medical emergency.

Initial management on-site or aboard a vessel involves administration of 100% oxygen, which accelerates nitrogen elimination through a process known as "nitrogen washout." Breathing pure oxygen displaces nitrogen from the alveoli, sharply reducing pulmonary nitrogen partial pressure in the lungs. This creates a diffusion gradient that draws nitrogen out of the blood and tissues into the lungs, allowing it to then be exhaled.

The patient should remain on their back (supine). Oral fluids are appropriate if the patient is alert and able to tolerate them. IV fluids are preferred if available. Definitive care is recompression therapy in a hyperbaric chamber, which should be initiated without delay. Early recompression—ideally within hours—yields the best outcomes.

While mild cases without neurologic symptoms may improve with oxygen therapy alone, this determination should only be made with input from medical control. A recent dive within 48 hours and compatible symptoms should always raise concern for DCS.

What is barotrauma as it relates to dive medicine?

Barotrauma is injury caused by pressure changes in gas-filled spaces of the body. The prefix *baro-* comes from the Greek word for pressure or weight. Unlike decompression sickness—which involves nitrogen bubbles forming in tissues—barotrauma happens when expanding gas stretches or ruptures tissue during ascent.

As a diver goes deeper, pressure increases and compresses gases in the body. On ascent, that pressure drops, and the gases expand. If the expanding gas can't escape—such as from the middle ear, sinuses, or lungs—it can damage surrounding tissue.

The middle ear is the most commonly affected area. If pressure isn't equalized through the eustachian tubes, it builds up and may cause pain or rupture the eardrum. Sinus barotrauma occurs when blocked sinus passages trap gas, leading to facial pressure or nosebleeds.

Pulmonary barotrauma is the most dangerous form. If a diver ascends without exhaling, expanding air can overinflate the lungs, causing rupture. This may lead to pneumothorax (collapsed lung) or, if gas enters blood vessels, arterial gas embolism (AGE)—a life-threatening condition that can block blood flow to the brain, heart, or other organs.

Barotrauma usually presents during or right after a dive. It can be distinguished from decompression sickness based on timing and symptoms. Most mild cases resolve with rest and pain control. Signs of lung or neurologic involvement—such as chest pain, shortness of breath, or confusion—require high-flow oxygen and immediate evacuation.

What is nitrogen narcosis?

As covered earlier, nitrogen from the breathing gas in a dive tank dissolves into the bloodstream and tissues under pressure—including the brain. At depth, rising nitrogen levels in the central nervous system begin to interfere with normal function, impairing the brain's ability to process information and respond appropriately.

The result is nitrogen narcosis, a condition typically seen below 30 meters (about 100 feet). It produces symptoms similar to alcohol intoxication—slowed thinking, impaired coordination, poor judgment, and, at times, confusion or anxiety. The deeper the dive, the more pronounced the effect.

The primary risk isn't the symptoms—but the fact that the diver often doesn't recognize them. Although narcosis resolves on ascent, it can lead to dangerous decisions at depth, including exceeding limits or missing signs of more serious problems.

Bites & Stings

How do I deal with bites and stings in the wilderness?

Bites and stings are common in wilderness settings, with outcomes ranging from mild irritation to life-threatening reactions. Effective management begins with identifying the type of injury, addressing the wound, minimizing complications, and evaluating the need for evacuation. Early, appropriate care can prevent a manageable issue from escalating into a medical emergency.

Scene safety comes first. Move away from swarming insects; avoid contact with venomous animals; and be alert for secondary hazards like falls, water exposure, or additional bites. Once the area is safe, clean the wound thoroughly with soap and water or an antiseptic such as povidone-iodine to lower the risk of infection. Remove any rings, bracelets, or watches from the affected limb before swelling begins. Immobilization and elevation may help reduce discomfort and swelling, depending on the injury.

For stings, visible stingers should be removed by gently scraping with a card or blunt-edged object. Avoid using tweezers or squeezing the site, as this can inject more venom into the tissue. Further management depends on the species involved, symptom severity, and whether systemic effects—such as allergic reactions or envenomation—are present.

Recognizing when evacuation is necessary is key to preventing serious complications far from help.

Are antibiotics necessary for all bites?

Bites from animals, humans, reptiles, or fish carry a high risk of infection. In most cases, antibiotics are indicated—especially for puncture wounds, bites to the hands or feet, or injuries involving significant tissue damage, where bacteria can spread rapidly.

Tetanus prophylaxis should be up to date before entering remote areas. Mammal bites also raise concern for rabies exposure, which requires *prompt* post-exposure treatment. In wilderness settings where access is limited, possible rabies exposure warrants *immediate* evacuation. *Read that again.*

Is it antivenin or antivenom?

Both terms are correct. *Antivenin* is an older term, while *antivenom* is more commonly used in modern medical literature. These products are made from antibodies harvested from animals—typically horses or sheep—that have been immunized with small amounts of venom. The resulting antibodies bind to and neutralize venom, helping to prevent or reduce systemic effects.

Antivenoms are usually region-specific and are produced for bites or stings from local species of snakes, spiders, scorpions, ticks, jellyfish, and other venomous animals. Availability varies widely by region and species.

Land

Spiders

Where do the most dangerous spiders live?

While most spider bites are harmless, a limited number of species worldwide are responsible for clinically significant envenomations. These can involve neurotoxic, cytotoxic, or systemic effects. Severity depends on species, geography, and access to medical care or antivenom.

North America

- Black widow spiders (*Latrodectus mactans*): Neurotoxic venom causes painful muscle cramping, abdominal rigidity and autonomic symptoms—like sweating and high blood pressure (latrodectism) Antivenom exists but is used selectively.
- Brown recluse spiders (*Loxosceles reclusa*): Cytotoxic venom can cause necrotic skin lesions. Systemic loxoscelism (e.g., hemolysis, renal injury) is rare but documented.

Central and South America

- Brazilian wandering spiders (*Phoneutria* spp.): Potent neurotoxic venom may lead to intense pain, nervous system instability, and respiratory distress.
- Chilean recluse (*Loxosceles laeta*): Similar but more severe than *L. reclusa*, with higher risk for systemic toxicity.

Europe and the Mediterranean

- Mediterranean black widow (*Latrodectus tredecimguttatus*): Causes painful muscle cramping and autonomic symptoms—like sweating and high blood pressure (latrodectism) similar to *L. mactans*, often affecting agricultural workers.

- Mediterranean recluse (*Loxosceles rufescens*): Associated with necrotic bites, although systemic effects are less frequent.

Africa

- Six-eyed sand spiders (*Sicarius* spp.): Rarely bite humans, but venom contains the toxic enzyme sphingomyelinase D, causing skin necrosis and possible systemic toxicity.
- Widow spiders (*Latrodectus* spp.): Neurotoxic effects similar to other *Latrodectus* species.

Asia

- Chinese bird spider (*Haplopelma* spp.): Anecdotal reports of neurotoxic symptoms exist, including muscle spasms and respiratory distress, but bites are rare.
- Indian ornamental tarantulas (*Poecilotheria* spp.): May cause localized pain and muscle cramping; systemic effects are uncommon.

Australia

- Sydney funnel-web spider (*Atrax robustus*): One of the world's most venomous spiders. Envenomation causes rapid-onset neurotoxicity, pulmonary edema, and death if untreated. Antivenom is effective and widely available.
- Northern tree funnel-web (*Hadronyche formidabilis*): Similar in clinical severity to *Atrax robustus*.
- Redback spider (*Latrodectus hasselti*): Causes latrodectism (intense muscle cramping, sweating, elevated heart rate, and widespread nerve overstimulation). Antivenom is readily available across urban areas.

Oceania and Pacific Islands

- Katipō spider (*Latrodectus katipo*): Endemic to New Zealand; rarely bites, but envenomation mimics other *Latrodectus* species.

- False widow spiders (*Steatoda* spp.): Bites may cause localized pain, muscle cramping, abdominal rigidity, and mild autonomic effects.

Who is most at risk for spider bites in the wilderness?

It's obvious, but wilderness travelers face a higher risk of spider bites when camping or hiking in areas where venomous species live.

Reaching into dark crevices, woodpiles, or under rocks, as well as sleeping directly on the ground without a barrier, increases exposure. Activities like collecting firewood, clearing brush, or building shelters without gloves raise the risk further. Spiders are more active at night, so bites are also more likely during evening activities or when sleeping in undisturbed areas.

To reduce the risk, wear gloves and long clothing when handling wood or debris, avoid reaching into dark areas, and shake out bedding, clothing, and shoes before use. Sleeping off the ground, checking under toilet seats—this is from experience—and using sealed tents or nets can help prevent contact. Awareness of local spider species and their preferred habitats is critical for prevention in spider-prone areas.

How are spider bites managed in the wilderness, and when is evacuation necessary?

Initial treatment includes washing the bite with soap and water, applying a cold pack for pain and swelling, immobilizing the limb, and using pain relievers like acetaminophen or ibuprofen. Cutting or sucking the wound is ineffective and can make things worse. Evacuation is necessary if systemic symptoms develop—such as muscle spasms, trouble breathing, fever, or confusion—or if the bite is suspected to be from a highly venomous species. Large necrotic wounds, signs of infection, or any concerning symptoms in children, the elderly, or those with medical conditions also warrant evacuation.

Ticks

What diseases can ticks transmit?

Tick-borne illnesses are a global concern, particularly in wooded, grassy, or brushy environments where ticks thrive. These blood-feeding parasites can transmit serious infections during attachment. In North America, the most common tick-borne diseases include Lyme disease, Rocky Mountain spotted fever (RMSF), and anaplasmosis—each caused by distinct bacterial pathogens.

Lyme disease, caused by the spirochete *Borrelia burgdorferi*, often begins with a flu-like illness and may feature a characteristic bull's-eye rash (erythema migrans). If untreated, it can progress to joint pain, neurologic complications, and cardiac involvement (Lyme carditis).

Rocky Mountain spotted fever, caused by *Rickettsia rickettsii*, is a classic example of a rickettsial illness, and among the most severe tick-borne infections in North America. It presents with high fever, headache, and rash, and may rapidly progress to multi-organ failure if not treated early.

Anaplasmosis, caused by *Anaplasma phagocytophilum*, infects white blood cells and leads to fever, chills, myalgias, and fatigue. In vulnerable individuals, it can result in respiratory compromise or bleeding disorders.

Many tick-borne bacteria—including *Rickettsia* and *Anaplasma* species—target either blood vessels or immune cells. In infections like RMSF, the bacteria invade the thin lining of blood vessels (endothelium), causing inflammation and leakage. This leads to symptoms like rash, low blood pressure, and organ dysfunction. In anaplasmosis, the bacteria hide inside a type of white blood cell (neutrophils), disrupting the immune response and triggering widespread inflammation. While symptoms often start out vague—fever, headache, fatigue—the underlying issues are direct hits to the body's circulation and immune regulation.

Globally, ticks transmit additional high-risk diseases. Tick-borne encephalitis virus (TBEV) is prevalent in parts of Europe and Asia, while Crimean-Congo hemorrhagic fever is found in Africa, Eastern Europe, and Central Asia. In sub-Saharan Africa and Australia, spotted fever group rickettsioses are a common cause of febrile illness and may become life-threatening if not treated promptly.

Because many of these infections present with nonspecific symptoms, early recognition of tick exposure is critical. Doxycycline is the first-line treatment for most bacterial tick-borne diseases, including rickettsial infections and anaplasmosis, is an important antibiotic to carry when in endemic areas and is most effective when started promptly.

How do you remove a tick?

Use fine-tipped tweezers to grasp the tick as close to the skin as possible and pull upward with steady, even pressure. Avoid twisting or jerking, which increases the chance of leaving mouthparts embedded in the skin. After removal, clean the bite site with soap and water or an antiseptic solution.

In the wilderness, disposal depends on what's available: dropping the tick into a fire, crushing it between two rocks, sealing it in a piece of tape, or feeding it to a passing ant colony—all are effective ways to ensure its disposal.

Is evacuation necessary for tick bites?

Most tick bites do not require evacuation. However, if symptoms of tick-borne illness develop—such as fever, rash, profound fatigue, or neurological changes like confusion—evacuation is warranted. Early antibiotic treatment, especially with doxycycline, is critical for diseases like Lyme and Rocky Mountain spotted fever, both of which can become severe or life-threatening if left untreated.

Prevention is equally—if not more important. The best defense is a combination of avoidance and vigilance: wear long clothing, use EPA-approved insect repellents containing DEET or permethrin, and perform thorough daily tick checks when traveling through high-risk areas.

Scorpions

What do I need to know about scorpions?

Scorpion stings range from painful but harmless to life-threatening, depending on the species and individual response. Most stings cause intense local pain, swelling, redness, and numbness. However, species in North Africa, the Middle East, and the southwestern U.S. can trigger systemic symptoms: muscle spasms, sweating, nausea, rapid heart rate, breathing difficulty, or—rarely—seizures and shock.

Scorpion venom contains neurotoxins that disrupt the sodium and potassium channels in nerves, keeping them firing when they should be at rest. This overstimulates muscles and the nervous system, affecting breathing or heart function.

Initial treatment includes cleaning the site, applying a cold pack (not direct ice), and immobilizing the limb at heart level. Use acetaminophen or ibuprofen for pain. Avoid aspirin due to increased bleeding risk.

Evacuate if systemic symptoms appear, especially in children, older adults, or anyone with underlying medical conditions. Evacuation is also recommended if symptoms persist for multiple hours, signs of infection develop, or the sting occurs in a region with high-risk species, where antivenom may be needed. Lastly, avoid outdated or harmful treatments like suction, electrical therapy, or tourniquets.

Snakes

Where are dangerous snakes found, and how common are snakebites?

Dangerous snakes are found on nearly every continent, with certain regions presenting higher risks due to their density and diversity of venomous species. In North America, rattlesnakes, coral snakes, copperheads, and cottonmouths are the primary threats—particularly in the southern U.S. Central and South America are home to species such as the fer-de-lance, bushmaster, and coral snake. In Africa, high-risk species include black mambas, puff adders, and spitting cobras. South and Southeast Asia are known for cobras, kraits, and Russell's vipers. My former home, Australia hosts some of the most venomous snakes globally, including the inland taipan, tiger snake, and eastern brown snake. Island regions of Southeast Asia and Oceania are inhabited by venomous sea snakes and banded kraits.

Each year, snakebites affect roughly 5 million people worldwide, with around 2 million cases of envenomation and over 100,000 deaths. The highest burden falls on rural, tropical, and subtropical regions, where access to medical care and antivenom is limited.

How can you identify venomous snakes in the field?

Identifying venomous snakes can be difficult, as there are no fully reliable physical characteristics. While some venomous species, such as pit vipers (e.g., rattlesnakes, copperheads), may have heat-sensing pits between the eyes and nostrils, and others may display triangular or diamond-shaped heads, these traits are not universal. Many venomous snakes have elliptical pupils, though the coral snake, for example, has round pupils. Venomous species may also exhibit warning behaviors like rattling (rattlesnakes) or hood flaring (cobras), but these behaviors aren't always consistent.

Although distinctive markings—such as the bright bands of coral snakes or the patterns on pit vipers—can sometimes help, mimics of these species can make identification unreliable. Ultimately, the best practice is to know what dangerous snakes are around and avoid handling any snake. Focus on prevention and avoidance.

How can snakebites be prevented?

To reduce the risk of snakebites, minimize exposure and stay alert to snake habitats. Wear protective clothing, such as high boots, long pants, and gaiters, during hikes in snake-prone areas. Like spider avoidance, refrain from reaching into holes, under rocks, or into thick brush and always shake out bedding, shoes, and clothing before use, as snakes may hide in these spaces. Stick to well-maintained trails and avoid dense vegetation where snakes may conceal themselves.

At night, use a flashlight or headlamp as snakes are more active after dark. Educating yourself and others about local snake species and their behaviors is key to preventing bites. If you encounter a snake, stay calm, back away slowly, and avoid sudden movements.

What are the symptoms of venomous snakebites?

Symptoms of a snakebite vary depending on the type of venom and generally fall into four broad categories:

- *Neurotoxic* venom, found in species like cobras, mambas, and kraits, interferes with the normal function of the nervous system. It typically works by blocking neurotransmitter receptors or preventing effective communication between nerves and muscles. This disruption can lead to symptoms such as ptosis (drooping eyelids), dysarthria (slurred speech), progressive muscle weakness, and, in severe cases, paralysis and respiratory failure due to diaphragm involvement.
- *Hemotoxic* venom, common in vipers and pit vipers, affects the blood and circulatory system. These venoms contain enzymes that disrupt clotting, damage blood vessels, and degrade tissue, leading bruising, swelling, and clotting abnormalities. If left untreated, hemotoxic envenomation can result in shock, severe internal hemorrhage, and organ damage.
- *Cytotoxic* venom, present in puff adders and some vipers, causes localized tissue destruction by breaking down cell membranes and proteins. This results in severe pain, swelling, blistering, and necrosis at the bite site. Without prompt treatment, the cytotoxic

effects can lead to permanent tissue damage, or even limb loss.

- Nonvenomous snakebites, while painful, typically cause localized swelling, redness, and puncture marks without systemic effects. However, all snakebites should be taken seriously, as misidentification of the species or unexpected reactions can complicate treatment.

Recognizing these categories helps determine the urgency of care and the best course of action, especially in remote settings.

How should a snakebite be managed in the wilderness?

Initial management focuses on patient stabilization and preparing for evacuation. Keep the patient calm and still, as movement can accelerate venom spread through the lymphatic system. Immobilize the affected limb with a splint or sling and position it at or slightly below heart level. Remove rings, watches, or tight clothing before swelling develops.

Gently clean the bite with soap and water. Avoid outdated or harmful interventions—cutting the wound, suctioning venom, applying ice, or using tourniquets are not effective and can cause additional damage.

Monitor for signs of systemic envenomation, including breathing difficulty, expanding swelling, altered mental status, or neurological symptoms. For pain, acetaminophen is preferred. Avoid NSAIDs like ibuprofen or aspirin due to the risk of bleeding.

Document the bite location, time, and progression of symptoms—this information is essential for receiving providers.

Lizards

Is this really a thing?

It shouldn't be—but is. Lizard bites generally fall into the category of "play stupid games, win stupid prizes." Most lizards will not bite unless provoked; but certain species, like the Gila monster and Komodo dragon, can deliver venomous and bacteria-laden bites that often lead to serious complications. These bites typically occur when the lizard is handled or threatened, often in the biodiverse regions such as tropical rainforests or arid deserts that they call home.

What venomous lizards should I know?

Only a small number of lizard species are venomous, but their bites can still cause serious complications—especially in remote or wilderness settings. The most well-known are the Gila monster (*Heloderma suspectum*) and the Mexican beaded lizard (*Heloderma horridum*), both native to North and Central America. These lizards deliver venom through uniquely grooved teeth while chewing, often resulting in prolonged bites that are difficult to disengage from. Envenomation may cause intense burning pain, swelling, nausea, and vomiting. Severe reactions can include loss of consciousness, respiratory distress, or shock if not managed promptly.

The Komodo dragon (*Varanus komodoensis*)—the largest venomous lizard on earth—poses a much greater threat due to its size, bite force, and venom effects. Native to Indonesia, its venom impairs blood clotting, increasing the risk of hemorrhage and hypovolemic shock. Combined with oral bacteria and the physical destruction from the bite itself, these injuries can rapidly progress to systemic infection and death. While rare, human attacks are well-documented and potentially fatal without urgent care.

Other monitor lizards (*Varanus* spp.) are found throughout Africa, South Asia, Southeast Asia, and northern Australia. While some species produce venom, their clinical significance remains unclear. Bites may still lead to infection, localized pain, or swelling—particularly if the wound is neglected or occurs in austere conditions. Most incidents involve humans attempting to handle, feed, or corner the animal.

Evacuation should be considered after any venomous lizard bite due to the risk of delayed symptoms, infection, or systemic involvement. Don't play with dinosaurs.

How do I treat a lizard bite?

Begin by thoroughly cleaning the wound with soap and water or an antiseptic solution (such as povidone-iodine, diluted hydrogen peroxide, or a weak bleach solution) to reduce the risk of infection. *This initial wound care is essential.* Avoid applying ice or using a tourniquet—both can worsen tissue damage.

Pain management should be approached carefully. Ibuprofen is generally avoided due to its potential to increase bleeding risk. Acetaminophen is a reasonable first-line option. In more severe cases, opioids may be needed for adequate pain control, and benzodiazepines can be used to manage muscle spasms, especially if there's envenomation with systemic effects.

There is no specific antivenom for lizard bites. Treatment focuses on symptom control, infection prevention, and monitoring for complications. Signs of systemic involvement—such as difficulty breathing, significant swelling, or shock—require prompt recognition. In most cases, evacuation is warranted for further evaluation and care.

Monkeys

Are monkeys dangerous?

Absolutely. Monkey bites carry significant medical risk due to the potential transmission of both viral and bacterial infections. In regions where monkeys live in close proximity to humans—such as parts of Asia, Africa, and tourist-heavy areas—zoonotic transmission is a serious concern. Diseases such as simian herpes virus (B virus), tuberculosis, and hepatitis B have all been documented in monkeys and can be transmitted through bites or scratches.

Bacterial infection is also common, as monkey bites often involve deep puncture wounds that introduce pathogens directly into tissue. These injuries can quickly become infected without prompt and appropriate wound care.

Rabies is the most critical concern. Rabies transmission from monkeys has been documented primarily in parts of Asia and Africa, where canine rabies remains endemic. In Central America, rabies is less common, but monkey bites are still considered a theoretical risk, especially in regions where rabies-infected dogs or bats are present.

Like any rabid mammal, an infected monkey can transmit the virus through saliva, typically via a bite or scratch. Even minor contact can be fatal if left untreated. Rabies is universally *fatal* once symptoms begin. Immediate wound cleaning and post-exposure prophylaxis (PEP) is essential—and should never be delayed.

Read that again.

Beyond infection, monkey bites can cause structural injury—damaging skin, muscle, or nerves, particularly on the hands, arms, or face. Monkeys may behave aggressively, especially when provoked or in competition for food, and their strength and speed often catch people off guard.

All monkey bites should be treated seriously, with a low threshold for evacuation—especially in areas where rabies risk is high or access to PEP is uncertain.

Bears

What should I do if I come across a bear?

Breathe. Do not run. Stand your ground, speak calmly, and back away slowly—without turning your back on the bear.

For brown bears like grizzlies: Play dead if attacked—face down, hands over your neck, pack on, legs spread. If the bear doesn't leave or becomes more aggressive, fight back—with everything you've got.

For black bears: Always fight back. Do not play dead.

What if I have bear spray or a firearm?

Spray should be deployed at 8-18 meters (25–60 feet). Aim low and sweep side to side. Spray is more effective than firearms in most encounters. When it comes to a gun, make it count. Only shoot if a good shot and at close range, aiming for the brainstem—low at the base of the skull. Otherwise, try to escape. A grizzly's skull can be 1.5 inches thick, with dense muscle and heavy hide over an angled skull making perfect placement of a high-powered round your only chance. Side shots just in front of the ear are apparently more effective. Poorly placed shots are rarely effective and may even worsen the attack.

What is the priority after a bear attack?

It's not the medical care of the patient. The immediate priority is responder and group safety. If the bear is still present or nearby, get distance. Break line of sight and avoid further provocation. *Do not attempt to render care until the threat is gone.*

What are the medical priorities?

This is the land-based equivalent of a white shark attack—sudden, violent, and treated in much the same way. Priorities become brutally simple—the patient will bleed out unless you act immediately and aggressively.

First, secure the scene. If the bear is still nearby, move. Stop bleeding as rapidly as possible and ignore everything else until you reach a safe location. The only thing worse than a bear attack victim is two victims.

Once the scene is safe, hemorrhage control remains the top priority. Bear maulings frequently involve the face, neck, arms, or thighs—areas where major bleeding can be rapidly fatal. Use direct pressure, hemostatic agents, and tourniquets as indicated. (See "Bleeding" or "Shark Attack.")

After bleeding is controlled, assess the airway. Facial trauma, soft tissue swelling, or neck injuries may compromise breathing. Clear the airway, reposition the patient, and assist ventilations if needed. Advanced procedures are rarely successful in wilderness settings and should not distract from basic interventions that stabilize the patient.

Fracture immobilization, hypothermia prevention, and rapid evacuation planning follow once bleeding and airway are addressed.

Anything else?

You know it. All bear bite wounds are high-risk for infection. If time and resources allow, copious irrigation is essential, followed by broad-spectrum antibiotics as soon as possible. Even minor-looking wounds often hide deep punctures, crushed muscle, or fractured bone beneath the surface.

All patients should be evacuated for surgical evaluation, debridement, and definitive care. Every attack should also be reported to wildlife authorities with accurate location and incident details to help prevent future encounters.

What about rabies?

Rabies in bears is rare but possible. If the attack was unprovoked, occurred during daylight, or involved abnormal behavior, post-exposure prophylaxis should be started. In bear attacks, it is reasonable to initiate the rabies vaccine series as soon as possible.

Big Cats

What should I do if I come across a big cat?

Big cats—mountain lions, pumas, jaguars, leopards, and lions—are ambush predators. Most attacks happen when a person is alone, quiet, or appears vulnerable. And relative to a cat, you're always vulnerable. If you find yourself in this situation, you were most likely being hunted. If you see one, do not run. Make yourself large, raise your arms, maintain eye contact, and back away slowly while speaking firmly. If the animal crouches, stares, or flicks its tail, it may be preparing to strike. If it charges, fight back—hard. Aim for the face and eyes. Use rocks, sticks, trekking poles—anything available. People have survived by fighting hard and staying aggressive. If you have bear spray, use it. While direct studies on big cats are limited, capsaicin affects all mammals and causes intense irritation to the eyes, throat, and airway. It has proven highly effective against bears and is recommended by the National Park Service and U.S. Fish and Wildlife Service for use on mountain lions.

What kinds of injuries should I expect?

Expect deep puncture wounds from the teeth and long slashing lacerations from the claws. Common injury sites include the head, neck, shoulders, back, and upper limbs. Victims may also be dragged or slammed, resulting in blunt trauma, fractures, or internal bleeding.

What are the treatment priorities in the field?

Again, ensure the scene is safe *before* beginning care. Hemorrhage control is the first priority—use direct pressure, hemostatic agents, or tourniquets as needed. Once bleeding is controlled, assess and manage the airway, especially in the presence of facial trauma or altered consciousness. Clear the airway, reposition the patient, and assist breathing if required. Focus on simple—life-saving measures over advanced procedures.

Anything else?

Yes. The oral flora of big cats includes *Pasteurella multocida*, *Staphylococcus*, *Streptococcus*, and a host of other bacteria. Their claws can introduce soil and fecal bacteria. Wounds should be irrigated thoroughly with clean water, or saline if available; left open; and loosely dressed. Do not close punctures in the field. If evacuation is delayed and antibiotics are available, start treatment. These wounds often require deep irrigation and formal debridement in an operating room. Evacuation is essential.

What about rabies?

Same deal as bears—the patient should start the post-exposure prophylaxis (PEP) series once they reach definitive care.

When should I evacuate?

All patients attacked by a big cat should be evacuated as soon as reasonably safe to do so. Even seemingly minor wounds can conceal deep injury, tendon or joint involvement, or dangerous infections. Immediate evacuation is critical if there is uncontrolled bleeding; injury to the face, neck, or airway; signs of systemic infection; or any suspicion of internal trauma. Surviving the attack is only the beginning—these patients often need surgery, antibiotics, and extensive follow-up care.

Water

Jellyfish

What should I know about jellyfish?

Jellyfish stings are one of the most common marine envenomations, with an estimated 150 million stings worldwide each year. While many cause only mild irritation, some species—such as the box jellyfish, Irukandji jellyfish, and Portuguese man o' war—can trigger severe pain, systemic reactions, or even cardiovascular collapse.

Environmental factors matter. Prevailing winds, tides, and currents often drive dangerous species closer to shore, increasing the risk for swimmers, waders, and beachgoers. In many regions, box jellyfish and Portuguese man o' war are carried into coastal waters by seasonal patterns. Understanding local conditions—and recognizing when risk is elevated—is just as important as knowing how to respond.

Jellyfish have been around for over 500 million years, and more than 100 species are capable of delivering venomous stings harmful to humans, making them the most dangerous of marine creatures. Severe envenomation can lead to intense pain, muscle spasms, breathing difficulties, paralysis, and even fatal reactions within minutes. Given the frequency and potential severity of encounters, understanding proper treatment is essential in wilderness and marine medicine.

Jellyfish are widely distributed across subtropical and tropical waters, including the Atlantic, Pacific, Asian, and Australian coasts. Their venom is delivered through thousands of specialized stinging cells called nematocysts, which can still fire even after the jellyfish is dead. Detached tentacles or washed-up jellyfish remain dangerous, making contact a risk even outside the water.

How dangerous are jellyfish stings?

Jellyfish stings range from mild irritation to life-threatening envenomation, depending on the species and venom exposure. Most stings cause intense burning pain, redness, swelling, and welts resembling tentacle marks. However, box jellyfish and Irukandji jellyfish can trigger nausea, vomiting, difficulty breathing, muscle spasms, chest pain, and even cardiac arrest within minutes. Detached tentacles can still sting, making even beached jellyfish or floating tentacles a risk.

Children, the elderly, and those with preexisting conditions are at higher risk for severe reactions. Immediate evacuation is necessary if the patient experiences trouble breathing, severe pain that does not improve, confusion, chest tightness, or signs of shock.

What is the best way to treat a jellyfish sting?

Immediately rinse the sting site with seawater—*never freshwater*, which will cause more venom to release. Use tweezers, chopsticks, or a credit card edge to remove visible tentacles, avoiding bare hands. Vinegar has shown mixed results—is ineffective for Portuguese man o' war—and is overall inferior to hot water. But if it's available, it may help reduce venom activation, won't hurt, and is worth trying.

The most effective treatment is hot water immersion 40-45°C (104-113°F) for 30-40 minutes, which denatures venom proteins and relieves pain. If hot water isn't available, a hot pack can serve as a subpar alternative. Acetaminophen or ibuprofen can help manage pain.

A 5% sodium bicarbonate solution (five teaspoons of baking soda per liter of seawater) has been proposed as a potential treatment for jellyfish stings. Laboratory results have been inconsistent—and from a research perspective, benefits appear limited. That said, it's unlikely to cause harm and may be reasonable to try if available.

Topical steroids (hydrocortisone or betamethasone-neomycin ointment) can help relieve skin irritation, and oral pain relievers or oral steroids may be needed for severe reactions.

While infinitely tempting, do not scrub, rub, or apply alcohol, ammonia, or urinate on the sting as these do not neutralize venom and can worsen the injury. Early treatment and close monitoring are critical, especially in remote settings where medical care is not immediately available. Severe or worsening pain that does not improve with initial treatment—especially hot- water immersion—warrants evacuation, as does any sign of shock such as pale skin, rapid pulse, or altered mental status.

What is Irukandji syndrome, and how is it managed?

Irukandji syndrome is a life-threatening condition caused by the venom of multiple jellyfish species in the Irukandji lineage. It is characterized by severe, diffuse pain; profuse sweating; nausea; vomiting; muscle cramps; and causes a dangerously *high* blood pressure and heart rate. The venom overstimulates the cardiovascular and nervous systems, potentially leading to fatal complications like heart failure or cardiovascular collapse. Immediate management includes pain control, monitoring vital signs, and evacuating the patient for advanced medical care.

Stingrays

Do stingrays "sting"?

Generally, no. Stingrays are found in both tropical marine and freshwater environments, with over 150 species worldwide. While generally nonaggressive, they defend themselves when threatened—typically by whipping their tail. Most injuries occur when someone accidentally steps on a stingray, resulting in a sting to the lower leg or foot.

Despite the name, stingrays don't "sting" in the usual sense. Their tails are equipped with sharp, often serrated barbs that can lacerate tissue and deliver venom. Unlike animals with venom glands, stingrays store venom in specialized secretory cells located in grooves along the spine. Freshwater stingrays tend to produce more toxic venom than their saltwater counterparts.

To reduce the risk of injury, shuffling the feet when walking in shallow water is a proven preventive technique. It alerts rays to your presence and gives them time to move. It's become second nature for me in tropical waters.

How do I treat a stingray injury?

Like jellyfish stings, hot water immersion is the first-line treatment for stingray injuries. The affected area should be immersed in water heated to 40–45°C (104–113°F) for 30–40 minutes, or until pain subsides. This should be done as soon as possible to help neutralize venom and reduce discomfort.

Proper wound care is equally important. Irrigate the wound thoroughly with seawater to remove sand, debris, and venom. If spine fragments are present, they must be removed—retained fragments delay healing and raise the risk of infection. The wound should not be closed. It should heal by secondary intention (from the inside out) to avoid sealing in bacteria.

Check and update tetanus status as needed. Watch for systemic symptoms like dizziness, muscle cramps, or seizures—these may indicate a more severe reaction. Evacuation is necessary if any of these signs develop.

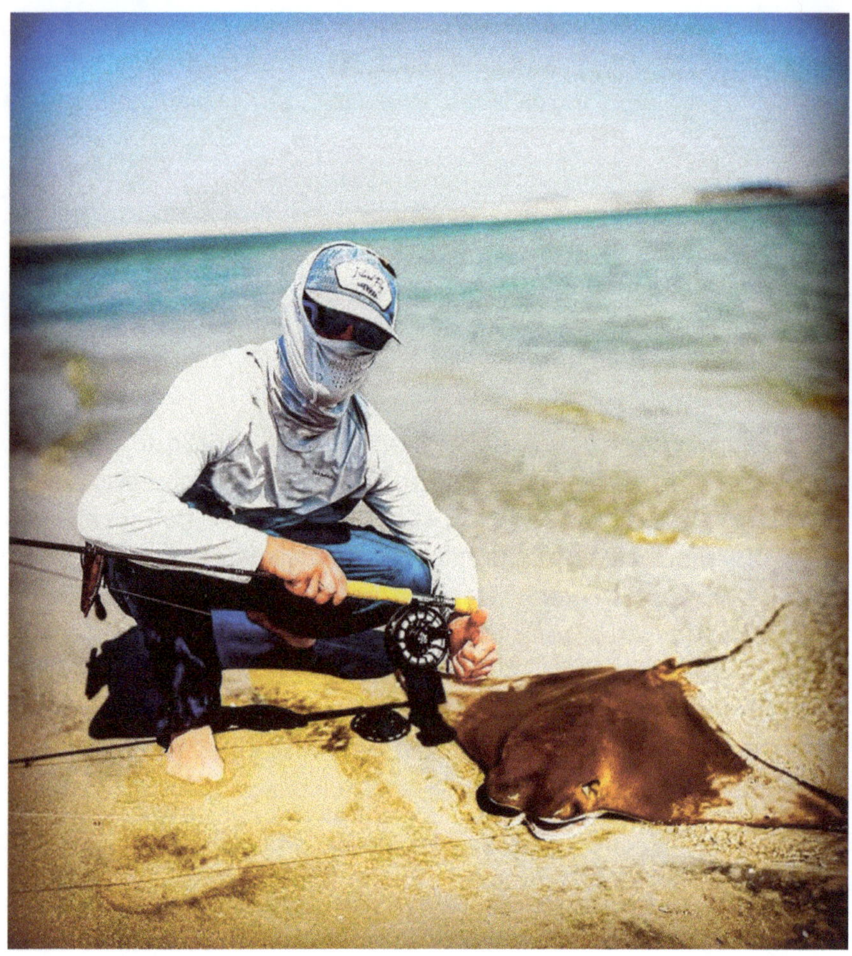

Cownose ray (Rhinoptera bonasus) caught on the fly in Brigantine, New Jersey. The venomous barb, located at the base of the tail, can inflict a serious injury if not handled with care. Photo courtesy of "Wild Bill" Benton.

Sea Urchins

What is a sea urchin, and what do guides need to know?

Sea urchins are spiny, globe-shaped marine animals found on rocky reefs, tidal pools, and coral beds worldwide. Their brittle spines can easily puncture skin—even through soft-soled shoes—making them a common hazard for waders and divers. Some species also have venomous spines or pedicellariae (small claw-like structures) that can inject venom, causing intense pain, swelling, and occasionally systemic symptoms.

Injuries often involve multiple puncture wounds with spines breaking off under the skin. Pain is immediate and sharp, followed by swelling and bruising. If venom is involved, symptoms may include burning, numbness, muscle weakness, or nausea. Infection is a common complication, especially when fragments remain embedded. Deep punctures in the foot can make walking difficult.

Treatment starts with careful removal of visible spines using tweezers—avoid pressure to prevent further breakage. Soak the area in hot water 40–45°C (104–113°F) for 30–40 minutes to reduce pain and neutralize venom. After soaking, scrub the wound with soap and clean water to lower infection risk. Do not dig out deep spines—many dissolve over time. If pain or swelling persists, medical removal may be needed.

Evacuation should be considered if spines are embedded near joints, tendons, or nerves, if infection develops, or if systemic symptoms appear. While rarely life-threatening, sea urchin injuries can lead to infection, chronic pain, or mobility issues without proper care.

Cone Snails

What's the deal with cone snails?

Cone snails (*Conus* species) are venomous marine snails found in tropical waters worldwide, including the Red Sea, Caribbean, Indian, and Pacific Oceans. These predatory snails use a harpoon-like tooth to inject venom that can instantly paralyze prey. Human stings typically occur when the snail is handled or disturbed, often during shell collection.

Cone snail venom is a complex mix of neurotoxic peptides that disrupt neuromuscular function. Envenomation can lead to paralysis, cardiovascular collapse, coma, and, in rare cases, death. With over 100,000 compounds in a single snail's venom and no effective antivenin available, treatment is entirely supportive.

Symptoms range from localized pain or numbness to life-threatening systemic effects. Prompt medical attention is essential, even if symptoms initially appear mild.

Are all cone snails dangerous?

Yes—at least treat all cone snails as potentially dangerous. While not all of the 500+ species produce venom lethal to humans, many do. The variability in venom toxicity makes these snails unpredictable. Some may cause only mild irritation; others can lead to paralysis or death. Given the risk, avoid direct contact entirely. Cone snails should never be handled or collected—unless you're buying one from an airport gift shop.

What should I do if a guest is stung?

This is bad. Immediate medical attention is critical. Stabilize the airway, breathing, and circulation, and initiate prompt evacuation. Symptoms can progress quickly and may be fatal within hours.

While waiting, consider pressure immobilization. Wrap the affected limb with a bandage starting at the distal end and working proximally, aiming to slow venom spread without cutting off circulation—check perfusion regularly and adjust as needed.

Hot water immersion ideally 40-45°C (104-113°F) may help relieve pain. While evidence is anecdotal and it's not universally effective, it may provide temporary relief—but it should never delay evacuation.

Even with care, the risk of death remains high. This underscores the need for rapid transport to advanced medical support. Preventing these injuries starts with clear education all around—cone snails aren't souvenirs. Don't touch them. Just leave them alone.

Stonefish

What is a stonefish?

Stonefish (*Synanceia* species) are among the ugliest and most venomous fish in the world. Native to shallow tropical waters across the Indo-Pacific, including northern Australia, Southeast Asia, the South Pacific, Indian Ocean, and Red Sea, they inhabit reefs, tidal flats, estuaries, and rocky nearshore zones. Often buried in sand or hidden among coral rubble, their rough, uneven skin and variable coloring (gray, brown, green, or reddish) make them nearly invisible.

Stonefish are short, thick-bodied (5–16 inches), with venomous dorsal spines. When stepped on, these spines are driven upward, injecting venom deep into tissue. Injuries typically involve the foot or ankle, and the spines can easily penetrate reef shoes or dive boots.

Pain is immediate and excruciating. Local swelling, tissue damage, and discoloration develop quickly. In severe cases, systemic effects may follow—vomiting, weakness, hypotension, or collapse. Untreated, stings may lead to tissue death and permanent damage.

Fatalities are rare, but this is a true medical emergency—especially in remote settings. The pain alone can be disabling, and the potential for systemic toxicity makes rapid recognition and evacuation essential.

This is a bad one.

What do I do when someone has been stung?

Pain is excruciating and begins within seconds. The affected limb should be immersed in the hottest water the patient can tolerate—ideally 40–45°C (104–113°F)—for at least 45 minutes, or until pain improves. This is the cornerstone of treatment for stonefish (and most marine envenomations). Hot water helps denature venom proteins and provides substantial relief.

In remote settings, embedded spines may need to be removed if they interfere with function, cause persistent bleeding, or block further care. Removal should be careful and deliberate to avoid leaving fragments behind. The wound should be irrigated thoroughly with potable water or diluted antiseptic and left open to heal by secondary intention—never sutured closed.

Antibiotics such as ciprofloxacin should be started early due to the high risk of marine infection, particularly from *Vibrio* and *Aeromonas* species. The limb should be immobilized, elevated, and loosely dressed. Pain management should be aggressive, and tetanus status confirmed.

Evacuation is necessary if pain persists despite hot water and analgesia, or if systemic symptoms develop—such as weakness, vomiting, dizziness, or respiratory difficulty. Antivenom is available in some countries and may be indicated in severe stings, particularly if pain is unrelenting or signs of systemic toxicity appear.

Sharks

What do guides need to know about shark attacks?

Shark attacks result in violent, high-energy trauma caused by crushing, tearing, and sawing forces from serrated teeth and powerful jaws. These injuries often involve massive hemorrhage, exposed bone, and, in many cases, complete amputation and joint disarticulation. Large sharks are capable of bite forces exceeding 4,000 psi—enough to crush a femur or sever a limb entirely. While direct measurements on large sharks are obviously limited, shark bite force is estimated to exceed that of a hippopotamus, polar bear, and even saltwater crocodile. The damage from a single bite is often catastrophic and rapidly fatal without immediate hemorrhage control.

Victims may present with isolated or multiple wounds, most commonly to the lower extremities. Injuries to the femoral artery are common and carry a very high mortality if not rapidly managed. In the largest clinical series to date, all recorded fatalities involved major vascular injury—most often *proximal* arterial disruption. Truncal injuries involving the chest, abdomen, or pelvis require immediate surgical intervention and are generally unsurvivable in wilderness settings.

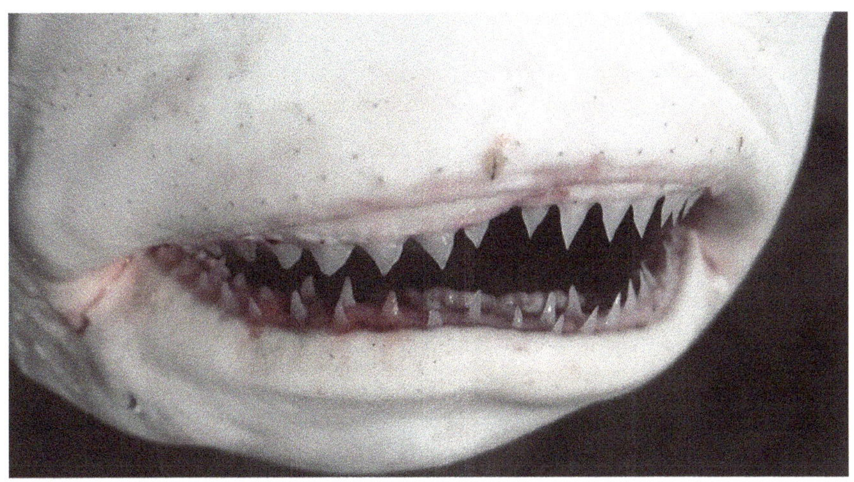

Dentition of a juvenile bull shark (Carcharhinus leucas) caught off Brigantine, New Jersey. Bull sharks are responsible for a significant number of unprovoked attacks worldwide. Their broad, serrated teeth are built for tearing flesh and can cause deep, ragged wounds with high infection potential. Image courtesy of the author.

How can I quickly assess the severity of a shark bite?

The *Durban Classification* provides a practical, field-relevant system for assessing survivability based on wound location and vascular involvement:

- Grade I: Injuries to major proximal arteries—such as the femoral artery in the upper thigh, the brachial artery near the shoulder, or any severe injury to the chest, abdomen, or pelvis. These are often fatal.
- Grade II: Injuries to distal major vessels—such as the lower femoral artery or the brachial artery near the elbow—or mild to moderate truncal trauma. Survivable if bleeding is controlled promptly.

- Grade III: Injuries limited to minor vessels, superficial structures, or distal extremities without significant vascular involvement. These patients generally survive with basic wound management.

If the wound is rapidly bleeding, visibly pulsing, or near the groin or axilla, assume a Grade I injury. If the abdomen or chest is involved, there is limited field care beyond basic airway, circulatory support and attempts at hemorrhage control. You can only do what you can do—this is a very bad day.

What is the immediate management following a shark attack?

Bleeding control is the only intervention that changes the outcome.

Hemorrhagic shock is the leading cause of death in shark attacks, and many victims could survive if bleeding is stopped early. A tourniquet should be applied—high and tight. If a commercial device isn't available, strong materials like a surfboard leash, wetsuit sleeve, or belt can be used—provided they generate enough pressure to fully occlude arterial flow. For wounds where a tourniquet can't be placed, such as in the groin or shoulder, continuous packing and firm direct pressure is the only option (see "Bleeding")

If the victim is still in the water, anything available should be used to create a barrier between them and the shark—board, fins, rods, bags. If the attack continues, targeting the snout, eyes, or gills may be the only effective way to break off the assault. Remaining calm and gaining enough distance to exit the water is critical.

Once on land, after bleeding is controlled and evacuation is underway, broad-spectrum antibiotics should be started immediately. Shark bites introduce aggressive bacteria from both oral flora and seawater, particularly *Vibrio* species. Ciprofloxacin is preferred in the field due to its broad coverage, oral formulation, and availability.

The patient should be kept flat, warm, and still. Hypothermia and shock are expected. CPR is rarely successful in this setting unless advanced life support and blood products are available. In cases involving major truncal injury, survival in the field is highly unlikely. If signs of life are present, the focus remains on hemorrhage control, comfort, and urgent evacuation.

What about minor shark bites?

Not all shark-related injuries involve massive trauma. Smaller bites, punctures, or abrasions—particularly from contact with a shark's abrasive skin—are common and require immediate attention. Shark skin is covered in dermal denticles, which can tear through exposed skin on contact.

Even minor wounds should be considered contaminated. The combination of shark oral flora and seawater exposure introduces pathogens like *Vibrio* and *Aeromonas* species, both known to cause aggressive soft tissue infections. Wounds should be irrigated thoroughly with clean water or a diluted antiseptic solution and should almost never be closed in the field. Primary closure increases the risk of trapping bacteria and causing deep tissue infection.

Antibiotics should be started immediately. As noted, ciprofloxacin remains the preferred option in the field due to its coverage of marine organisms. The wound should be loosely dressed and monitored closely. Injuries involving joints, tendons, or rapidly spreading redness or swelling warrant evacuation—even if the wound appears superficial.

Sea Snakes

Are sea snakes dangerous?

Yes. All sea snakes are highly venomous, possessing a potent neurotoxin that can cause life-threatening effects. While up to 50% of bites are dry, true envenomation can result in paralysis, muscle breakdown (rhabdomyolysis), kidney failure, and severe cardiovascular complications.

Early signs may include blurred or double vision and difficulty swallowing, often progressing to respiratory failure. The venom also causes widespread muscle tissue breakdown, leading to elevated serum potassium levels (hyperkalemia), which further increases the risk of renal failure and cardiac arrest.

What should you do if someone is bitten by a sea snake?

Immediate action is critical. Keep the patient calm and still to slow venom spread. Immobilize the affected limb with a splint or pressure bandage. Clean the wound gently with soap and water to reduce infection risk.

Monitor for muscle weakness, paralysis, or dark urine, and be alert for signs of rapid deterioration. Evacuation to a medical facility is essential, as antivenom is the definitive treatment and is often available in regions where sea snakes are endemic.

Avoid outdated interventions such as suction, incision, or tourniquets—these do more harm than good. During evacuation, focus on pain management and maintaining hydration to support circulation and reduce complications.

Are sea snake bites avoidable?

In almost all cases, yes. Sea snakes rarely bite unless provoked. Most incidents happen when they're deliberately handled or caught. The best prevention is simple: Don't touch them. Bites are rare, but the consequences can be severe. Caution and common sense go a long way in avoiding trouble.

Special Mentions: The Candiru Fish and Ciguatera Poisoning

What is the candiru fish?

The candiru is a small parasitic catfish native to the Amazon River basin, infamous for its alleged ability to enter the human urethra during urination. According to legend, it follows the urine stream, anchors itself with backward-facing spines, and causes intense pain and bleeding. While the story has persisted in Amazonian folklore, scientific evidence is lacking. A 2001 study by Spotte et al., published in *Environmental Biology of Fishes*, found little support for urine-attraction behavior, effectively challenging the long-standing accounts. A shame, really—I've been spreading the rumor for decades.

Traditional remedies include herbal teas thought to repel the fish or aid in its removal. Anecdotal reports mention high-dose vitamin C to acidify the urine, though these practices lack any scientific backing or documented success. Still, they reflect the ingenuity—or at least the imagination—of local communities and early explorers.

Prevention is simple: Avoid urinating in freshwater and wear protective swimwear when wading in the Amazon. For most travelers, the candiru remains more myth than threat, but the folklore offers a glimpse into the rich intersection of culture, caution, and curiosity in remote environments.

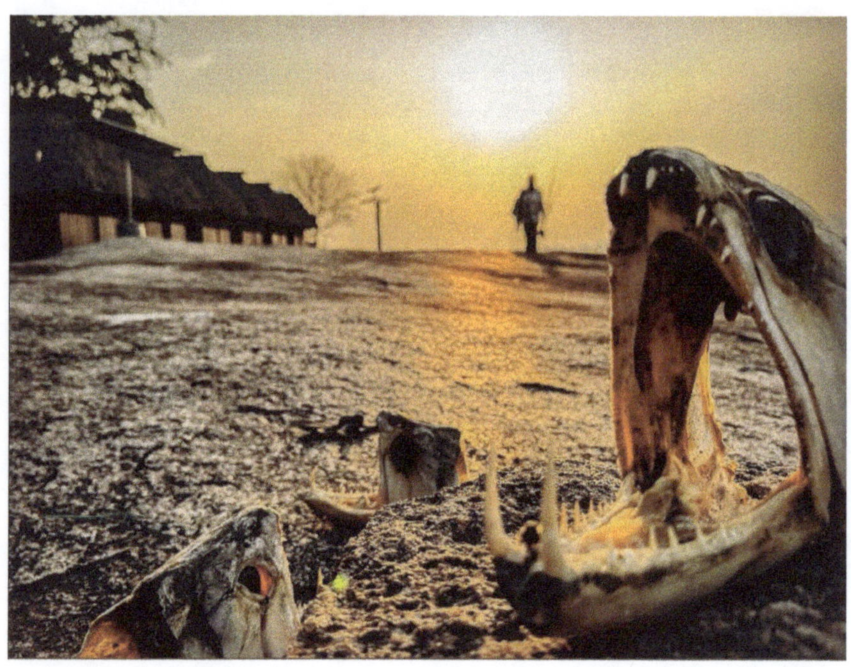

Jaw of the payara (*Hydrolycuss scomberoides*), photographed in the Colombian Amazon. Known as the "vampire fish," its oversized fangs are built for impaling prey. The payara is another reminder that Amazon waters hold a multitude of risks. Bites from this species can cause deep puncture wounds that are difficult to irrigate and prone to infection. Image courtesy of the author.

What's Ciguatera poisoning?

Ciguatera is a marine toxin illness caused by eating reef fish that have accumulated ciguatoxins from microscopic algae. It's the most common fish-related food poisoning worldwide, found in tropical and subtropical waters—including the Caribbean, Pacific Islands, Indian Ocean, and coastal areas of Florida and the Gulf of Mexico. Risk increases with fish size and position in the food chain. Barracuda, grouper, snapper, jack, and moray eel are among the highest-risk species. While smaller reef fish are considered lower risk, no fish from a ciguatera-endemic region is completely safe. Ciguatoxin is odorless; tasteless; heat-stable; and unaffected by cooking, freezing, or drying.

Symptoms usually appear within 24 hours. Early signs include nausea, vomiting, and diarrhea, followed by neurological symptoms like numbness, tingling, burning sensations, and a distinctive reversal of hot and cold perception. Severe cases may involve slow heart rate, low blood pressure, and profound fatigue. Symptoms can last for days to weeks—sometimes longer—and are rarely fatal.

There's no specific test or antidote. Diagnosis is clinical: If neurological symptoms develop after eating reef fish, assume ciguatera. Treat dehydration with oral rehydration solutions rather than plain water to replace both fluids and electrolytes. Acetaminophen or ibuprofen may ease discomfort. Avoid alcohol, caffeine, and all fish for several weeks, as these can worsen or prolong symptoms. Prevent cold exposure during recovery as sensory reversals can be intensely painful. Evacuate if the patient has ongoing vomiting, cardiovascular involvement, or severe weakness.

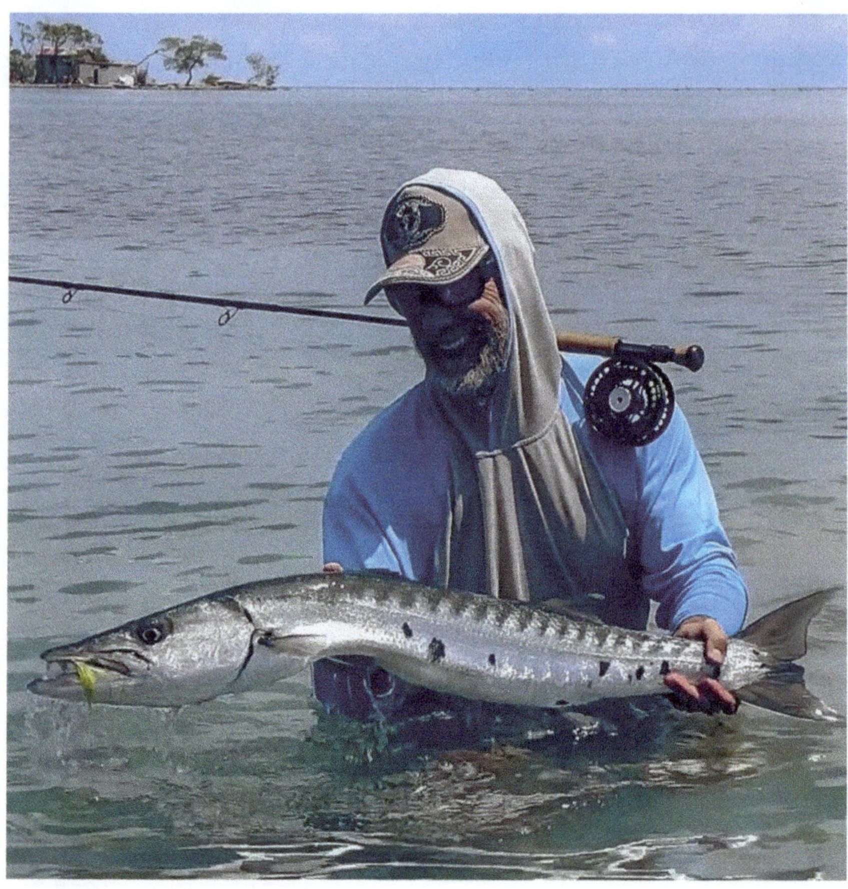

The author with a solid barracuda taken on the fly on an expedition off the east coast of Nicaragua. Larger individuals like this become more likely to carry ciguatoxins, as the risk of ciguatera poisoning increases with size and age. Image courtesy of the author.

Red Flag Framework: Environmental Emergencies

What's an easy way to remember what signs and symptoms warrant evacuation using the Red Flag Framework?

For Environmental Emergencies: **CHILL**

- **C**hanges in mental status - Confusion, seizures, or unresponsiveness (e.g., heat stroke, hypothermia, lightning strike, poisons, stings)

- **H**igh or low body temperatures - Hypothermia (shivering, cold, pale skin) or hyperthermia (flushed skin, rapid pulse, confusion)
- **I**mpaired breathing - Gasping, wheezing, or respiratory distress (e.g., near-drowning, anaphylaxis, smoke inhalation)
- **L**ightning-related injuries - Burns, cardiac issues, or altered mental status
- **L**ife-threatening reactions - Chest pain; swelling; vomiting; or collapse from stings, bites, or envenomation

Any of these signs indicate a potentially serious condition, requiring immediate evaluation and possible evacuation. When in doubt, follow the Red Flag Framework: CHILL = Evacuate.

Stung in the Sea of Cortez

The road in had been hell. Dust thick enough to choke on, heat pressing in from all sides—the kind that made the air shimmer. The washboard ruts rattled everything—truck, gear, bones. The kind of road that shakes you so hard it feels like your kidneys might drop out of your body. We'd been driving for hours, and by the time we hit the coast, nothing else mattered. The Sea of Cortez stretched out in front of us—turquoise and endless, shimmering under the brutal sun. Wind had picked up, whitecaps slapping against the shore. Just needed to cool off.

I waded in, let the salt pull the sweat and dust from my skin. Then it hit.

Like a live wire to the chest. A bolt of pain, sharp and immediate, cutting through muscle and down my arm. My body locked up. My heart hammered—too fast, out of rhythm. Breath shallow, hands shaking. The world shrank.

Heart attack. That was the only thing that made sense.

I stumbled toward shore, feet burning against the sand, vision closing in at the edges. The horizon swayed. I made it back to the palapa and collapsed into a chair, chest heaving. The ocean stretched out in front of me, unmoved.

Then I saw them—red, angry welts crawling across my chest and arm, the skin swollen and tight. Not a heart attack. A sting.

The pain didn't let up. Nausea hit in waves—dragging me under. My skin had shifted from sun-darkened tan to something else—something wrong. A sick olive hue, like the color had drained out of me. A retired dermatologist wandered by, took one look, and I watched as he quickly reached the end of his medical reasoning. Whatever he had planned to say died before it left his lips. He studied me again, exhaled through his nose, and settled on, "Bud, you don't look good."

Yeah—thanks.

He had steroids back at his place. Figured they couldn't hurt. I wasn't in a position to argue. At that point, I'd have swallowed a burnt feather dipped in goat's milk if a local shaman told me it would help. The hours stretched. My body stayed locked in a fog of pain and nausea, my gut a mess, my head spinning. My buddies hovered, talking in low voices—the mood shifting from jokes to something closer to concern. When they finally brought the tequila, it tasted like gasoline—but at least I was still breathing.

Later, when I could finally sit up without feeling like I was going to puke all over myself, I started piecing it together. This was vaguely familiar. I'd been here before—years back, surfing Angourie Point in northern New South Wales, Australia. That one stung like hell, but a few cold beers knocked it down and life went on. This was different. This had wrecked me.

What I didn't know then—but I do now—is that hot-water immersion would have been the best move: 40–45°C (104–113°F) for at least 20 minutes. Heat neutralizes the venom, dulls the pain. Vinegar? Not for a Portuguese man o' war. Wouldn't have hurt—but wouldn't have helped either. The real priority should have been getting the tentacles off—without touching them, and definitely without rinsing with fresh water, which only makes the stingers fire off more venom.

It took days for life to crawl back to normal. My arm throbbed. My chest ached. The whole thing burned way longer than it should have. Portuguese man o' war. Not always deadly—just never predictable.

Just got lucky.

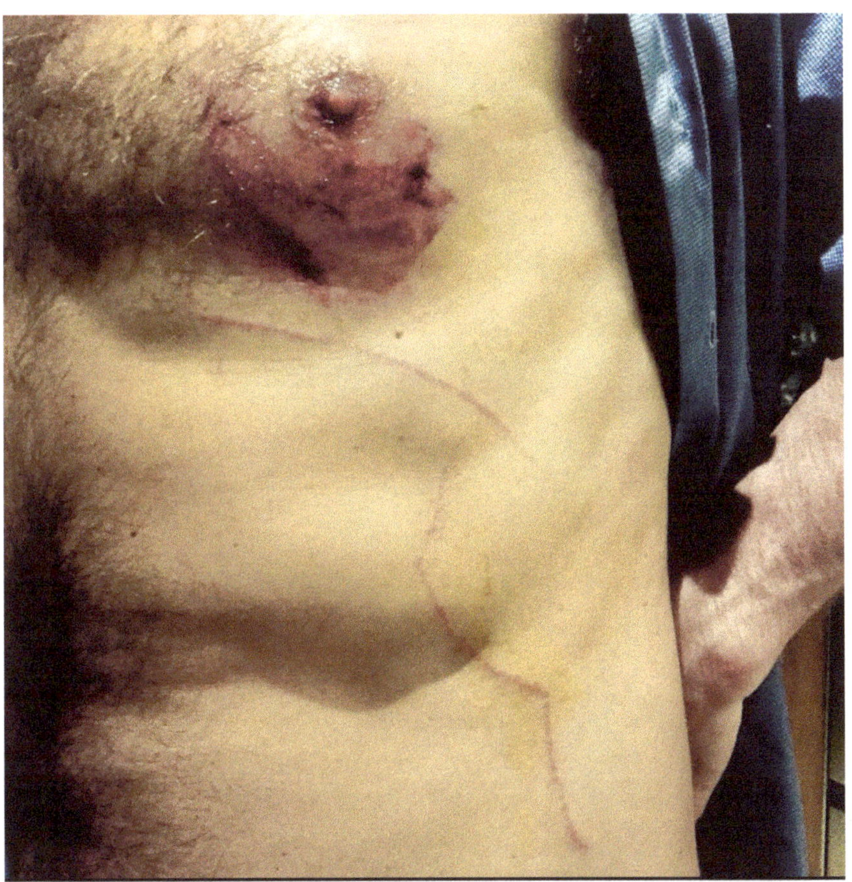

The author's chest and abdomen following a severe Portuguese man o' war sting in the Sea of Cortez off Baja. Note the early skin sloughing around the nipple, with whip-like linear welts tracking across the torso. Image courtesy of the author.

Infectious & Travel-Related Diseases

Overview

Why is there so much content on infectious disease in this book?

Because infectious disease remains one of the most common, underestimated, and operationally disruptive threats encountered in remote environments. For guides and travelers heading into remote corners of the world, tropical diseases are an unavoidable part of the experience. From malaria to guinea worm, these conditions serve as a reminder that the beauty of nature often comes with hidden risks. Their inclusion in this book isn't just about practical preparedness—it reflects the reality of venturing into places where disease, ecology, and even human history are deeply intertwined.

Understanding these diseases isn't just about knowing what to do in an emergency; it's about respecting the environments and cultures we move through. These diseases are part of the landscape, just like the rivers, oceans, forests, and mountains that draw us to explore. A background in infectious disease and epidemiology gives a framework—not to avoid these places, but to move through them with purpose and respect.

As a precautionary mention, vaccines and preventive medications play a *critical* role in mitigating the risk of contracting many infectious diseases. For travelers, staying up to date on vaccinations and following appropriate prophylaxis guidelines can mean the difference between staying healthy and—well—not.

What do I need to know to avoid serious infectious diseases in the wilderness?

If you only remember one thing—okay, two things—focus on mosquito protection and clean drinking water. Most serious infectious diseases worldwide are either vector borne (like malaria, dengue, zika, and yellow fever) or waterborne (like cholera, giardia, and typhoid). Always use reliable mosquito repellents, sleep under nets when necessary, and avoid untreated water. In higher-risk areas, research region-specific vaccines, carry prophylactic medications, and follow basic sanitation principles. What follows is a breakdown of major infectious diseases by region—a quick reference followed by a more in-depth discussion of high-risk, adventure-relevant diseases. The goal is to help you recognize the most important threats in the regions where guides, responders, and travelers are most likely to spend time. Godspeed.

South and Central America

- Mosquito-borne: dengue, Zika, yellow fever, malaria
- Other insect vectors: Chagas disease (kissing bugs), leishmaniasis (sandflies), tick-borne rickettsiosis
- Waterborne: leptospirosis, schistosomiasis
- Foodborne: typhoid, cholera, hepatitis A
- Other risks: rabies (bats, stray dogs), hantavirus (rodents), cutaneous myiasis (botfly larvae)

Africa

- Mosquito-borne: malaria, yellow fever, Rift Valley fever, dengue
- Tick-borne: African tick bite fever, Crimean-Congo hemorrhagic fever
- Other insect vectors: onchocerciasis (blackflies), African trypanosomiasis (tsetse flies), leishmaniasis (sandflies)
- Waterborne: schistosomiasis, leptospirosis, cholera, typhoid
- Body fluid exposure: Ebola, Marburg virus, Lassa fever

- Other risks: rabies, meningococcal meningitis (sub-Saharan "meningitis belt")

Southeast Asia & Oceania

- Mosquito-borne: malaria, dengue, Zika, Japanese encephalitis, chikungunya
- Tick-borne: Tick typhus, Lyme-like illnesses (emerging reports in Southeast Asia)
- Other insect vectors: Leishmaniasis (sandflies), scrub typhus (mites)
- Waterborne: leptospirosis, cholera, typhoid
- Other risks: Melioidosis (soil/water exposure), rabies, hepatitis A and E

The Caribbean

- Mosquito-borne: dengue, Zika, chikungunya, malaria (rare but present in some areas)
- Tick-borne: rare, but local transmission of rickettsial infections has been reported
- Waterborne: leptospirosis, typhoid, cholera
- Foodborne: hepatitis A, travelers' diarrhea
- Other risks: ciguatera poisoning (reef fish)

Indian Subcontinent

- Mosquito-borne: Malaria, dengue, Japanese encephalitis, chikungunya
- Tick-borne: Kyasanur Forest disease (India), tick typhus
- Other insect vectors: leishmaniasis (sandflies), scrub typhus (mites)
- Waterborne: typhoid, cholera, leptospirosis
- Other risks: tuberculosis (high prevalence), rabies, hepatitis A and E

Middle East

- Mosquito-borne: dengue, malaria (in some regions)
- Tick-borne: Crimean-Congo hemorrhagic fever
- Other insect vectors: leishmaniasis (sandflies)

- Waterborne: schistosomiasis, cholera, typhoid
- Other risks: MERS (camel exposure), hepatitis A and E

Alaska & Northern Rivers

- Waterborne: giardiasis, cryptosporidiosis
- Tick-borne: tularemia, tick-borne relapsing fever (rare but possible)
- Mosquito-borne: West Nile virus
- Other risks: rabies (foxes, bats), tularemia (also via deer flies or water)

Pacific Islands (e.g., Tahiti, Fiji)

- Mosquito-borne: dengue, Zika, chikungunya
- Tick-borne: Not commonly reported
- Waterborne: leptospirosis, hepatitis A, travelers' diarrhea
- Other risks: ciguatera poisoning (reef fish), strongyloidiasis (soil penetration through bare feet)

How effective are travel-related vaccines?

Travel-related vaccines are crucial tools in preventing serious infections during international travel. Their effectiveness varies depending on the disease, vaccine type, and individual immune response. Some vaccines offer near-total immunity, while others significantly reduce the risk of severe infection. Here's an overview of key travel-related vaccines and their effectiveness:

Vaccine	Effectiveness	Duration
Yellow Fever	99%+	Lifetime
Hepatitis A	95% (1 dose), nearly 100% (booster)	Lifetime with booster
Typhoid (Injectable)	50%–80%	2 years
Typhoid (Oral)	70%	Up to 5 years
Rabies (Pre–Exposure)	100% when combined with post–exposure treatment	Requires boosters if at risk
Japanese Encephalitis	96%	At least 5 years
Cholera	60%–85%	2 years, best in first 6 months
Meningococcal Meningitis	90%+	5+ years
Polio (IPV)	Nearly 100%	Lifetime
Influenza	40%–60%	Seasonal, annual booster recommended
COVID–19 (mRNA)	90% against severe disease	Varies, boosters needed
MMR (Measles, Mumps, Rubella)	97% (2 doses)	Lifetime
Tetanus (Td/ Tdap)	100% with full series	Booster every 10 years
Malaria Prophylaxis	90%+ (medications, not a vaccine)	Depends on continued use
Pneumococcal Vaccine	60%–80%	At least 5 years
Shingles (Shingrix)	90%+	Long-term after 2 doses

Incorporating vaccine recommendations into pre-trip planning is a fundamental responsibility of guides and expedition leaders. Ensuring that guests are informed about necessary immunizations not only safeguards their health but also contributes to the well-being of the entire group *and the communities they visit.* Proactive vaccination planning helps prevent the introduction and spread of infectious diseases across borders. For the latest travel vaccine recommendations, consult the CDC Travelers' Health website: https: //wwwnc.cdc.gov/travel

Okay, but are vaccines safe?

Hold my beer. Vaccination remains one of the greatest public health achievements in medical history. In just the past 50 years, immunization efforts have saved an estimated 154 million lives—nearly half the U.S. population and almost four times the population of Canada. The impact is undeniable: polio, once a global threat, has been reduced by over 99% worldwide thanks to vaccination efforts. Smallpox, a disease that killed millions, was declared eradicated in 1980 after an aggressive global vaccination campaign. Despite this success, vaccines continue to spark debate, largely fueled by misinformation, not evidence.

Now, no medical intervention is without risk, and vaccines are no exception. But the risks associated with vaccination are remarkably low. Guillain-Barré Syndrome after a seasonal flu shot occurs at a rate of roughly 1 per million doses.

Severe allergic reactions (anaphylaxis) following *any* vaccination is similarly rare, with an estimated incidence of 1.3 cases per million doses.

Not to poke a skunk, but a current, widely discussed concern is myocarditis following mRNA COVID-19 vaccination—particularly in younger males. The most recent data estimate rates of approximately 10 cases per million after the first dose and 75 per million after the second, in males aged 12–17. Most reported cases are mild and resolve quickly with little or no treatment. For comparison, the risk of myocarditis following *unvaccinated* COVID-19 infection in the same population is estimated at over 450 cases per million—more than six times higher.

For context, the lifetime odds of dying in a motor vehicle crash in the U.S. are about 1 in 93, and the risk of death from general anesthesia is approximately 1 in 100,000. In contrast, serious vaccine complications are measured in single cases per *million*—orders of magnitude less likely than many accepted risks in everyday life and medicine.

Think of vaccines like seat belts. Rib fractures and internal injuries can and do occur with seat belt use—especially in high-impact crashes—but no one questions their role in saving lives. The same principle applies to vaccines: rare side effects exist, but the benefits overwhelmingly outweigh the risks. Vaccines dramatically reduce the chance of severe disease, hospitalization, and death. The goal isn't perfection—it's protection. A vaccine may not prevent all infections, just like a seat belt may not prevent all injuries. But both are designed to prevent the worst-case outcomes, and that matters—especially in remote environments where access to healthcare is limited or nonexistent.

For guides and expedition leaders, vaccine planning is part of risk management. Contracting a preventable disease in the field affects more than just the patient—it can compromise the entire group. Having your group up to date on vaccinations isn't about politics or opinion. It's about preparation, responsibility, and protecting the people you lead.

What is DEET, and is it safe to use?

DEET (N,N-diethyl-meta-toluamide) is a highly effective insect repellent developed by the U.S. Army in the 1940s to protect troops in mosquito-heavy environments. It works by masking the human scent, making it harder for mosquitoes, ticks, and biting flies to detect and locate their prey. DEET is considered the gold standard for repelling disease-carrying insects like those that transmit malaria, dengue, Zika, and Lyme disease. It comes in concentrations ranging from

10% to 100%, with 20–30% typically providing 6–8 hours of protection—enough for most wilderness and travel settings.

When used properly, DEET is safe. Mild skin irritation or rare allergic reactions can occur, but the protection it offers far outweighs these minor risks. It can damage plastics, synthetic fabrics, and varnished surfaces, especially at high concentrations, so it's best applied sparingly to exposed skin and clothing—avoiding eyes, mucous membranes, and broken skin. For children, lower concentrations (10–30%) are recommended, and it should not be applied to their hands. DEET is also considered safe for use during pregnancy and breastfeeding when used as directed. While alternatives like picaridin and oil of lemon eucalyptus are available and may offer some protection, DEET remains the most reliable choice in high-risk areas.

Are infectious diseases or injuries a bigger threat to adventure travelers?

By far, infectious diseases are the bigger threat, especially for travelers heading to Africa, Oceania, the Caribbean, or Latin America. Almost 80% of travelers returning from developing countries report an acute health issue, with the majority being infections. Travelers' diarrhea alone hits over 50% of travelers, while malaria, dengue, and parasitic infections remain common diagnoses. By comparison, injuries affect only up to 7% of travelers. While cuts, sprains, and fractures often make for memorable stories, they pale next to infections.

Do I need to remember all of these diseases to stay safe?

Nope—and you probably won't remember most of the names anyway—which is fine. What matters more is knowing how they spread. *If you understand the transmission route, you can avoid most of the risk.*

For guides and wilderness responders, knowing how a disease spreads is more useful than knowing what it's called.

Pathogens don't appear out of nowhere—they follow specific pathways. Risk depends on the environment, the activity, and how people interact with both. Most diseases relevant to wilderness and international travel fall into a few key transmission categories: *Animals and the Air, Insects, Food & Water, and the Environment.*

Understanding those pathways helps you anticipate exposure, adjust behavior, and take smart precautions. What follows isn't exhaustive—it's a focused breakdown of the most relevant diseases, grouped by how they spread and what actually matters in the places you're likely to be.

Transmission: Animals & the Air

Mpox

Can I catch monkeypox from a monkey?

Not likely. Mpox, formerly known as monkeypox, is a viral infection caused by the *Monkeypox virus*—a close relative of the smallpox virus, within the *Orthopoxvirus* genus. The disease was first identified in lab monkeys in 1958, but wild rodents—such as Gambian pouched rats and dormice—are believed to be the primary animal reservoirs. Human infection occurs through direct contact with infected animal fluids, skins, or tissue—usually during hunting, handling, or consuming wild game in endemic regions of Central and West Africa. Human-to-human transmission occurs through direct contact with sores, scabs, or bodily fluids, as well as via contaminated bedding, clothing, or prolonged face-to-face exposure to respiratory droplets from an infected person.

Once the virus enters through broken skin, mucous membranes, or the respiratory tract, it spreads through the lymphatic system and bloodstream, eventually reaching the skin. Early symptoms include fever, fatigue, muscle aches, and swollen lymph nodes. This is followed by a rash that progresses from flat spots to fluid-filled blisters and scabs. The presence of lymph node swelling (lymphadenopathy) helps distinguish mpox from smallpox and chickenpox. Most infections are mild and resolve within 2–4 weeks, but severe cases can involve the eyes, airway swelling, or secondary infections. Treatment is supportive—focused on hydration, wound care, and pain control. Evacuate any patient with facial swelling, vision changes, respiratory symptoms, or signs of systemic illness.

Nipah

What do bats, mangoes, and pigs have to do with a viral outbreak?

Not a happy story but a classic teaching point in epidemiology. Nipah virus is a deadly zoonotic pathogen found in parts of South and Southeast Asia. It is carried by fruit bats and can spread to humans through contaminated fruit, raw palm sap, or close contact with infected animals, particularly pigs. In a 1998 Malaysian outbreak, fruit bats were drawn to mango orchards planted near pig farms, where they dropped their partially eaten fruit and excrement into pig feed. The pigs consumed this contaminated material, became infected, and served as amplifier hosts—rapidly spreading the virus to farm workers and resulting in over 100 human deaths. Subsequent outbreaks in Bangladesh and India have shown even higher case fatality rates and more direct human-to-human transmission, especially in the later stages of illness.

Once inside the body, Nipah virus spreads through the bloodstream and crosses into the central nervous system, where it causes brain inflammation(encephalitis)—leading to confusion, seizures, coma, and frequently death. The virus can also damage blood vessels in the lungs, resulting in respiratory distress and hypoxia(low oxygen levels). There is no antiviral treatment. Care is supportive, with a focus on managing the airway and neurologic complications. In the field, any individual with known exposure who develops fever accompanied by altered mental status or respiratory symptoms should be considered high risk and evacuated immediately.

Rabies

Can rabies turn people into zombies?

Not exactly—but not far off. Rabies is a viral infection caused by a rhabdovirus that attacks the central nervous system of mammals, including humans. It is almost always transmitted through the bite or scratch of an infected animal, with the virus present in the animal's saliva. In North America, rabies is most commonly carried by bats, raccoons, skunks, and foxes. Globally, dogs account for 99% of human deaths—nearly 60,000 each year. Once symptoms begin, rabies is universally fatal. This bears repeating: *there is no cure after symptom onset*. However, postexposure prophylaxis (PEP), if given early, is nearly 100% effective.

The virus travels along peripheral nerves toward the brain, where it causes inflammation, dysfunction, and eventually widespread, catastrophic damage. In the field, if a guest is bitten by a suspicious animal (bat, dogs, cats, fox, monkey, skunk, racoon) in a rabies-endemic area or by any animal acting abnormally, you have little choice but to assume the worst. Immediately irrigate the wound with soap, water, and antiseptic, then evacuate for PEP: rabies immune globulin (RIG) plus a vaccine series. In animals, rabies causes aggression, confusion, drooling, and hindquarter paralysis. In humans, early symptoms include fever, tingling at the wound, and fatigue—progressing to agitation, hydrophobia, paralysis, and death. No, rabies doesn't turn people into zombies, but it's as close as nature gets. Approaching stray dogs or unknown animals in a foreign country may feel like compassion, but the risks far outweigh the sentiment. Locals don't pet, feed, or cuddle them for a reason; and ignoring that reality is more reckless than kind.

Hanta

Why is mouse urine so dangerous?

Hantavirus refers to a group of rodent-borne viruses in the family Hantaviridae that can cause severe, often life-threatening illness in humans. In the Americas, *Sin Nombre* virus causes Hantavirus Pulmonary Syndrome (HPS), a rapidly progressive form of respiratory failure. In Europe and Asia, related viruses such as *Puumala, Seoul, and Hantaan* are responsible for Hemorrhagic Fever with Renal Syndrome (HFRS), which primarily affects the kidneys.

Infection occurs through *inhalation* of aerosolized particles from infected rodent urine, droppings, or saliva—especially in enclosed or poorly ventilated areas. Each strain is tied to a specific rodent host, and transmission does not require direct contact or bites.

Inside the body, the virus damages small blood vessels, causing them to leak fluid into the lungs or cause inflammation in the kidneys. This leads to pulmonary edema, hypoxia, and respiratory failure in HPS or acute kidney injury in HFRS. There is no antiviral treatment. Management is supportive and may require ICU-level care with oxygen therapy, fluid balance, and mechanical ventilation. Prevention relies on rodent control, sealing structures, ventilating confined spaces before entry, and using proper PPE during cleanup. Evacuate if symptoms escalate rapidly, especially with respiratory distress or signs of kidney failure.

Avian Flu

What's bird flu got to do with a chicken farm in Australia?

I worked on a farm there for a while. It was wild—and the full story probably belongs around a campfire or in the next book. Let's just say it involved feathers, chaos, and more than a few questionable life choices. Thankfully, none of them involved infectious disease.

Australia isn't part of the avian flu story—but much of the rest of the world hasn't been so lucky. Poultry and pathogens go hand in hand, and bird flu remains a serious concern in both animal and human health. Avian influenza is caused by strains of the influenza A virus—most notably H5N1 and H7N9—that primarily infect birds but occasionally jump to humans.

Most human infections result from close contact with infected poultry, bird droppings, or contaminated surfaces, especially in live bird markets or during slaughter. Though rare, human cases are serious and have caused fatal outbreaks across Asia, the Middle East, Africa, and Europe. Transmission between humans is limited but possible with close, sustained contact.

Once inhaled, the virus targets the lower respiratory tract, causing aggressive inflammation and damage to lung tissue. This can rapidly progress to viral pneumonia, acute respiratory distress syndrome (ARDS), and multiorgan failure. Symptoms typically begin with high fever, cough, and shortness of breath and may worsen within 48–72 hours. Antivirals such as oseltamivir may be helpful if started early, but treatment is mostly supportive. Evacuate immediately if a guide or traveler develops respiratory symptoms following bird exposure in a known outbreak area—early evacuation to definitive care is critical.

Tuberculosis

What should guides know about TB?

Tuberculosis (TB) is a highly contagious respiratory disease caused by *Mycobacterium tuberculosis*, responsible for an estimated 10 million new cases and over a million deaths annually. It spreads through airborne droplets released by coughing, sneezing, or speaking—making enclosed, poorly ventilated spaces like buses, planes, or hostels high-risk environments. TB most often targets the lungs, with symptoms that include a persistent cough, weight loss, fever, night sweats, and fatigue—typically progressing over weeks, not days.

Once inhaled, TB bacteria reach the alveoli and are taken up by macrophages. The bacteria survive inside these immune cells and trigger a localized immune response, forming granulomas—clusters of immune cells and fibrous tissue that contain *but don't eliminate* the infection. If the immune system weakens, the bacteria can reactivate, causing lung lesions and systemic symptoms. Treatment requires multiple antibiotics for 6–9 months, typically including isoniazid, rifampin, and pyrazinamide. Evacuate any patient with a prolonged cough (especially if bloody), unexplained fever, or significant weight loss, particularly after exposure in a high-incidence region. Prevention includes avoiding prolonged exposure in enclosed spaces, wearing a hospital-grade mask in high-risk areas, and seeking prompt evaluation if symptoms develop.

Anthrax

What's anthrax?

Anthrax is a bacterial disease caused by *Bacillus anthracis*, a spore-forming organism that can persist in soil for decades. Infection occurs through contact with contaminated animal hides, meat, or soil—primarily in Africa, the Middle East, Central Asia, and occasionally the western United States. There are three forms: cutaneous (via skin contact), inhalational (via aerosolized spores), and gastrointestinal (via ingestion of contaminated meat). The route of entry determines the clinical presentation, but all forms can progress rapidly without treatment.

Once inside the body, *B. anthracis* releases toxins that disrupt immune signaling, cause fluid leakage, and destroy cells. Cutaneous anthrax typically begins as a painless sore that becomes a black eschar surrounded by significant swelling. Inhalational anthrax starts with nonspecific flu-like symptoms but progresses quickly to chest pain, respiratory failure, and shock. Early treatment with antibiotics—such as ciprofloxacin or doxycycline—is essential. Evacuate immediately if there is a suspicious skin lesion following contact with animal products or if respiratory symptoms and chest pain develop in a known exposure zone.

Hendra Virus

Should you be afraid to go to the Melbourne Cup?

Definitely not. That's Australia's most prestigious horse race, and those animals are often cared for better than most humans. Still, Hendra virus disease—a rare but deadly zoonotic infection caused by *Hendra henipavirus*, endemic to Australia—is a reminder that even the most well-loved animals can harbor hidden risks under the right ecological conditions.

Hendra circulates in fruit bats (flying foxes), but human cases have only occurred through close contact with infected horses, which act as intermediate hosts. Horses are thought to become infected by ingesting feed or water contaminated with bat urine, saliva, or birth fluids. The virus was first identified during a 1994 outbreak near Brisbane that killed horses and their handlers. Transmission to humans typically occurs through exposure to respiratory secretions or body fluids from sick horses.

Inside the body, Hendra virus infects blood vessels and rapidly spreads, damaging the lungs and central nervous system. Patients may develop cough, shortness of breath, fever, confusion, or seizures—often progressing quickly to respiratory or neurologic failure. There is no antiviral therapy. Management is supportive and often requires ICU-level care. Guides working around horses in endemic areas should treat any illness following exposure as a medical emergency. Evacuate immediately if respiratory distress or neurologic symptoms occur after suspected contact with a sick animal.

Ebola

Is Ebola still a thing?

Very much so. *Ebolavirus* and its cousin *Marburgvirus* are related viruses that cause deadly hemorrhagic fevers—Ebola and Marburg Virus disease respectively. Both are found in sub-Saharan Africa and are believed to originate in fruit bats, with human outbreaks starting through contact with infected animals—often primate body fluids. Once human-to-human transmission begins, the virus spreads rapidly through contact with blood, vomit, feces, or other fluids from symptomatic individuals. Healthcare settings, funerals, or poor hygiene environments are common sites of spread. Outbreaks are rare but severe, with fatality rates between 25% and 90%, depending on the strain and access to care.

The virus causes widespread damage by attacking immune cells and the lining of blood vessels. As blood vessels lose their ability to contain fluids, patients develop severe dehydration, low blood pressure, and internal bleeding. At the same time, the body's clotting system becomes unbalanced, increasing the risk of bleeding and shock. Symptoms begin with fever, weakness, and gastrointestinal issues—then progress to bleeding, confusion, and collapse. There is no antiviral treatment. Care is supportive: fluids, monitoring, and organ support as needed. Any patient with fever and rapid decline after possible exposure should be evacuated immediately. Prevention depends on strict hygiene, avoiding wildlife exposure, and never touching sick individuals without protection.

As a sidenote, if you want something to truly worry about from an epidemiological perspective, viral hemorrhagic fevers (VHFs) are strong contenders. These severe, often fatal diseases—while rare—are devastating and pose real risks in remote international settings.

Lassa Fever

Are there any other viral hemorrhagic fevers we should know about?

Yep. Lassa fever is a viral hemorrhagic illness caused by the *Lassa virus*, endemic to West Africa—think Sierra Leone and Nigeria. It spreads to humans through exposure to food, water, or surfaces contaminated with urine or droppings from infected rats—the primary reservoir. Person-to-person transmission can also occur through direct contact with bodily fluids, particularly in healthcare settings or during home care without proper protective equipment. Outbreaks are most common in Nigeria, Sierra Leone, Liberia, and Guinea, often peaking during the dry season when rodent-human contact increases.

Once inside the body, the virus multiplies in immune cells and spreads through the bloodstream, targeting the liver, spleen, and vascular tissue. This leads to fever, weakness, sore throat, chest pain, and, in severe cases, bleeding, low blood pressure, and fluid loss. Lassa fever can also cause deafness in survivors due to inflammation of the auditory nerves. Treatment is primarily supportive, though early use of ribavirin may reduce severity. Evacuation is indicated if patients develop persistent fever, altered mental status, bleeding, or signs of systemic compromise. Prevention depends on rodent control, proper food storage, and minimizing exposure to body fluids during suspected outbreaks.

MERS

Are camels safe?

Usually. Middle East Respiratory Syndrome (MERS) is caused by *MERS-CoV*, a coronavirus first identified in Saudi Arabia in 2012. The virus is believed to have originated in bats but spread to humans through dromedary camels, which act as the primary reservoir. Human-to-human transmission occurs through close contact, especially in households and healthcare settings with inadequate infection control. MERS is rare but carries a high case fatality rate—approximately 35% in reported cases.

MERS targets the lower respiratory tract, leading to fever, cough, and shortness of breath. In severe cases, it progresses to pneumonia, acute respiratory distress syndrome (ARDS), and multi-organ dysfunction. The virus damages lung tissue and the lining of small blood vessels, leading to fluid leakage into the air sacs of the lungs. This disrupts oxygen exchange and can also affect kidney function in severe cases. There is no antiviral treatment—management is supportive and may require oxygen therapy, IV fluids, or mechanical ventilation. Evacuate immediately if a traveler develops respiratory symptoms after camel contact or time in an outbreak area. In remote settings, respiratory distress following desert travel or animal exposure should always raise clinical concern.

COVID-19 & Flu

How are COVID-19 and the flu similar?

COVID-19, caused by the *SARS-CoV-2 virus*, and influenza, caused by the *influenza A and B viruses*, are both highly contagious respiratory illnesses with overlapping symptoms. While most cases are mild, both diseases carry case fatality rates ranging from approximately 0.1% to 2%, depending on age, underlying health conditions, and access to medical care.

Common features include fever, cough, fatigue, muscle aches, and shortness of breath. Influenza tends to present with a sudden, intense onset, while COVID-19 often develops more gradually. Both can impair physical performance and recovery in wilderness settings, where dehydration, altitude, and exertion compound their effects. Transmission occurs through respiratory droplets and contaminated surfaces, making group travel, tents, and lodges high-risk environments. Vaccination, hand hygiene, improved ventilation, and avoiding shared gear remain the most practical methods of prevention.

In the field, there's no practical way to tell COVID-19 and influenza apart, and clinically, it doesn't matter as the field management is the same: rest, hydration, and symptom control. Oral rehydration solutions are preferred over plain water, particularly in COVID-19 patients, where low sodium levels (hyponatremia) have been reported in up to 40% of severe cases.

Antipyretics such as acetaminophen or ibuprofen help reduce fever and discomfort. Antivirals like oseltamivir (Tamiflu) or nirmatrelvir/ritonavir (Paxlovid) may reduce severity if started within 48 hours—but are rarely available in remote areas. Evacuate any patient with progressive respiratory distress, altered mental status, cyanosis, or signs of shock. While influenza typically follows a seasonal pattern, COVID-19 continues to evolve unpredictably. Guides should also remain aware of zoonotic strains of flu—like H5N1 (avian) or H1N1 (swine), particularly in areas with bird or pig exposure.

Transmission: Insects

Rift Valley Fever

Where's the Rift Valley?

The Rift Valley cuts through East Africa—from Ethiopia down through Kenya and Tanzania, into Mozambique and Malawi. It's a landscape of tectonic upheaval, ancient lakes, fertile plains, and fossil-rich soil—often called the "cradle of humanity". But it's also a place of dense human-animal interaction, where livestock, wildlife, and mosquitoes overlap in ways that make it a natural incubator for emerging disease.

Rift Valley fever is a mosquito-borne viral disease caused by the *Rift Valley fever virus* (RVFV), a virus in the *Bunyaviridae* family. It primarily affects livestock, but humans can become infected through mosquito bites or direct contact with animal tissue during butchering or slaughter. Outbreaks are typically linked to heavy rainfall or flooding and have been reported in East Africa, the Arabian Peninsula, and parts of southern Africa. Infection in humans ranges from mild febrile illness to severe complications.

The virus targets liver and eye tissue, leading to liver inflammation and retinal damage. Clinical symptoms include fever, headache, photophobia, eye pain, and, in some cases, blurred vision. Severe disease may progress to hepatitis, encephalitis, or permanent vision loss. Retinal scarring occurs in up to 10% of symptomatic cases. There is no antiviral treatment. Management is supportive with fluids, fever control, and close monitoring. Evacuate any patient with confusion, jaundice, bleeding, or visual changes following mosquito exposure or contact with livestock in endemic areas.

Typhus

Are typhus and typhoid the same thing?

Nope. Despite the similar names, typhus has nothing to do with typhoid. Typhus refers to a group of diseases caused by *Rickettsia* bacteria and spread by arthropods—typically body lice, fleas, mites, or ticks, depending on the type. It's often associated with overcrowding, poor sanitation, and close contact with vectors. Typhoid, by contrast, is a completely different illness caused by *Salmonella typhi* and transmitted through contaminated food or water.

Epidemic typhus (transmitted by body lice) is most common in overcrowded or unsanitary settings; murine typhus (spread by rat fleas) occurs sporadically worldwide; and scrub typhus (carried by chigger mites) is endemic in Southeast Asia and parts of Oceania. Symptoms typically begin 1–2 weeks after exposure with high fever, severe headache, myalgias, and a spotted rash. In older adults or immunocompromised patients, the disease can progress to delirium, hypotension, and multiorgan dysfunction.

The bacteria invade blood vessel cells, triggering widespread inflammation, vascular leakage, and, in severe cases, organ ischemia. Doxycycline remains the treatment of choice and is effective even when started after symptom onset. There is no vaccine, so prevention depends entirely on insect control: DEET-based repellents, permethrin-treated clothing, and avoiding close contact in high-risk environments. Evacuate for any patient with high fever and altered mental status or signs of circulatory collapse. In remote travel or disaster zones, typhus should remain on the differential anytime fever and rash appear together, especially in someone recently exposed to rodents, body lice, or dense populations.

Malaria

Is malaria the most influential disease in history?

That depends on your perspective but it's a strong contender. Malaria is a parasitic infection caused by *Plasmodium* species—most commonly *Plasmodium falciparum, P. vivax, P. ovale, P. malariae, and P. knowlesi*—transmitted through the bite of infected Anopheles mosquitoes. Once injected via mosquito saliva, the parasites migrate to the liver, multiply, then reenter the bloodstream and invade red blood cells. Their synchronized rupture of the red blood cells causes the hallmark waves of fever, chills, fatigue, and headache. Malaria remains one of the world's deadliest infectious diseases, responsible for an estimated 250 million cases and over 600,000 deaths in 2022. Young children, pregnant women, and the elderly are especially vulnerable due to weaker immunity, particularly in sub-Saharan Africa, Southeast Asia, and parts of South America.

In its severe form, malaria can lead to cerebral involvement, acute kidney injury, and multiorgan failure. In cerebral malaria, infected red blood cells adhere to small vessels in the brain, limiting oxygen delivery and triggering seizures, coma, or death—sometimes within hours. Immediate treatment with artemisinin-based combination therapies (ACTs) is essential. Preventive measures include DEET-based repellents, insecticide-treated bed nets, and antimalarial prophylaxis for travelers. Any fever following time in an endemic area should be treated as malaria until proven otherwise. Evacuate if confusion, jaundice, respiratory distress, or hemodynamic instability is present.

Field note: Bitter kola (*Garcinia kola*), used in West African traditional medicine, is sometimes chewed in remote settings for its reported effects against *P. falciparum*, the parasite behind severe malaria. Its main compound, *kolaviron*, shows antioxidant, anti-inflammatory, and antiparasitic properties and may disrupt parasite metabolism in red blood cells. While *not* a substitute for proven treatment for malaria, it is highly valued for its stimulating and digestive effects. Though traditionally regional, bitter kola is now widely available through global retailers. Human safety data are limited, and high doses may carry risks, but it remains a traditional remedy worth knowing in austere environments.

Field Notes from the Mosquito Wars

Malaria hasn't just shaped medicine—it's shaped history. In 1802, Napoleon sent 50,000 troops to retake Haiti following the Haitian Revolution—a successful slave uprising that overthrew French colonial rule. But malaria and yellow fever decimated his forces, forcing a retreat and ultimately leading to the sale of the Louisiana Territory to the United States. Disease didn't just win a battle—it redrew the map of North America.

Not long after, quinine—extracted from the bark of the Andean cinchona tree—became standard issue for British troops in India to fight malaria. It works by disrupting the parasite's ability to digest hemoglobin, a process essential to its survival inside red blood cells. Bitter and barely drinkable on its own, quinine was made more tolerable when mixed with soda water, sugar, and lime—a remedy largely reserved for officers who had access to such luxuries. Since gin was already part of the daily ration, the gin and tonic was born: part antimalarial, part imperial tradition, and eventually, a global cocktail success story.

Plague

Is the Black Death still a thing?

It is absolutely still a thing. Caused by the bacterium *Yersinia pestis*, it triggered the 14th-century pandemic that killed tens of millions across Europe between 1347 and 1351. Today, the same infection (plague) still occurs in parts of Africa, Asia, South America, and the western United States. It's usually spread by the bite of infected fleas carried by rodents but can also be transmitted through contact with infected animal tissue or, in rare cases, by inhaling droplets from someone with the pneumonic form of plague.

In the body, the bacteria spread through the lymph nodes and bloodstream. Infected lymph nodes swell and become inflamed, forming the painful lumps known as buboes, the hallmark of bubonic plague. As the infection progresses, it can damage blood vessels, interfere with normal clotting, and trigger widespread inflammation. This leads to bleeding, tissue death, and, in severe cases, shock or organ failure. Bubonic plague presents with sudden fever, chills, and swollen lymph nodes. Septicemic plague involves the bloodstream and causes bleeding, necrotic skin, and collapse. Pneumonic plague affects the lungs and can spread between people through coughing or sneezing.

Plague is treatable if caught early. Doxycycline is the antibiotics of choice. Delayed treatment increases the risk of severe illness or death. Prevention includes rodent control, "flea avoidance," and protective clothing in outbreak zones. Evacuate any patient with sudden fever, painful lymph nodes, bleeding, breathing trouble, or signs of shock after possible exposure.

Chikungunya

What's Chikungunya?

Chikungunya is a mosquito-borne viral illness caused by chikungunya virus, transmitted by *Aedes aegypti* and *Aedes albopictus*—the same bloodsuckers responsible for spreading dengue and Zika. The name chikungunya comes from the Makonde word meaning "that which bends up," a reference to the stooped posture caused by severe joint pain; it originates from the Makonde people of East Africa, where the virus was first identified during a 1952 outbreak in Tanzania.

After a short incubation period, illness begins abruptly with high fever, rash, headache, and intense joint pain—especially in the hands, wrists, and ankles. Though the virus clears quickly, the body's inflammatory response can linger, leading to fatigue and joint pain that may last for weeks or even months. There is no antiviral treatment; care is supportive with fluids, rest, and pain control. Co-infection with dengue can occur in regions where both viruses circulate and may complicate diagnosis or recovery. Infants, older adults, and those with chronic illness are at greater risk for severe or prolonged symptoms. Evacuation is rarely necessary unless symptoms interfere with basic functioning or oral hydration.

Yellow Fever

Does Yellow Fever make you yellow?

Only if you're unlucky. Yellow fever is a viral hemorrhagic disease caused by the Yellow Fever Virus (YFV), a *flavivirus* transmitted by mosquitoes—mainly *Aedes aegypti* in cities and *Haemagogus* species in jungle environments. The virus is endemic to tropical regions of Africa and South America, where outbreaks can cause high mortality. Symptoms begin 3–6 days after infection and include fever, chills, muscle aches, headache, nausea, and vomiting. While most people recover at this stage, about 15% progress to a toxic phase with high fever, abdominal pain, vomiting blood, and bleeding from mucous membranes. Mortality in this stage exceeds 50%, even with care.

The "yellow" in yellow fever comes from jaundice, which occurs when liver cells are damaged and cannot process bilirubin, a yellow pigment formed from the recycling of red blood cells. As bilirubin accumulates in the blood, it deposits in the skin and eyes, producing the yellow tint. In severe cases, liver injury is compounded by clotting dysfunction, kidney failure, and cardiovascular collapse. There is no antiviral treatment. Care is supportive. Evacuate any patient who shows signs of worsening fever, jaundice, bleeding, or altered mental status. *Prevention is highly effective: One dose of the yellow fever vaccine provides lifelong immunity and is required for travel to certain endemic countries.* DEET, long sleeves, and mosquito netting remain essential. This is one of the deadliest mosquito-borne illnesses—but also one of the most preventable.

Sleeping Sickness

Does sleeping sickness actually make you sleepy?

At least. African sleeping sickness, or African trypanosomiasis, is a parasitic disease caused by *Trypanosoma brucei*, transmitted by the bite of infected tsetse flies. It is found in rural areas of sub-Saharan Africa, especially near rivers, game reserves, and brushland. There are two forms: *T. b. gambiense* causes a slow-progressing illness in West and Central Africa, while *T. b. rhodesiense*, found in East and Southern Africa, leads to a more acute, aggressive disease. After a bite, the parasite spreads through the bloodstream and lymphatic system, eventually crossing into the central nervous system. Early symptoms include fever, headache, joint pain, and swollen lymph nodes. As the parasite invades the brain and spinal cord, neurologic signs develop—confusion, personality changes, daytime sleepiness, nighttime insomnia, tremors, and progressive neurologic decline. Without treatment, the disease is uniformly fatal.

Treatment depends on the stage. Early infections are treated with oral medications like pentamidine or suramin, while CNS involvement requires more intensive drugs—often available only at referral centers. Prevention includes avoiding tsetse fly habitats, wearing long neutral-colored clothing, and using insect repellents (though tsetse flies are less deterred by DEET than other vectors). Evacuate any traveler with prolonged fever, mental status changes, or unexplained neurologic symptoms after travel in endemic regions.

Dengue

What's "breakbone" fever?

Dengue fever is caused by the *Dengue Virus*, a flavivirus transmitted by the infamous *Aedes aegypti* mosquito—of yellow fever and Zika fame. It affects an estimated 390 million people each year, with about 100 million developing symptomatic illness requiring medical care. Symptoms begin 4–10 days after a bite and often include high fever, headache, retro-orbital eye pain, rash, and severe muscle and joint pain—earning dengue its nickname: "breakbone fever." It is most common in Southeast Asia, the Pacific Islands, Central and South America, and the Caribbean, with outbreaks peaking during the rainy season when mosquito populations increase.

The virus damages the small blood vessels (capillaries) and alters the body's immune response, increasing the risk of plasma leakage, bleeding, and circulatory collapse. Treatment is supportive—hydration is critical, and acetaminophen is preferred for fever control. NSAIDs should be avoided due to the increased risk of bleeding. Early warning signs of severe dengue include persistent vomiting, abdominal pain, or a sudden drop in body temperature—any of which may indicate impending shock. Preventive measures include eliminating standing water, using DEET-based repellents, protective clothing, and sleeping under insecticide-treated nets. Evacuate if bleeding, hypotension, or signs of organ dysfunction develop.

Zika

What's Zika?

Zika virus, a mosquito-borne flavivirus transmitted by *Aedes* mosquitoes, was first identified in the Zika Forest of Uganda in 1947. Today, it's found across tropical and subtropical regions, including South America, Southeast Asia, the Caribbean, and parts of Africa. The virus drew international attention during the 2015–2016 outbreak in Brazil due to its link to microcephaly and severe brain underdevelopment in infants exposed in utero. With that said, the vast majority of cases are mild, presenting with low-grade fever, rash, conjunctivitis, headache, and muscle pain. In rare instances, Zika can trigger Guillain-Barré syndrome, an autoimmune condition that causes progressive muscle weakness and even paralysis.

The virus appears to target brain and placental tissue, disrupting fetal brain development and triggering the inflammation of peripheral nerves in adults. There is no specific antiviral treatment. Management is supportive, focused on rest, fluids, and symptom control. Prevention is essential, especially for those who are pregnant or planning pregnancy. Avoiding travel to endemic areas, using DEET-based repellents, wearing long clothing, and removing standing water all reduce risk. Evacuate any patient who develops neurologic symptoms or has confirmed exposure during pregnancy, as complications may arise after symptoms resolve.

Leishmaniasis

Are sandflies dangerous?

If they're mentioned in this book—probably. Leishmaniasis is a parasitic disease caused by species of the *Leishmania* parasite, transmitted through the bite of infected female sandflies. It is found in parts of South America, Africa, the

Middle East, Asia, and southern Europe. There are three main forms: cutaneous leishmaniasis (typically caused by *L. major*, *L. tropica*, or *L. mexicana*), which produces skin ulcers that begin as painless bumps and develop into open sores; mucocutaneous leishmaniasis (commonly from *L. braziliensis*), which spreads to the mucous membranes of the nose, mouth, or throat; and visceral leishmaniasis (caused by *L. donovani* and *L. infantum*), which affects internal organs and is often fatal if untreated. The parasite invades and multiplies inside immune cells—primarily macrophages—leading to localized inflammation, disfigurement, and, in the visceral form, suppression of bone marrow function and immune response. Treatment depends on the type and severity of illness: some cutaneous cases resolve on their own, but mucocutaneous and visceral forms require intravenous antiparasitic therapy. Evacuation is warranted for worsening lesions, airway involvement, or systemic symptoms like fever and weight loss. Sandflies are small, quiet, and most active from dusk to dawn, so DEET-based repellents, long clothing, and permethrin-treated bed nets are key to prevention.

Japanese Encephalitis

Is Japanese encephalitis found only in Japan?

No, but the Japanese macaque, also known as the snow monkey, is. It's probably the only monkey in the world that enjoys soaking in hot springs—but I digress.

Japanese encephalitis (JE) is a mosquito-borne viral disease caused by the *Japanese Encephalitis Virus* (JEV), a *flavivirus* spread primarily by *Culex* mosquitoes in rural parts of Southeast Asia, South Asia, and the Western Pacific. Despite its name, JE is not limited to Japan. Pigs and waterbirds serve as amplifying hosts, particularly in rice-farming regions where human exposure is common. Most infections are mild or asymptomatic, but in severe cases, the virus crosses the blood-brain barrier and triggers inflammation in the brain. This can result in high fever, confusion, seizures, paralysis, or coma. While most infections are asymptomatic, in those who develop clinical disease, mortality rates can reach 30%. Among survivors, up to half are left with permanent neurologic damage, including cognitive deficits and movement disorders.

There is no antiviral treatment. Supportive care focuses on managing fever, controlling seizures, maintaining hydration, and monitoring for neurologic deterioration. Evacuation is critical at the first sign of altered mental status or central nervous system involvement. Prevention includes vaccination for travelers to endemic regions and strict mosquito precautions: DEET-based repellents, long clothing, insecticide-treated bed nets, and minimizing outdoor exposure at dusk and dawn. In high-risk areas, survival depends entirely on prevention and early recognition.

Botfly

What is a botfly?

The human botfly (*Dermatobia hominis*) is a parasitic insect found in humid, tropical regions from Mexico to Argentina. To reproduce, it doesn't lay eggs directly on a host—instead, it hijacks other insects—typically mosquitoes or biting flies—as delivery systems. When one of these carrier insects bites a person, the warmth of human skin triggers the botfly eggs to hatch. The larvae then burrow painlessly into the skin, often without detection, and begin feeding on tissue beneath the surface while breathing through a small pore.

As the larva matures, it causes localized inflammation and a raised, boil-like swelling. While some recommend suffocating the larva by sealing the breathing hole with petroleum jelly or tape, the preferred method—both by most patients and providers—is to make a small incision directly over the burrow and extract the larva intact. This approach minimizes tissue trauma and shortens the course of irritation. After removal, the wound should be thoroughly cleaned to prevent secondary infection. Evacuate if extraction fails or signs of deeper infection or systemic illness develop. Prevention includes using DEET-based repellents, permethrin-treated clothing, and avoiding insect bites. In endemic areas, ironing line-dried clothes can destroy eggs before they hatch. Though unpleasant, botfly infestations are typically a minor field issue when identified early and handled properly.

Chagas Disease

What's a "kissing bug"?

Hold on for this one. Chagas disease is a parasitic infection caused by *Trypanosoma cruzi*, transmitted primarily by triatomine insects—commonly called "kissing bugs." These blood-feeding insects bite humans on the face while they sleep, then defecate near the site. The parasite isn't in the bite—it's in the feces. When the person scratches or rubs the area, the parasite enters through the mucous membranes or broken skin. That's how *Trypanosoma cruzi* gets into the bloodstream and causes Chagas disease. Kissing bugs live in cracks of mud, thatch, or adobe in rural Central and South America. Less commonly, transmission can occur through blood transfusion, organ transplant, contaminated food or drink, or from mother to child during pregnancy.

Inside the body, the parasite spreads through the bloodstream and infects muscle and nerve cells—particularly in the heart, brain, and digestive tract—causing inflammation and long-term tissue damage. The disease has two phases. The acute phase causes fever, lymph node swelling, and localized inflammation at the bite site—sometimes presenting as Romana's sign (eyelid swelling). Many cases go unnoticed; but myocarditis, encephalitis, or meningitis may develop. The chronic phase may lie dormant for decades before causing serious cardiac or gastrointestinal complications. There is no cure for chronic disease. Early treatment with benznidazole or nifurtimox is essential. Evacuate if fever, chest pain, fainting, eye swelling, or neurologic symptoms occur. Prevention hinges on sealed housing, treated bed nets, DEET, and avoiding food contamination in endemic zones.

Tickborne Diseases

What are the notable tickborne diseases in North America?

Several medically significant tickborne diseases are found across North America, each with its own regional distribution and clinical profile.

- In North America, several tickborne diseases pose significant risks in wilderness settings, especially when prompt diagnosis and treatment are delayed. Rocky Mountain spotted fever (RMSF), caused by *Rickettsia rickettsii* and transmitted by the American dog tick (*Dermacentor variabilis*), is most prevalent in the south central and southeastern United States, with the majority of cases reported from North Carolina, Oklahoma, Arkansas, Tennessee, and Missouri. It typically presents with sudden onset of fever, headache, muscle aches, and a characteristic spotty purple rash that may spreads from the wrists and ankles to the trunk. Without prompt antibiotic treatment, RMSF can rapidly progress to severe illness or rarely death.
- Ehrlichiosis, primarily caused by *Ehrlichia chaffeensis* and transmitted by the lone star tick (*Amblyomma americanum*), is most commonly reported in Missouri, Arkansas, and Oklahoma. Patients often experience fever, headache, fatigue, and muscle aches. Severe cases may involve confusion or difficulty breathing.
- Lyme disease, caused by *Borrelia burgdorferi* and spread by the blacklegged tick (*Ixodes scapularis*), is concentrated in the Northeast, upper Midwest, and parts of the Pacific Northwest. Early symptoms include a distinctive bull's-eye rash, fever, and joint pain. If untreated, it can lead to neurologic and cardiac complications.
- Tularemia, caused by *Francisella tularensis*, is most common in Arkansas, Kansas, Missouri, and Oklahoma, accounting for 50% of U.S. cases. It can be

contracted through tick bites or handling infected animals, presenting with skin ulcers, swollen lymph nodes, and, in severe cases, pneumonia.

- Babesiosis, caused by *Babesia microti* and transmitted by *Ixodes scapularis*, is most prevalent in the Northeast and upper Midwest. It resembles malaria, with symptoms like fever, chills, and dark urine, and is particularly dangerous for the elderly or immunocompromised.
- Powassan virus, though rare, is a severe tickborne illness found in the northeastern U.S. and Great Lakes region. Transmitted by *Ixodes* ticks, it can cause rapid-onset encephalitis, leading to confusion, seizures, and potentially long-term neurologic damage. There is no specific treatment, only supportive care.

In the field, any patient exhibiting fever, rash, neurologic symptoms, or signs of systemic illness following a tick bite in these regions should be evacuated promptly and started on empiric doxycycline therapy when appropriate. For all of these diseases, delayed therapy is the strongest predictor of poor outcomes. Prevention hinges on tick checks, insect repellents (like DEET or permethrin-treated clothing), and removing ticks promptly and completely.

What are some international tickborne disease to worry about?

Internationally, several tickborne diseases stand out for their severity and potential to become life threatening in remote settings.

- Crimean-Congo fever, caused by a nairovirus, is found across Eastern Europe, Central Asia, the Middle East, and parts of sub-Saharan Africa. It's one of the few tickborne viruses that can spread person to person, often through blood contact. Patients may start with fever, muscle aches, and dizziness, but quickly deteriorate with spontaneous bleeding, low blood pressure, and shock. The virus damages the lining of blood vessels, causing capillary leak and systemic collapse. There is no proven antiviral therapy. Treatment is supportive only.

- Tick-borne encephalitis, caused by a flavivirus, is endemic in Central and Eastern Europe, the Baltics, Russia, and some parts of China. It often presents in two phases: a mild viral illness followed by sudden onset of neurologic symptoms like confusion, imbalance, or seizures. The virus targets the brain and spinal cord, sometimes causing permanent neurologic damage. Again, there's no specific treatment. Supportive care and rapid evacuation are essential.
- Omsk hemorrhagic fever, also caused by a flavivirus, occurs in southwestern Siberia and is primarily associated with muskrats and Dermacentor ticks. It shares features with both diseases above, including vomiting, fever, and neurologic decline. All three viral diseases require aggressive supportive care, isolation if possible, and immediate evacuation if severe symptoms develop.
- In contrast, African tick bite fever, caused by *Rickettsia africae*, is a bacterial infection that is found throughout sub-Saharan Africa and parts of the Caribbean and is especially common among travelers on safari or working in rural areas. A unique feature is the presence of multiple eschars—dark, crusted sores at tick bite sites—along with fever, fatigue, and swollen lymph nodes. The bacteria infect the inner lining of blood vessels, leading to localized inflammation and systemic symptoms. Doxycycline is highly effective if started early, making empirical treatment reasonable in any stable patient with compatible symptoms and exposure history.

Prevention for all of these diseases starts with minimizing exposure to ticks: wear long clothing, treat gear with permethrin, use DEET-based repellents, and perform daily tick checks. A vaccine is available in Europe for tick-borne encephalitis and should be considered for prolonged stays in endemic regions. In expedition medicine, early suspicion, prompt treatment (often with doxycycline), and rapid evacuation for viral syndromes are your best tools to reduce mortality.

Transmission: Food & Water

Giardia

Are clear mountain streams safe to drink from?

Usually not. Giardiasis is an intestinal infection caused by the protozoan parasite *Giardia lamblia*, transmitted through water, food, or surfaces contaminated with, often animal feces. The parasite's cyst form is highly resilient, surviving in cold, untreated water sources—making it one of the most common causes of waterborne illness in wilderness environments. Infection occurs when cysts are ingested and transform into trophozoites in the small intestine, where they adhere to the lining and disrupt nutrient absorption. Outdoor travelers, campers, and guides are at particular risk when drinking untreated stream or lake water, even from seemingly pristine sources.

Symptoms typically appear 1–2 weeks after exposure and include watery or greasy diarrhea, bloating, flatulence, cramps, fatigue, and sulfuric-smelling stools. Prolonged cases may lead to weight loss, dehydration, and chronic gastrointestinal symptoms like postinfectious irritable bowel syndrome. Treatment involves rehydration and antiprotozoals such as metronidazole or tinidazole. Prevention starts with boiling, filtering, or chemically treating all water in the backcountry. Hand hygiene is critical, particularly after toileting or handling food. Evacuate if symptoms persist beyond a week, oral intake fails, or dehydration becomes severe.

Cholera

How did a UN peacekeeping mission cause an epidemic?

After the 2010 earthquake in Haiti, a cholera outbreak struck a population already devastated by collapsed infrastructure and limited access to clean water. Cholera was introduced by United Nations peacekeepers from Nepal and spread rapidly through rivers and water systems used for drinking, cooking, and bathing. Over the following years, more than 800,000 people were infected and an estimated 10,000 died, overwhelming Haiti's already fragile healthcare system and highlighting how quickly cholera can escalate, *especially* in post-disaster settings.

Cholera, caused by the bacterium *Vibrio cholerae*, is a severe diarrheal illness spread through contaminated water, food, or unwashed hands—particularly in areas with poor sanitation or following natural disasters. It remains a global health threat, with millions of cases causing over 100,000 deaths annually. Symptoms often begin suddenly and include profuse watery diarrhea, vomiting, and intense dehydration. Without rapid fluid replacement, patients can progress to shock and death within hours. Treatment is centered on aggressive oral rehydration. Intravenous fluids and antibiotics (doxycycline or ciprofloxacin) are needed in severe cases. Patients with persistent vomiting, confusion, or signs of circulatory collapse should be evacuated immediately. Prevention depends on clean drinking water, proper sanitation, good hygiene practices, and vaccination in high-risk areas for emergency use.

Of historical interest, cholera's place in modern public health traces back to Dr. John Snow's investigation of an 1854 outbreak in London. At the time, most physicians believed disease spread through "bad air," or miasma. Snow instead suspected contaminated water, and by mapping illness patterns, traced the outbreak to a single water pump in central London. After he persuaded local officials to remove the pump handle, new cases declined sharply. This event marked a turning point in epidemiology and disease control, and it still serves as a model for how direct observation and timely public health action can stop the spread of deadly disease. Cool story and definitely worth the read.

Guinea Worm

What is Guinea worm disease?

Guinea worm disease is a parasitic infection caused by *Dracunculus medinensis*, typically acquired by drinking untreated water contaminated with infected copepods (tiny freshwater crustaceans known as "water fleas"). After ingestion, the copepods die in the stomach, releasing larvae that penetrate the intestinal wall and migrate into body tissues. Over the course of 8 to 12 months, the adult female worm—sometimes over a meter long—travels through connective tissue and eventually breaks through the skin, usually on the lower legs or feet. This causes a painful, burning blister followed by the gradual appearance of the worm at the skin's surface. The surrounding tissue becomes inflamed and swollen, often leaving the person unable to walk or perform daily activities. There is no medication that kills the worm. Removal is a slow, exquisitely painful process, typically accomplished by gently pulling the worm out over *several days or weeks*, wrapping it around a clean stick or gauze a little at a time. Forceful removal risks breaking the worm, which can lead to severe inflammation and infection from the retained fragments. Wound care is essential, and signs of infection must be watched closely. Evacuation is rarely required unless there is evidence of abscess, cellulitis, or systemic illness.

Global eradication efforts have reduced the number of cases by more than 99%, but Guinea worm disease still occurs in remote regions of South Sudan, Chad, Mali, and Ethiopia. Because humans are the only known reservoir, prevention depends entirely on interrupting the transmission cycle. Simple interventions—like filtering drinking water through cloth, boiling untreated water, and avoiding stagnant surface sources—remain the most effective tools. For wilderness teams or guides operating in endemic areas, it's critical to treat *all* surface water as potentially unsafe. While the disease is no longer widespread, it remains a painful and prolonged medical challenge when contracted.

Fried Rice Syndrome

What is "Fried Rice Syndrome"?

"Fried rice syndrome" refers to food poisoning caused by *Bacillus cereus*, a spore-forming bacterium that thrives in starchy foods—especially cooked rice. The spores survive cooking, then germinate and produce a toxin if the rice is left unrefrigerated for more than a few hours. Symptoms typically begin within 1–5 hours and include sudden nausea, vomiting, abdominal cramping, and sometimes mild diarrhea. The illness is brief but intense and is commonly linked to buffet-style or leftover rice dishes with poor temperature control. In wilderness settings without refrigeration, cooked rice should be eaten immediately or kept hot above 60°C (140°F). *Once the toxin is present, reheating does not inactivate it.*

The heat-stable toxin stimulates the vagus nerve, triggering vomiting through central and gastrointestinal pathways. Treatment is supportive: oral fluids, rest, and electrolyte replacement. Antibiotics are *not* indicated, as symptoms are due to a toxin, not an active infection. Evacuation is rarely needed but should be considered if vomiting lasts beyond 24 hours, if signs of dehydration develop, or if the patient is unable to tolerate oral intake. Prevention is straightforward: Cool cooked rice rapidly; store it below 40°F (4°C); and avoid holding it in warm, stagnant containers for extended periods.

Typhoid

Who was "Typhoid Mary"?

We'll get to Mary in a minute. First the disease. Typhoid fever is a serious bacterial infection caused by *Salmonella typhi*, transmitted through food or water contaminated with human waste. It is most prevalent in regions with poor sanitation, particularly South Asia, sub-Saharan Africa, and parts of Latin America. Symptoms begin gradually over 1–3 weeks, starting with fever, malaise, abdominal pain, and headache. Constipation is common early, followed by diarrhea in later stages. Without treatment, the bacteria can invade the intestinal wall, causing perforation, hemorrhage, and sepsis. The bacteria penetrate intestinal lymph tissue (Peyer's patches), enter the bloodstream, and spread to the liver, spleen, and bone marrow—causing a prolonged febrile illness. Treatment in the field includes oral antibiotics such as ciprofloxacin, and severe cases require IV fluids and advanced monitoring. Evacuation is indicated for persistent vomiting, worsening abdominal pain, altered mental status, or GI bleeding. Prevention includes typhoid vaccination, treated drinking water, avoiding raw or undercooked food, and strict hand hygiene.

One of the most infamous outbreaks in U.S. history was traced to Mary Mallon—"Typhoid Mary"—an *asymptomatic* carrier who worked as a cook in New York in the early 1900s. She is believed to have infected at least 50 people and was forcibly quarantined for nearly three decades. Her case remains a cautionary tale of asymptomatic transmission and the public health consequences of foodborne illness—and ultimately helped drive better hygiene practices and food safety regulations.

Hepatitis A

What should guides know about Hepatitis A?

Hepatitis A is a highly contagious liver infection caused by the hepatitis A virus (HAV), transmitted via the fecal-oral route. It spreads through contaminated food, water, or surfaces—especially in areas with inadequate sanitation or during outbreaks. Travelers to endemic regions are most at risk when consuming raw or undercooked food, untreated water, or unwashed produce. The virus survives well in the environment and is easily transmitted by poor hand hygiene or handling contaminated items. Oyster lovers beware: Shellfish harvested from sewage-contaminated waters is a common culprit.

HAV targets hepatocytes (liver cells), triggering a pronounced immune response that inflames the liver and disrupts bile processing. Symptoms usually appear 2–6 weeks after exposure and include fever, nausea, fatigue, abdominal discomfort, jaundice, dark urine, and pale stools. There is no antiviral treatment. Management is supportive with hydration, rest, and monitoring. Most cases resolve fully, but the illness can last weeks to months. Evacuation is indicated if the patient develops persistent vomiting, jaundice, or altered mental status. Vaccination offers reliable protection and is recommended for all travelers to high-risk areas. Prevention hinges on handwashing, avoiding raw foods, and drinking only boiled or treated water.

Botulism

What should I know about botulism?

Botulism is a rare but potentially fatal illness caused by *Clostridium botulinum*, a bacterium that produces a powerful neurotoxin under anaerobic (low oxygen) conditions. It typically results from ingesting improperly canned, preserved, or stored food—especially in wilderness settings where food safety protocols may be "relaxed." Once consumed, the toxin blocks nerve signals to the muscles, causing progressive muscle weakness and paralysis. Early symptoms include blurred vision, slurred speech, drooping eyelids, and difficulty swallowing, progressing to muscle weakness and potentially respiratory failure. Improper food handling in remote environments increases risk, particularly with home-canned items; vacuum-sealed packages; or any can that appears damaged, leaking, or bulging. The bulge forms when spores germinate and release gas inside of the sealed containers. Field suspicion should be high if multiple individuals develop descending neurologic symptoms after sharing a meal. Unfortunately, there is no role for antibiotics in foodborne botulism. Immediate evacuation is critical for airway protection and antitoxin administration. Prevention hinges on strict food hygiene, boiling low-acid foods—like vegetables, rice, and meats—before storage and discarding questionable items without hesitation.

Worms

Are street vendors safe?

Sometimes. Tapeworms are parasitic flatworms transmitted through undercooked or contaminated meat—especially pork (*Taenia solium*), beef (*Taenia saginata*), fish (*Diphyllobothrium latum*), or via water contaminated with feces. *Echinococcus* species, more invasive than others, are typically contracted through exposure to the feces of infected canids—such as dogs, foxes, or wolves. Once ingested, larvae mature in the intestines and can grow several *meters* in length, anchoring to the gut wall and absorbing nutrients. Most infections are asymptomatic at first. Over time, symptoms may include abdominal discomfort, diarrhea, or unexplained weight loss.

This story worsens when larvae migrate outside the GI tract. *T. solium* and *Echinococcus* can form cysts in the brain (neurocysticercosis), liver, or lungs—leading to seizures, hydrocephalus, or organ damage. Treatment includes antiparasitic drugs such as praziquantel or albendazole, which are widely available—even in many developing regions where these infections are most common. Surgery may be needed for invasive disease. Evacuate for neurologic symptoms or systemic involvement. In the field, prevention is key: Avoid undercooked meat, boil or filter water, and practice good hygiene. Diagnosis in remote areas is difficult, so if there's concern, evacuation is probably the best call.

Can worms cause cancer?

In some cases, yes. Certain parasitic worms have been directly linked to specific human cancers. One of the most well-known is *Schistosoma haematobium*, a blood fluke that causes urinary schistosomiasis and has been associated with bladder cancer in chronically infected individuals.

Infection begins with freshwater exposure in areas where human waste contaminates lakes or rivers. *Schistosoma* eggs released in urine or feces hatch in the water into free-swimming larvae called miracidia, which infect freshwater snails. Inside the snail, the parasite multiplies and transforms into cercariae, a new larval stage that's released back into the water.

These cercariae can penetrate intact human skin during swimming, bathing, or even brief contact with contaminated water. Once inside the body, they travel through the bloodstream to the liver, mature into adult worms, and then migrate to veins near the bladder or intestines. There, they reproduce and release eggs.

Some eggs are passed in urine or stool, continuing the transmission cycle. Others get stuck in body tissues, where they cause ongoing irritation and inflammation. Over time, this repeated immune response can cause scarring and structural damage, particularly in the bladder. In rare cases, this chronic injury has been linked to the development of bladder cancer.

Symptoms depend on the stage of infection and the location of the trapped eggs. Early signs may include rash, fever, abdominal pain, or bloody urine. With prolonged or repeated exposure, complications can progress to kidney problems, liver damage, or cancer.

Praziquantel is the standard treatment and effectively kills adult worms, but it doesn't prevent reinfection. Prevention depends on avoiding freshwater in endemic areas, drying off immediately after contact, and using protective footwear or clothing.

Evacuation should be considered if urinary bleeding or systemic symptoms develop after freshwater exposure in high-risk regions.

Field Note:

It's also worth noting that another group of parasitic worms has been linked to cancer: the liver flukes *Opisthorchis viverrini* and *Clonorchis sinensis*. These infections are associated with bile duct cancer but are geographically limited to parts of Southeast Asia, where raw or undercooked freshwater fish are commonly eaten.

For most wilderness responders, the risk is essentially zero—*unless* operating in those regions and regularly consuming local freshwater fish. I've yet to meet many guides or expedition travelers in Southeast Asia who rely on raw river fish as a staple. But now you know.

Transmission: The Environment

Trachoma

They didn't mention chlamydia in the eye in health class, did they?

Probably, but not this topic. Trachoma is a chronic eye infection caused by the bacterium *Chlamydia trachomatis* and remains the leading infectious cause of preventable blindness worldwide. It spreads through direct contact with infected secretions—typically by sharing towels, clothing, or bedding—or via flies like *Musca sorbens*, which are drawn to moisture around the eyes and nose and transfer bacteria between people. Trachoma thrives in hot, dusty environments with poor sanitation, affecting rural areas in Africa, Asia, Latin America, the Middle East, and Australia. Early signs include eye irritation, redness, tearing, and mild discharge.

The bacteria trigger recurrent inflammation of the *inner* eyelid (conjunctiva), which leads to scarring that causes the lashes to turn *inward*—a condition known as trichiasis. As lashes scrape the cornea, they cause chronic mechanical injury that results in ulceration, clouding, and eventual blindness. The vision loss is due to scarring and abrasion, not direct bacterial damage. The best field treatment is a single oral dose of azithromycin. Evacuate for visible trichiasis, corneal damage, or any changes in vision.

And no, this isn't the sexually transmitted strain you learned about in health classes. Trachoma is caused by an *ocular* strain of *Chlamydia* and spreads through poor hygiene and contact, *not sexual activity*.

Scabies

What is scabies?

Scabies is a highly contagious skin infestation caused by microscopic mites (*Sarcoptes scabiei*) that burrow into the outer layers of the skin to lay their eggs. The mites are tiny—about 0.3 to 0.4 mm—and not visible without magnification. What you do see are the effects: intense itching (especially at night); small red bumps; and fine, wavy burrow lines, often between the fingers, on the wrists, in the groin, or around the waistband. These symptoms result from the body's reaction to the mite's eggs, feces, and saliva. Scabies spreads through prolonged skin-to-skin contact or shared bedding and clothing, making it a concern in expedition environments where people often sleep in close quarters. Unfortunately, hygiene alone won't eliminate the mites. Some have tried petroleum-based ointments like Vaseline in an attempt to suffocate surface mites, but this offers only temporary relief. The adult mites, their eggs, and developing larvae remain protected under the skin; so the life cycle continues.

If scabies is suspected, isolate bedding, limit contact, and—depending on your setting—arrange for evacuation. Treatment requires permethrin 5% cream or oral ivermectin, given in two doses 7-14 days apart. Without proper medication, the infestation will unfortunately persist.

Brain-Eating Amoeba

Is the "brain-eating amoeba" a real thing?

Unfortunately, yes. *Naegleria fowleri* is a free-living amoeba found in warm, stagnant freshwater such as lakes, hot springs, and even poorly maintained pools. Infection occurs when contaminated water is forcefully inhaled through the nose—typically during swimming or diving—allowing the organism to travel up the olfactory nerve into the brain. Once in the central nervous system, the amoeba uses specialized surface structures to break down and digest surrounding brain tissue, while also releasing destructive enzymes that degrade cell membranes and contribute to severe inflammation, nerve damage, and tissue death. The result is primary amebic meningoencephalitis (PAM), a rapidly progressive and nearly always fatal brain infection. Early symptoms mimic bacterial meningitis—headache, fever, nausea, and stiff neck—but quickly progress to confusion, seizures, coma, and death, often within 5 to 10 days.

To date, there is no reliably effective therapy. Early recognition and ICU-level supportive care are critical, but survival remains exceedingly rare. Prevention is the only reliable strategy: Avoid swimming in warm, stagnant water, especially during hot weather, and do not forcibly submerge the head or stir up sediment in suspect environments. For guides and travelers in endemic areas, any nasal exposure to untreated freshwater should be considered high risk.

Chicago Disease

What's Chicago Disease?

Blastomycosis was once called "Chicago Disease" because so many early cases were clustered around the city and the Great Lakes region. Blastomycosis is a fungal infection caused by *Blastomyces dermatitidis*, which thrives in moist soil and decaying vegetation near rivers, lakes, and forested regions of the southeastern and midwestern United States. Infection occurs when spores are inhaled—often during trail clearing, excavation, or logging in endemic areas. Most exposures are unnoticed at the time, with symptoms developing days to weeks later.

Once inhaled, the spores convert to yeast in the lungs, provoking inflammation that can resemble pneumonia or lung cancer. Symptoms range from mild cough and low-grade fever to severe pulmonary illness. In disseminated cases, the fungus spreads to skin, bones, or the genitourinary tract. Antifungal treatment is necessary, usually with itraconazole or amphotericin B in severe cases. Evacuate if respiratory symptoms persist or worsen after known exposure, especially with systemic signs such as weight loss, skin lesions, or joint pain.

Valley Fever

What's Valley Fever?

Coccidioidomycosis is a fungal infection caused by *Coccidioides* species, found in arid, dusty soils of the southwestern United States, Mexico, and parts of Central and South America. Infection occurs when fungal spores are inhaled during activities that disturb soil—such as hiking, construction, or cave exploration. Also known as "Valley Fever," the illness is endemic to desert regions and often overlooked in field settings.

Once inhaled, the spores settle in the lungs and begin to grow, triggering an immune response and causing inflammation in the surrounding lung tissue.

Most cases present with low-grade fever, dry cough, fatigue, and chest discomfort; but some progress to pneumonia or disseminated infection involving skin, bones, or the central nervous system. Immunocompromised individuals and those with prolonged symptoms may require antifungal therapy, typically fluconazole. Evacuate if the patient has persistent fever, respiratory decline, or signs of systemic spread after exposure in an endemic zone.

Caver's Disease

What's Caver's Disease?

Histoplasmosis is a fungal infection caused by *Histoplasma capsulatum*, found in soil "enriched" with bird or bat droppings—especially in caves, old buildings, and roosting areas. The disease is most prevalent in the Ohio and Mississippi River valleys, Central and South America, and areas with significant cave tourism or excavation. It's often referred to as "Caver's Disease" due to its frequent association with spelunking and guano-rich environments. Infection occurs through inhalation of airborne spores released during soil or dust disturbance.

In the lungs, the spores convert to yeast, triggering an immune response that can mimic viral pneumonia. Most infections are mild or asymptomatic, but symptoms may include fever, chest pain, cough, and fatigue. In immunocompromised individuals or with high spore exposure, the disease can disseminate to other organs, requiring systemic antifungal treatment with itraconazole or amphotericin B. Evacuate if symptoms persist or worsen after cave or demolition exposure—particularly if respiratory distress, weight loss, or night sweats develop.

Leptospirosis

What if I need one more reason to avoid swimming in warm, lowland rivers?

You got it. Leptospirosis is a bacterial infection caused by *Leptospira* species, transmitted through water contaminated with urine from infected animals—especially rodents, livestock, and wild mammals. The bacteria enter the body through cuts, mucous membranes, or prolonged exposure to contaminated water even across intact skin. It's most common in tropical climates, flood-prone regions, and areas with poor sanitation. Once in the bloodstream, *Leptospira* spread rapidly to multiple organs. The bacteria damage the linings of small blood vessels, leading to capillary leak, tissue swelling, and impaired oxygen exchange. They also target the liver and kidneys directly, causing cellular injury, inflammation, and, in severe cases, multi-organ failure.

Symptoms typically appear 2–14 days after exposure and often follow a biphasic pattern. The initial phase includes sudden fever, chills, headache, muscle pain (especially in the calves), and redness of the eyes without discharge (known as conjunctival suffusion). Some cases resolve without complication, but others progress to Weil's Disease, a more severe form characterized by jaundice, kidney failure, bleeding, and low blood pressure. A particularly deadly variant, leptospiral pulmonary hemorrhage syndrome (LPHS), involves bleeding into the lungs, leading to respiratory distress and collapse. Early antibiotic treatment—usually with doxycycline or penicillin—can reduce the risk of complications, but severe cases may require intensive care management. Evacuate for persistent fever, jaundice, decreased urine output, confusion, bleeding, or shortness of breath. Prevention includes avoiding contact with potentially contaminated water sources, using protective footwear in flooded or muddy environments, and considering doxycycline prophylaxis during high-risk exposures.

What is meant by the phrase "the viruses always win"?

This phrase speaks to the unmatched ability of viruses to adapt, spread, and thrive. Viruses mutate faster than humans can counter, often outpacing immune defenses and ultimately rendering medical treatments ineffective. They're not even alive by traditional definitions: Viruses don't grow or reproduce on their own. Instead, they hijack the cellular machinery of humans, animals, fungi, plants, and even other microbes. Despite advances in medicine, viruses continue to exploit our gaps in surveillance, shifts in global travel, and changes in human behavior. In remote regions, the risk of exposure to emerging or exotic pathogens remains high. Although roughly 260 animal-borne viruses are known to infect humans, current estimates suggest that nearly 2 million zoonotic viruses still exist, waiting to be discovered.

Red Flag Framework: Infectious Diseases

What's an easy way to remember what signs and symptoms warrant evacuation using the Red Flag Framework?

For Infectious Disease Emergencies: **FIERCE**

- **F**ever-Persistent, high fever 38.3°C/101°F), rigors, or fever with confusion or altered awareness
- **I**mpaired function - Weakness, inability to walk, jaundice, confusion, seizure, or collapse
- **E**scalating symptoms - Worsening swelling, redness, rash, vomiting, or diarrhea despite basic treatment
- **R**espiratory symptoms - Shortness of breath, cough with fever, or signs of pulmonary distress
- **C**irculatory changes - Rapid heart rate, low blood pressure, cool extremities, or decreased urine output
- **E**xposure history - Known or likely exposure to contaminated water, insect bites, animal contact, sick people, or recent travel through high-risk areas

Any of these signs indicate a potentially serious condition, requiring immediate evaluation and possible evacuation. When in doubt, follow the Red Flag Framework: FIERCE = Evacuate.

Shared Miles

Bob and I have been surfing side by side for almost 30 years. Back when Costa Rica was still rugged "Centro

America"—before surf reports and GPS—before you could pull up a satellite image and know what a surf break looked like without getting your feet wet. We chased waves across the globe, slept in the dirt in the Western Sahara, stretched hammocks between trucks in remote Australia, lived cheap, traveled hard, and figured it out as we went. He's the kind of guy who's been to more countries than most people have even heard of.

So, when he called me from Jakarta complaining about a nasty case of "Bali belly," neither of us thought too much of it. Traveler's diarrhea is usually just an inconvenience. Hydrate, rest, carry on.

Then he called again from San Francisco. The cramping hadn't let up, and now he was short of breath and starting to have chest pains—a new twist. But foodborne illness can drag on, beat you up for a while. Usually there's not much to do but stay on top of fluids and wait it out.

A day later, another call—this time from Denver—he couldn't lie flat. Breathing hurt. He knew he was in a bad way.

By the time he walked into the hospital, things had gone from bad to worse. Within hours, he was in the ICU, then straight to the cardiac cath lab. Every indicator—blood work, scans, symptoms—pointed to a heart attack. Except it wasn't.

The infection had made its way into the muscle of his heart, triggering inflammation that mimicked a classic cardiac event.

It took nearly three weeks before we got the answer: Salmonella-induced myocarditis.

This was one of those rare cases where an infection that usually just makes you regret not investing in toilet paper and Gatorade jumps to the bloodstream, attacking distant organs—like the heart. Left untreated—especially in the developing world—it might have killed him.

Instead of staying in his gut, the Salmonella bacteria invaded his bloodstream, triggering a systemic inflammatory response and hitting key organs like his heart and kidneys. The right antibiotics, the right support, and time pulled him back—but it took days in the ICU and months of recovery. The kind of recovery where you measure progress in stairs climbed and deep breaths taken.

Traveler's diarrhea is usually nothing more than an inconvenience. You hydrate, rest, eat some toast, take Pepto, and let it pass. But when it starts showing different cards—chest pain, shortness of breath, exhaustion—it's no longer just about rehydrating. That's when you start antibiotics. When the infection has left the gut and is affecting other organ systems, fluids and electrolytes aren't going to cut it—and the sooner you act, the better your odds.

Bob was thankfully already on his way out of the developing world when things went south. If he hadn't been, this story might have ended differently.

Medical Emergencies

Overview

Why is a strong grasp of medical issues critical in remote settings?

In wilderness medicine education, trauma often takes center stage, but medical emergencies are just as common and frequently more difficult to recognize. Traumatic injuries typically present with obvious signs, while medical conditions tend to develop gradually and without clear external cues.

Epidemiologic data from U.S. wilderness rescue operations show that illness alone accounts for nearly half of all nonfatal incidents, and reviews of expedition evacuations consistently find that medical conditions—most often dehydration, gastrointestinal illness, allergic reactions, or infection—are responsible for the majority of wilderness evacuations. Regardless of the setting, medical problems degrade group function, impair decision-making, and turn routine logistics into operational risks.

Sugar Highs & Lows: Diabetes

What is diabetes?

To understand diabetes, we first need to understand how the body uses fuel at the cellular level. For most cells—especially in the brain and muscles—glucose is the main energy source. When we eat, foods containing starches and sugars (collectively known as carbohydrates) are broken down into glucose, which then enters the bloodstream. In response to this rise in blood sugar, the pancreas releases insulin—a hormone that acts like a key, unlocking cells so glucose can enter and be converted into usable energy, primarily in the form of ATP (adenosine triphosphate).

In diabetes, this process breaks down. Either the body doesn't produce enough insulin, or the cells stop responding to it effectively (insulin resistance). As a result, glucose remains in the bloodstream, leading to high blood sugar levels while cells remain starved for fuel.

Type 1 diabetes (insulin-dependent) is an autoimmune disease in which the immune system mistakenly attacks and destroys the insulin-producing beta cells of the pancreas. Without insulin, glucose cannot enter cells, and blood sugar levels can rise dangerously. People with type 1 diabetes must take insulin regularly to survive. They are particularly vulnerable to rapid swings in blood sugar, and missing even a single dose of insulin can lead to a life-threatening complication called diabetic ketoacidosis (DKA).

Type 2 diabetes (non–insulin-dependent) is far more common. In this form, the body still produces insulin, but cells become resistant to its effects—a condition known as insulin resistance. Glucose can't efficiently enter cells despite the presence of insulin, leading to rising blood sugar levels. Over time, the pancreas may also produce less insulin. Type 2 diabetes is often managed with oral medications like metformin, which lowers blood sugar by decreasing the liver's glucose output and improving insulin sensitivity in tissues.

How does diabetes become dangerous in the field, and what are the key emergencies to recognize?

Diabetes becomes dangerous when blood sugar swings too far in either direction—too low (hypoglycemia) or too high (hyperglycemia). In remote or wilderness settings, these shifts can occur rapidly and may go unnoticed until symptoms are severe. The greatest risks arise from missed meals, prolonged physical exertion, illness, vomiting, or disrupted access to insulin. In the field, the two most critical complications to recognize are hypoglycemia and diabetic ketoacidosis (DKA), both of which can progress quickly and become life-threatening if not managed early.

What happens during hypoglycemia, and how is it treated?

Hypoglycemia occurs when blood sugar drops too low to meet the body's energy needs—especially in the brain, which relies almost entirely on glucose. Unlike muscles or the liver, the brain can't store fuel and can't use fat directly, since fatty acids don't cross the blood-brain barrier. In fact, under conditions of prolonged glucose deprivation—such as fasting or starvation—the liver converts fats into ketones: small molecules made from fatty acids that serve as an emergency fuel for the brain. But that shift takes time, often several days. In sudden hypoglycemia—like what can happen with excessive insulin use or poor diabetes control—there's no time for the liver to adapt, and without glucose, brain function rapidly deteriorates, leading to confusion, seizures, or even coma.

Early symptoms include shakiness, sweating, irritability, dizziness, and fatigue. As levels fall, confusion, slurred speech, poor coordination, or unconsciousness may follow. Common field triggers include missed meals, overexertion, vomiting, alcohol use, or excess insulin.

If the person is awake and can swallow, give fast sugar—juice, candy, glucose tablets, sugar packets, or honey. Symptoms should improve within minutes. Follow with a meal or snack to help stabilize levels.

If the person can't reliably swallow, sugar sources like honey, glucose gel, or table sugar can be placed inside the cheek or under the tongue. These are absorbed through the mucous membranes and can serve as a useful bridge in remote settings.

What's the difference between hyperglycemia and diabetic ketoacidosis (DKA)?

Not all high blood sugar is an emergency. People with diabetes may develop mild hyperglycemia from missed medication, illness, dehydration, or eating more carbohydrates than usual. If the person is alert, able to eat and drink, and not vomiting, this is usually manageable in place. Encourage hydration, support their usual medication routine, and monitor for worsening symptoms.

Diabetic ketoacidosis (DKA) is a different animal. It most often occurs in people with type 1 diabetes who don't have enough circulating insulin. Without insulin, glucose can't move into cells, so the body thinks it's starving—despite high sugar levels in the blood. In response, it turns to fat for energy. But burning fat releases acidic byproducts called ketones. As ketones accumulate, they lower the blood pH, leading to a dangerous state known as metabolic acidosis.

To compensate, the body starts breathing faster and deeper in an effort to blow off carbon dioxide—a natural acid in the blood—and raise the pH. This respiratory pattern, known as Kussmaul respirations, is not just rapid but deep and labored, and it signals serious metabolic stress. Meanwhile, the excess glucose pulls water into the urine through a process called osmotic diuresis. This explains the frequent urination (polyuria) often seen in diabetics. The kidneys dump large amounts of fluid and electrolytes—especially sodium and potassium—leading to severe dehydration and worsening organ function.

As DKA progresses, symptoms may include dry mouth, excessive thirst, nausea, vomiting, abdominal pain, weakness, confusion, and eventually coma. The breath may have a sweet or fruity odor due to volatile ketones being exhaled.

How can I manage high sugars in the field?

In both uncomplicated hyperglycemia and diabetic ketoacidosis (DKA), fluid loss is the primary concern. Elevated blood glucose causes osmotic diuresis, drawing water into the urine and leading to dehydration and reduced circulating blood volume. As volume decreases, tissue perfusion declines. Without adequate oxygen delivery, cells shift to anaerobic metabolism, producing lactic acid. This adds to the existing acidosis caused by ketones and worsens the overall metabolic state.

The combined effects of dehydration, acidosis, and electrolyte loss result in progressive physiological deterioration. Breathing becomes deep and labored (Kussmaul respirations) as the body attempts to blow off carbon dioxide to correct the pH imbalance. Vomiting may worsen fluid depletion, and significant losses of sodium and potassium further impair organ function.

If the patient is alert and able to swallow, steady oral hydration with water or electrolyte fluids is the most appropriate field intervention. If prescribed insulin is available and the patient is oriented and capable of self-administration, assistance may be appropriate. However, insulin should not be initiated or adjusted in any patient showing signs of confusion, vomiting, or clinical instability.

Early evacuation is warranted if DKA is suspected. Indicators such as vomiting, altered mental status, deep or labored respirations, or a known history of insulin dependence should prompt immediate arrangements for transport. Oral fluids may provide temporary support during evacuation but do not replace definitive care.

If urine test strips ("dipsticks") are available, they can help confirm the diagnosis. These strips are a worthwhile addition to a wilderness medical kit, widely available without a prescription, and capable of detecting ketones, acidic byproducts of fat metabolism that rise when insulin is lacking. A positive test supports the clinical impression, but the decision to evacuate should be based on the overall presentation, not test results alone.

What if I can't tell if it's low or high blood sugar?

When in doubt, give sugar. Hypoglycemia can lead to seizures, coma, and irreversible brain damage if not treated promptly. It's also easier to reverse in the field than hyperglycemia or DKA. Administering sugar will not significantly worsen hyperglycemia or DKA in the short term, but it may save the life of someone who is hypoglycemic.

If symptoms improve within minutes, hypoglycemia was likely the cause. If there is no improvement or symptoms worsen, DKA should be suspected and evacuation initiated. In the absence of a glucometer or lab testing, it is safer to assume low blood sugar and treat early.

The Thyroid

What if a guest forgets their thyroid medication on a trip?

The thyroid is a small butterfly-shaped gland in the neck that plays a central role in regulating metabolism. It produces two key hormones—thyroxine (T4) and triiodothyronine (T3)—which help set the body's metabolic "idle speed," influencing how quickly cells convert nutrients into usable energy. These hormones affect nearly every organ system, helping to regulate body temperature, heart rate, brain function, and digestion.

If a guest forgets their thyroid medication for a week, the impact depends on their underlying condition: hypothyroidism (underactive thyroid) or hyperthyroidism (overactive thyroid).

In hypothyroidism, thyroid hormone levels are already low, and daily medication (typically levothyroxine, a synthetic form of T4) is used to restore normal metabolic function. Missing doses for a few days may lead to symptoms such as fatigue, cold intolerance, or constipation, as the body's metabolic rate slows in response. However, because thyroid hormones—particularly T4—have a long half-life (about 7 days), serious complications like myxedema coma (a rare, life-threatening suppression of bodily functions) are extremely unlikely after a short interruption.

In hyperthyroidism, the concern is excess hormone. Medications used to manage it work by reducing hormone production or blocking its effects. Skipping them may allow thyroid activity to increase, potentially triggering symptoms such as anxiety, rapid heartbeat, heat intolerance, or restlessness. Severe outcomes like thyroid storm—characterized by fever, confusion, and extreme tachycardia—typically result from prolonged medication lapses, sudden withdrawal from high-dose treatment, or concurrent illness or trauma.

A week without thyroid medication is rarely a medical emergency, though some symptoms may return or worsen. Observation is generally appropriate, and evacuation should only be considered if symptoms interfere with safety or essential function. During pre-trip planning, guests should be reminded to pack extra medication and store it in a secure, accessible location to avoid unnecessary disruptions.

Red Flag Framework: Endocrine Emergencies

What's an easy way to remember what signs and symptoms warrant evacuation using the Red Flag Framework?

For the endocrine system: **GLAND**

- **G**lucose imbalance: signs of hypoglycemia (confusion, sweating, trembling) or hyperglycemia (severe thirst, frequent urination, fatigue)
- **L**ethargy or altered mental status (e.g., hypoglycemia, hyperglycemia, or adrenal crisis)
- **A**cidosis: fruity breath, extreme dehydration, nausea, or rapid breathing (ketoacidosis)
- **N**eurological symptoms: seizures, confusion, or unresponsiveness associated with severe hypo-or hyperglycemia
- **D**ehydration or electrolyte imbalances causing muscle cramps, weakness, or cardiac symptoms

Any of these signs indicate a potentially serious condition, requiring immediate evaluation and possible evacuation. When in doubt, follow the Red Flag Framework: GLAND = Evacuate.

Fainting in the Wilderness

What is syncope?

Syncope (sing-kuh—pee), or fainting, is a temporary loss of consciousness caused by reduced blood flow to the brain. In the wilderness, understanding *why* someone faints helps determine whether it's a minor issue or a sign of something more serious. The circulatory system functions like a network of pipes delivering oxygen and nutrients. If pressure in these "pipes" drops—due to dehydration, vasodilation, blood loss or other causes—blood flow to the brain decreases, leading to syncope.

Dehydration and diarrhea are common culprits, as they reduce overall blood volume, making it harder for circulation to maintain adequate pressure, especially when standing up quickly. Heat exhaustion compounds the problem by causing blood vessels to dilate in an attempt to cool the body, further lowering blood pressure. Low blood sugar can also trigger fainting, as the brain lacks the necessary fuel to function properly. Emotional stress or pain can stimulate the vagus nerve, slowing the heart rate and dilating blood vessels, leading to a sudden drop in blood pressure and loss of consciousness.

Most fainting episodes from these causes are brief and not life-threatening, but guides should remain alert for more serious conditions such as cardiac events or strokes. If syncope is accompanied by chest pain, confusion, or difficulty speaking, evacuation to advanced medical care is critical.

How should a guide handle fainting in the wilderness?

When a person faints in the wilderness, the immediate priority is to restore blood flow to the brain. They should be laid flat with legs elevated to improve circulation and stabilize blood pressure. Once consciousness returns, hydration and blood sugar levels should be assessed, as both dehydration and hypoglycemia are common contributors in remote environments. Small sips of water or electrolyte solution can help, and if low blood sugar is suspected, a sugary snack, honey, or glucose should be provided. The individual should be allowed to rest and rise slowly, as sudden movement may trigger another episode.

Evacuation should be considered when concerning signs suggest an underlying medical problem. Persistent or worsening dizziness, confusion, slurred speech, gait instability, or focal neurologic deficits raise suspicion for central nervous system causes such as stroke. Chest pain, palpitations, shortness of breath, or abnormal vital signs may indicate cardiac or pulmonary issues requiring urgent care. Failure to improve after hydration and rest, particularly in the context of heat illness or a known medical history (e.g., arrhythmia, seizure, stroke), also lowers the threshold for evacuation. If red flags are present or the condition does not resolve, evacuation should not be delayed.

Dehydration

What do I need to know about dehydration?

Dehydration happens when the body loses more fluid than it takes in, disrupting vital functions. In the wilderness, heat, exertion, and limited access to clean water make dehydration a constant risk. The body compensates by releasing antidiuretic hormone (ADH) to reduce urine output and aldosterone to retain sodium, which helps hold onto water and stabilize blood pressure. When dehydration sets in, blood volume drops, forcing the heart to work harder to maintain circulation. This impairs temperature regulation, increasing the risk of heat-related illness.

Electrolyte imbalances further complicate dehydration. Sodium, potassium, and other minerals are essential for nerve, muscle, and heart function. When these levels drop, symptoms can escalate from mild thirst and fatigue to muscle cramps, dizziness, confusion, and even chest pain. In severe cases, dehydration can lead to kidney failure, seizures, shock, and even death—making early recognition and treatment critical.

How can I recognize and prevent dehydration?

Early signs of dehydration include thirst, dry mouth, headache, concentrated urine, and fatigue. As it worsens, symptoms may progress to rapid heart rate, dizziness, confusion, and eventually unconsciousness. Monitoring urine color is a simple field tool—pale yellow suggests adequate hydration, while dark urine signals a need for fluids.

Prevention starts with consistent fluid intake, especially in heat or during exertion. When water is scarce, rationing and finding alternative sources are critical. Electrolyte replacement matters just as much as water—sodium and other minerals help the body retain fluids and prevent further loss. In the backcountry, recognizing early signs and responding promptly can prevent dehydration from becoming a serious medical emergency.

What is a good rehydration recipe, and how does it compare to commercial sports drinks?

In wilderness settings, having a reliable oral rehydration solution (ORS) is essential for managing dehydration from illness, heat, or prolonged exertion. A simple, effective homemade ORS can be made by mixing 1 liter of clean water with ½ teaspoon (about 3 grams) of table salt and 6 teaspoons (roughly 30 grams) of sugar. This formula supports sodium-glucose co-transport in the intestines, enhancing water absorption. It closely mirrors the World Health Organization's recommended ORS used globally to treat dehydration from diarrhea, vomiting, or other medical causes.

Commercial sports drink powders, such as Gatorade Thirst Quencher Powder™, are formulated for healthy individuals losing fluid through sweat—not for medical dehydration. A 12-ounce serving provides about 150 mg of sodium and 21 grams of sugar. Scaled to a liter, this yields approximately 430 mg sodium and 60 grams of sugar—lower in sodium and higher in sugar than WHO standards. This reduced sodium is intentional: most sweat losses are modest and can be replaced with normal food and fluids.

By contrast, dehydration from vomiting, diarrhea, or metabolic stress requires a carefully balanced sodium-to-glucose ratio to optimize fluid uptake and restore volume. While sports drinks may help with hydration during exertion, they are inadequate substitutes for true ORS in medical emergencies.

What if the patient can't drink?

In rare, critical situations—when severe dehydration is present, oral fluids aren't an option due to vomiting, confusion, or unconsciousness, and no medical support is available—rectal hydration (proctoclysis) may be the only practical option. Though rarely used in modern clinical care, it is a legitimate consideration in remote settings without access to IV therapy. It works by leveraging the colon's natural ability to absorb water and electrolytes.

Under normal conditions, the colon (large intestine) absorbs fluid and salts from indigestible material, helping to form solid waste and maintain the body's fluid balance. In emergencies, this same function can be used to deliver a rehydration solution when drinking isn't possible. Absorption is limited—typically around 300 mL per hour in adults—but even modest volumes can help support circulation and buy time for evacuation or other definitive care.

To perform rectal hydration:

- Prepare the solution: Mix a clean rehydration solution, like an oral rehydration solution (ORS), and warm it to body temperature to reduce discomfort.

- Set up the equipment: Use a clean container, such as a hydration bladder, connected to a narrow, *soft*, flexible tube.
- Position the person: Have them lie on their left side; this position helps the fluid stay in the left part of the colon, where absorption is effective.
- Insert the tube: Apply a lubricant to the tube and gently insert it about 7.5–10 cm (3–4 inches) into the rectum.
- Administer the fluid: Let the fluid flow in by gravity; do not force it.

After the procedure, closely watch for signs of improvement, such as increased alertness, stable vital signs, and normal urination. In wilderness situations, using the colon's ability to absorb water can be a lifesaving way to treat severe dehydration when other methods aren't available.

When should a dehydrated patient be evacuated?

Evacuation is necessary if symptoms worsen despite rehydration efforts. Signs that warrant immediate evacuation include persistent vomiting, confusion, an inability to stay awake, low blood pressure, rapid breathing, or no urine output for an extended period. As dehydration progresses, the body struggles to maintain circulation and organ function, making early intervention critical. As these symptoms develop, delaying transport increases the risk of organ failure or death. In wilderness settings, dehydration can become a life-threatening condition that must be recognized early and treated aggressively.

Can a person drink seawater in an emergency?

Hell to the no. Drinking seawater in an emergency will surely make dehydration worse. It contains roughly 11 grams of sodium per liter—more than six times the sodium found in the World Health Organization's oral rehydration solution

(ORS), which is carefully balanced to help the body *absorb* fluid.

Here's the problem: to excrete excess sodium, the kidneys need water—lots of it. But sodium can't leave the body on its own; it has to be diluted first. When you drink seawater, the sodium content is far higher than what the kidneys can safely process. To manage the salt load, the body pulls water from its own reserves. Fluid shifts out of cells, into the bloodstream, and eventually to the kidneys, where it helps dilute the excess sodium so it can be flushed out in the urine.

But this comes at a steep cost: your cells dehydrate in the process. With every sip of seawater, you end up with *less* usable water in your system than before. As dehydration progresses, symptoms like fatigue, dizziness, confusion, and kidney injury emerge. Without access to freshwater, the cycle accelerates—driving the body toward organ failure and death.

Historical accounts reinforce this storyline. In the 1816 wreck of the French frigate *Méduse*, survivors adrift at sea resorted to drinking seawater. Rather than prolonging survival, it led to rapid physical and mental decline, hallucinations, mutiny, and eventually cannibalism. The scandal erupted into a national crisis, and public outrage over the tragedy contributed to the July Revolution of 1830, which overthrew King Charles X of France and ended his absolute rule in favor of a constitutional monarchy. Though it fell short of full democracy, the revolution marked a major shift toward representative government and helped spark liberal reform movements across Europe, leaving a lasting impact on modern global politics.

Stroke & Seizures

What is a stroke?

A stroke, or cerebrovascular accident (CVA), occurs when blood flow to the brain is disrupted by either a blockage (ischemic stroke) or bleeding (hemorrhagic stroke). Ischemic strokes, which account for nearly 90% of cases, result from blood clots in narrowed arteries, depriving brain tissue of oxygen. Hemorrhagic strokes, though less common, tend to be more severe, occurring when a blood vessel ruptures and causes bleeding in the brain.

While strokes are rare in wilderness settings, they can happen, especially in individuals with risk factors like hypertension, diabetes, or atrial fibrillation. Recognizing symptoms early is critical, as delayed care can lead to permanent neurological damage.

What are the risk factors for stroke?

Stroke risk increases with age, but the major contributors include high blood pressure, diabetes, smoking, high cholesterol, atrial fibrillation, obesity, and a history of stroke or transient ischemic attacks (TIAs). A TIA, or mini-stroke, causes temporary stroke-like symptoms that resolve within minutes to hours and serve as a critical warning sign for future stroke risk.

In wilderness settings, additional factors can elevate stroke risk even in those without prior history—dehydration and physical exertion increase blood viscosity and cardiovascular strain. High-altitude exposure may cause hypoxia and fluctuations in blood pressure. Cold environments trigger vasoconstriction, which can raise blood pressure and promote clot formation. Guides should pay close attention to clients with known or suspected risk factors, as these vulnerabilities often remain hidden until symptoms appear. Early recognition and prompt evacuation are essential. Timely treatment offers the best chance to minimize long-term neurologic damage.

What are the symptoms of a stroke, and how can guides recognize them?

Strokes typically present with sudden neurological changes, including weakness, numbness, or paralysis, usually on one side of the body. Speech may become difficult, with slurring, confusion, or an inability to find words. Vision can be affected, with sudden changes in acuity or loss of sight in one or both eyes. Some strokes, particularly hemorrhagic ones, cause severe headaches, while others result in a loss of balance, poor coordination, or difficulty walking.

Guides can quickly assess for a stroke using the FAST acronym:

- Face: Ask the person to smile—does one side droop?
- Arm: Have them raise both arms—does one drift downward or feel weak?
- Speech: Ask them to repeat a simple phrase—do they slur words or struggle to speak?
- Time: If any of these signs are present, seek medical help immediately.

How is a stroke managed in the wilderness?

Stroke management in the wilderness focuses on supportive care and urgent evacuation. The patient should be positioned with their head slightly elevated to reduce pressure on the brain while ensuring a clear airway. Keeping them calm and warm is essential, as stress and unnecessary movement can worsen symptoms. If dehydration is suspected and the patient can swallow safely without coughing, small sips of water may be offered, but fluids should never be forced.

Because strokes can mimic other conditions like hypoglycemia, administering a fast-acting sugar source such as glucose tablets or honey is a reasonable step if symptoms align with low blood sugar. If symptoms resolve immediately after sugar administration, ongoing monitoring, hydration, food, and rest become the priority. If symptoms persist, the situation should be treated as a suspected stroke, and evacuation should be initiated as quickly as possible.

While commonly used in hospitals to treat ischemic strokes, aspirin should not be given in the wilderness setting, as there is no reliable way to determine whether a stroke is ischemic (caused by a clot) or hemorrhagic (caused by bleeding) in the field. If the stroke is hemorrhagic, aspirin can worsen bleeding by impairing platelet function, making it harder for the body to form a clot and stop the hemorrhage. Without imaging to confirm the cause, giving aspirin carries significant risk and should be avoided.

All cases of sudden neurological symptoms must be considered medical emergencies. Ischemic strokes may benefit from clot-dissolving medications (thrombolytics) if given within a few hours, while hemorrhagic strokes may require surgical intervention. The faster a stroke is recognized and the patient evacuated, the better the chance of minimizing permanent damage or death.

What is a seizure, and how should it be managed?

A seizure is a sudden surge of electrical activity in the brain that disrupts normal function, leading to changes in behavior, movement, or consciousness. Seizures in the wilderness can occur due to head injuries, infections, metabolic imbalances, or noncompliance with medication in those with epilepsy. They vary in severity, from brief lapses in awareness to generalized convulsions.

Most seizures stop on their own within one to two minutes and can be managed with supportive care. However, if a seizure lasts longer than five minutes or multiple seizures occur without full recovery in between, the condition is known as status epilepticus. In a wilderness setting, this is a life-threatening emergency, as prolonged seizures can lead to brain damage, respiratory failure, or death.

In the wilderness, any seizure should be treated as a serious event due to limited access to medical care and the risks of complications such as hypoxia, aspiration, or additional injury. If a person with a known seizure disorder has a breakthrough seizure, evacuation is necessary unless there is a clear and non-life-threatening explanation, such as missing a dose of anti-epileptic medication. Even in known epilepsy patients, all seizures in the field are considered abnormal and warrant evacuation to ensure the patient receives appropriate medical evaluation.

Immediate care in the field should focus on safety: protecting the airway, preventing injury, and monitoring the patient until evacuation can be arranged. The priority is to stabilize the patient and get them to definitive care as quickly as possible.

Headaches

What do I need to know about headaches?

Headaches are among the most common medical complaints in the wilderness and can range from minor discomfort to signs of life-threatening conditions. Typical causes include dehydration, exertion, tension, altitude sickness, stress, sinus pressure, alcohol use, and underlying disorders such as migraines. Less common but more serious causes include stroke, intracranial hemorrhage, or central nervous system infections such as meningitis.

Assessment begins with the headache's onset, duration, intensity, and associated symptoms. Ask whether the individual has experienced similar headaches before, what treatments have worked in the past, and whether this episode differs from their usual pattern. If the headache is mild and consistent with a known history of past headaches, basic field management is often sufficient. Rehydration is a priority, as dehydration is a frequent trigger. Over-the-counter medications like ibuprofen or acetaminophen may reduce pain, and caffeine can be useful in cases of tension headaches or migraines. Rest in a cool, quiet environment may also help relieve symptoms.

However, it is critical to identify red flags that suggest a more serious cause. Headaches accompanied by neurological changes, fever, stiff neck, visual disturbances, altered mental status, or sudden severe onset require immediate evacuation and advanced medical evaluation.

Who is at high risk for life-threatening headaches?

Individuals taking anticoagulants (blood thinners) are at increased risk of intracranial hemorrhage, while those with cancer, HIV, or other causes of immunosuppression are more prone to brain infections. Pregnant women and people over 50 experiencing new or unusual headaches may be at risk for severe blood-pressure emergencies or vascular disease.

Environmental and behavioral factors such as drug or alcohol use, rapid altitude changes, or prolonged physical exertion can further increase risk.

What are the signs of a high-risk headache?

A high-risk headache is one that suggests a serious underlying condition requiring urgent medical attention. A sudden, severe headache that reaches maximum intensity within seconds, described as “thunderclap” presentation or “the worst headache of my life” presentation may indicate a subarachnoid hemorrhage caused by a ruptured aneurysm, which can rapidly lead to brain damage or death.

Headaches associated with persistent nausea or vomiting, confusion, seizures, or changes in consciousness raise concern for increased pressure inside the skull due to brain swelling, bleeding, infection, or a tumor. Vision disturbances, such as double vision, blind spots, or loss of vision, may signal pressure on the optic nerve or compromised blood flow to the brain.

Neck stiffness, pain with the “chin-to-chest” maneuver, fever, and sensitivity to light, especially when accompanied by confusion, suggest meningitis, a severe infection of the brain’s protective layers that can deteriorate quickly without treatment. Progressive neurological symptoms such as weakness, numbness, facial drooping, difficulty speaking, or loss of coordination strongly suggest stroke or intracranial hemorrhage and require immediate intervention.

A headache that worsens with coughing, straining, or lying flat may indicate increased intracranial pressure. A headache following head trauma should always be taken seriously, particularly in those on anticoagulants, as they are at higher risk for subdural or epidural hematoma. Any of these warning signs warrant immediate evacuation, as delaying treatment increases the risk of permanent damage or death.

How should headaches be managed in the wilderness?

For mild headaches without red flag symptoms, management focuses on hydration, rest, and symptom relief. Even mild dehydration can trigger headaches, so rehydration should be prioritized early. Over-the-counter medications such as ibuprofen or acetaminophen may help, provided there are no contraindications. Resting in a shaded, quiet environment can reduce sensory input and promote recovery. Avoiding alcohol and limiting caffeine may help prevent worsening symptoms, though caffeine *can* be beneficial in certain cases like migraines or tension headaches.

If altitude illness is suspected, descending to a lower elevation is the most effective intervention. Supplemental oxygen, if available, can further reduce symptoms. Most uncomplicated headaches improve with these basic measures, but persistent or worsening symptoms should prompt reassessment and possible evacuation.

A headache warrants immediate evacuation if it is associated with neurologic symptoms (such as confusion, weakness, visual changes, or seizure), persistent vomiting, fever, or neck stiffness. A sudden, severe headache with no identifiable cause should always be treated as an emergency, as it may indicate subarachnoid hemorrhage or elevated intracranial pressure.

Any severe headache following trauma, especially in individuals on blood thinners, raises concern for intracranial bleeding, such as a subdural or epidural hematoma. These conditions involve blood collecting between the brain and skull, compressing brain tissue and potentially leading to rapid neurological decline. Fever, neck rigidity, and a worsening overall condition may indicate meningitis or other serious infection. If broad-spectrum antibiotics are available and meningitis is suspected, they should be given. Antibiotics do not replace the need for evacuation and any delays in evacuation place the patient at significant risk.

Red Flag Framework: Neurological Emergencies

What's an easy way to remember what signs and symptoms warrant evacuation using the Red Flag Framework?

The Red Flag Framework for neurological emergencies is **HEADS UP**.

- **H**eadache (severe or sudden onset)
- **E**yes (vision changes or loss)
- **A**symmetry in the face (facial droop)
- **D**izziness or difficulty balancing
- **S**peech difficulties (slurred or incomprehensible)
- **U**ncontrolled movements (tremors, twitching, or seizures)
- **P**ersonality or mental status changes (confusion, lethargy)

Any of these signs indicate a potentially serious condition, requiring immediate evaluation and possible evacuation. When in doubt, follow the Red Flag Framework: HEADS UP = Evacuate.

Teeth and Gums

What is the essential anatomy for managing wilderness dental emergencies?

Understanding dental pain begins with the structure of the tooth and surrounding tissues. The crown—the visible part above the gum line—is coated in enamel, the hardest substance in the body, which protects the inner layers from damage and infection. Beneath it lies dentin, a porous, sensitive tissue that responds to temperature and pressure; when exposed by fracture or decay, it can cause sharp pain. At the center is the pulp, which houses nerves, blood vessels, and connective tissue. Because the pulp is encased in rigid walls, any inflammation or infection—whether from trauma or cavities—increases internal pressure and intensifies pain. If the infection spreads beyond the tooth into nearby bone or soft tissue, it may form an abscess, causing swelling, redness, and pus that often requires drainage and antibiotics.

Below the gum line, the tooth roots are anchored into the jaw by the periodontal ligament, which cushions movement and stabilizes the tooth. The gums and surrounding tissue provide a protective barrier but are prone to inflammation from trauma, poor hygiene, or systemic illness. Gum infections may mimic tooth pain, presenting with swelling, tenderness, or difficulty opening the mouth if the infection spreads.

In the field, recognizing the difference is key: pulp pain is usually sharp and triggered by temperature or chewing, while gum infections tend to produce dull, throbbing discomfort with localized swelling. Identifying the source helps guide treatment decisions—whether simple pain control and hygiene will suffice or whether urgent evacuation is needed for a progressing infection.

How should dental problems be managed in the wilderness?

Dental problems in the wilderness require both practical management and a clear understanding of when to evacuate. Begin with a focused assessment: have the patient rinse with warm water to clear debris and allow for inspection of the teeth, gums, and surrounding tissues. Look for signs of trauma, swelling, exposed dentin, or developing abscess. Pain is best managed with a combination of ibuprofen and acetaminophen, which work through different pathways to reduce inflammation and discomfort more effectively than either alone. If a tooth is chipped or fractured, the priority is to protect the exposed area. Cyanoacrylate glue, softened wax, or commercial dental materials can be used to seal the surface; in a pinch, softened chewing gum may provide a temporary barrier. Deeper fractures that expose the pulp increase infection risk and warrant antibiotics, close observation and even evacuation.

Warm salt rinses can help reduce mild swelling and support healing and should be repeated several times a day. If an abscess becomes fluctuant, an incision and drainage may relieve the pressure, followed by continued saline or diluted hydrogen peroxide rinses. However, any signs of facial swelling, fever, or systemic illness suggest a spreading infection and requires prompt evacuation.

If a permanent tooth is completely knocked out, rinse it gently with clean water—never scrub—and attempt to reinsert it into the socket within 30 minutes if possible. The socket may be rinsed as well. Once replaced, the tooth can be stabilized by splinting it to neighboring teeth using glue, wax, or a dental splint if available. If reinsertion isn't feasible, store the tooth in saline or the patient's own saliva—never dry—and evacuate promptly. Baby teeth should not be reimplanted. Persistent bleeding, uncontrolled pain, or progressive facial swelling are all red flags. Infections in the face and oral cavity can escalate quickly and become life-threatening without early intervention. Watch facial infections carefully.

What if a tooth is knocked out?

If a permanent (adult) tooth is completely avulsed, rinse it gently with clean water—do not scrub—and attempt to reinsert it into the socket as soon as possible, ideally within 30 minutes. Rinse the socket if needed. Stabilize the tooth by splinting it to adjacent teeth using cyanoacrylate glue, wax, or dental material. If reinsertion isn't possible, store the tooth in saline or in the patient's saliva-not dry—and evacuate promptly. Baby teeth should not be reimplanted.

Evacuate any patient with persistent bleeding, uncontrolled pain, visible facial swelling, or signs of systemic infection. Infections involving the face and oral cavity can spread quickly into deeper tissues and become life-threatening without timely care.

Can dental infections become life-threatening?

All infections can become life-threatening when left unmanaged. Untreated dental infections can spread beyond the tooth, leading to severe and sometimes fatal complications. Bacteria can invade surrounding soft tissues and bone, causing osteomyelitis, an infection of the jawbone, or Ludwig's angina, a rapidly progressing infection of the floor of the mouth that can invade and obstruct the airway. These conditions require immediate medical intervention.

Serious dental infections typically present with escalating pain, fever, and noticeable swelling that may spread to the side of the face or under the jaw. Any signs of deep tissue involvement, such as difficulty swallowing, voice changes, or rapidly worsening swelling, indicate that the infection is advancing. Early treatment with broad-spectrum antibiotics and, if an abscess is present, incision and drainage can help control the infection. However, if symptoms do not improve or show signs of spreading, immediate evacuation is necessary, as these patients can deteriorate quickly, particularly in remote settings where medical care is delayed.

What if I forget toothpaste?

Without toothpaste, basic oral health in the wilderness relies on managing pH and disrupting bacterial growth. *Streptococcus mutans*—the main culprit behind cavities—feeds on sugars and produces acid, which lowers mouth pH and erodes enamel. To counter this, aim to keep the mouth neutral or slightly alkaline. Brushing or rinsing with baking soda (sodium bicarbonate) is highly effective, as it neutralizes acid and provides gentle abrasion to remove plaque. Salt (sodium chloride) is mildly alkaline, and it can help reduce bacterial load, ease gum inflammation, and support short-term oral hygiene. Chewable calcium carbonate antacids also buffer acidity and may aid enamel repair. Avoiding sugar is critical, as it fuels acid-producing bacteria. Even without toothpaste, regular rinsing and mechanical cleaning—using floss, a cloth, or an improvised brush—can help prevent decay.

No Harbor for the Sick

We'd been running the outer islands of Indonesia for days, threading the mothership through reefs and jungle-covered atolls that had been untouched for millennia. After a long crossing from Sumatra, we had settled into the rhythm—early mornings, long days on the water, evenings spent trading stories under equatorial skies. Then, one morning, the ship's captain didn't show.

That wasn't like him.

We found him still in his bunk, sheets damp with sweat, skin taking on a sickly, greenish pallor that comes when the body is losing ground. His breath carried the unmistakable stench of infection. His left cheek was swollen, skin stretched tight. Just above his upper molars, a firm, painful abscess bulged against his gumline.

He tried to wave us off. Said he'd be fine. He wasn't fine.

Tom, a solid orthopedic surgeon, and me, fresh out of my general surgery training—neither of us exactly dentists, but we'd spent enough time in ERs and operating rooms to know when something needed to be cut. Teeth weren't our specialty, but we knew one thing: you don't treat an abscess with antibiotics alone. Infections like this don't just fade away. You have to let the evil humors out.

The captain wasn't thrilled, but there wasn't much choice. We gave him the choices–drain it now or let it fester and risk something worse. He gave a slow nod.

The scalpel blade bit into the tense, shining skin of the gums, directly over the most fluctuant part of the abscess. The second the skin split, thick, foul-smelling pus spilled out, pooling against his lower teeth before he leaned over the trash bin. His shoulders slackened. The pressure that had been building for days was finally gone. We had him rinse with a mix of hydrogen peroxide and water, flushing out the remaining debris until the fluid ran clear.

The source was immediately obvious—a cracked molar. The infection had invaded the tooth and worked its way into the surrounding soft tissue. It had been brewing for days, maybe longer.

We started him on broad-spectrum antibiotics and pushed fluids hard to replace what the infection had taken from him. By dinnertime, his color was back, his energy returning. Three days later, when some residual swelling returned, we reopened the site, drained what remained, and kept him on antibiotics until we hit a mainland port where he could get real dental care. Dental infections, like any infection, can become life-threatening if ignored. Left unchecked, they can spread—leading to airway compromise, deep-space infections, or sepsis.

In remote environments, where help is far away and delays are dangerous, you just may have to intervene to keep things from getting worse.

Allergic Reactions

What is an allergic reaction?

An allergic reaction occurs when the immune system misidentifies a harmless substance as a threat and overreacts. This exaggerated response can happen within minutes or take hours to develop, depending on the immune pathway involved. Immediate reactions are driven by IgE antibodies, which activate immune cells to release histamine and other chemical messengers. These cause symptoms like itching, hives, swelling, and–in severe cases–tightening of the airways and a drop in blood pressure. Delayed reactions, such as rashes from poison ivy, involve different immune pathways and develop more gradually.

Common triggers include foods (especially nuts and shellfish), insect stings, medications, and environmental allergens like pollen or animal dander. Symptoms can range from mild–like nasal congestion and itchy skin–to life-threatening, with airway swelling and circulatory collapse.

In remote settings, early recognition and prompt management are essential, as allergic reactions can progress rapidly and access to definitive care is, by definition, delayed.

How should allergic reactions be managed in the wilderness?

Even mild allergic reactions should be treated promptly, as they can escalate unpredictably. Oral antihistamines are the first line of defense. These medications block histamine receptors—specifically the H1 receptors found in skin, blood vessels, and mucous membranes—to reduce symptoms like itching, swelling, and hives. Newer agents like loratadine or cetirizine cause less drowsiness than older options like diphenhydramine and still control symptoms effectively. Adding an H2 blocker, such as famotidine, can provide additional relief by targeting histamine receptors in the stomach and skin, dampening the overall response.

If wheezing or respiratory symptoms appear, albuterol can be used to relax the smooth muscle surrounding the airways, improving airflow and reducing shortness of breath. Corticosteroids like prednisone help suppress the broader immune response by interfering with inflammatory signaling pathways. While they don't act immediately, they're valuable for preventing symptom rebound or progression hours later.

Any signs of airway involvement, low blood pressure, or altered consciousness require immediate evacuation. In the wilderness, close monitoring is essential—even mild reactions can become dangerous without warning.

What is anaphylaxis, and why is it so dangerous?

Anaphylaxis is a severe, systemic allergic reaction that can become life-threatening within minutes. It begins when someone who's been sensitized to a specific allergen—like insect venom, food proteins, or medications—is re-exposed. The immune system misidentifies the substance as dangerous and launches an exaggerated, body-wide response.

The reaction is driven by powerful chemical mediators released from immune cells found in the skin, lungs, and gastrointestinal tract, as well as others circulating in the bloodstream. These mediators cause blood vessels to dilate and leak, smooth muscles to constrict, and secretions to increase—all of which can lead to airway swelling, low blood pressure, hives, nausea, and difficulty breathing.

Together, these mediators explain why anaphylaxis affects so many systems at once. You get airway swelling, wheezing, and low oxygen from bronchial constriction; dizziness and shock from falling blood pressure; nausea and vomiting from intestinal muscle contraction. The body is flooded with immune signals meant to fight danger, but they're now going overboard and threatening survival.

This is why early recognition matters. Anaphylaxis isn't a slow, progressive allergic reaction—it's a sudden immune cascade that spirals quickly if untreated.

How does epinephrine work for anaphylaxis?

Epinephrine is the first-line treatment for anaphylaxis because it directly counteracts the life-threatening effects of a severe allergic reaction. It works by stimulating both alpha- and beta-adrenergic receptors in the body. Activation of *alpha* receptors causes blood vessels to constrict, which raises dangerously low blood pressure and helps reduce swelling. Stimulation of *beta* receptors relaxes the smooth muscles lining the airways, easing breathing, and also helps the heart beat more effectively to maintain circulation. These combined effects help stabilize the patient quickly. Epinephrine must be injected, as it breaks down too quickly to be useful if taken by mouth. Auto-injectors like EpiPen, Jext, or Anapen deliver the medication into the thigh muscle, allowing for rapid absorption. Because symptoms can return as the drug wears off, a second dose may be needed. In wilderness or remote settings, it's critical to carry at least two auto-injectors and to use the first one without delay as early treatment significantly improves outcomes.

Who is at risk for severe allergic reactions?

Individuals with a history of anaphylaxis are at the highest risk for recurrence. Those with asthma; a strong family history of severe allergies; or frequent exposure to high-risk allergens, such as insect venom, certain foods, or medications, are particularly vulnerable. These individuals should always carry an epinephrine auto-injector and know how to use it properly.

What are the key takeaways for guides?

Recognizing allergic reactions early and responding quickly can mean the difference between life and death. Epinephrine should be administered at the first sign of anaphylaxis. Delays can be fatal. Antihistamines and corticosteroids may help control symptoms but should never replace epinephrine when anaphylaxis is suspected.

Prevention starts with education. Clients should be aware of allergen avoidance strategies, carry their prescribed medications, and know how to use an epinephrine auto-injector. Guides should never hesitate to administer epinephrine if anaphylaxis is suspected, as waiting too long increases the risk of severe complications. In any suspected case, it is safer to treat early than to risk a fatal delay.

The Guts

What should a guide understand about abdominal pain?

Abdominal pain is one of the most complex complaints in wilderness medicine. The abdomen houses multiple organs, each with distinct functions, and an unfortunate tendency for their symptoms to overlap. Some causes are minor. Others are life-threatening. Guides don't need to pinpoint the exact source, but a basic understanding of anatomy helps recognize patterns and make informed decisions about monitoring in the field versus evacuation. Pain may be sharp or vague, intermittent or progressive. Some conditions improve with rest or hydration. Others, like internal bleeding or bowel obstruction, require more urgent evacuation. Knowing which organs lie beneath the pain adds context and supports better decision-making in the field.

Abdominal Pain: Surface Location & Likely Source

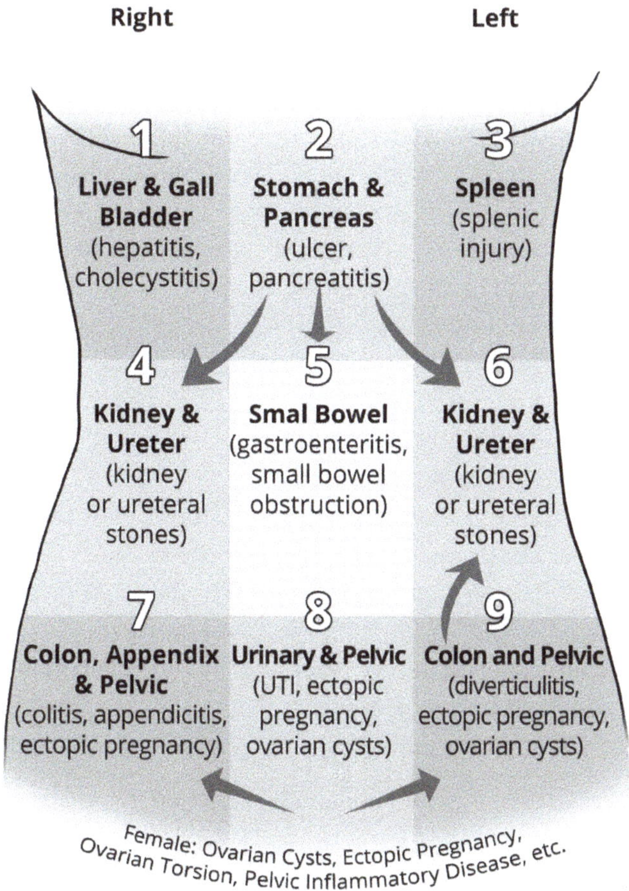

What does the stomach do, and how can it cause pain?

The stomach is a muscular sac that uses acid and digestive enzymes to break down food. It churns food into a semiliquid mixture called chyme, which then moves into the small intestine. The stomach lining is protected by mucus, bicarbonate, and other natural defenses that prevent the acid from damaging its tissue. When these defenses are weakened by stress, alcohol, NSAIDs, or infection with *Helicobacter pylori*, ulcers can form. Ulcers cause burning or gnawing pain, often worse on an empty stomach or after acidic foods. If an ulcer erodes into a blood vessel, it can cause significant bleeding. If it perforates the stomach wall, it becomes a surgical emergency.

What's the difference between the small and large intestine?

The small intestine continues digestion after food leaves the stomach. It receives partially digested material mixed with bile from the liver and enzymes from the pancreas. This is where most nutrient absorption occurs. The small intestine runs through much of the central abdomen and moves contents forward to the colon using wave-like contractions. Pain from the small bowel is usually crampy and diffuse.

A small bowel obstruction occurs when part of the intestine is physically blocked by scar tissue, a hernia, or twisting itself (volvulus). It's similar to a garden hose with a kink: Pressure builds behind the blockage while nothing moves forward. This leads to bloating, pain, nausea, vomiting, and the absence of bowel movements or gas. If the blockage is complete and prolonged, pressure can compromise the blood supply to the bowel wall and cause bowel-wall injury including perforation.

The large intestine, or colon, absorbs water and forms stool. It moves slowly and runs along the outer edges of the abdomen. Pain from the colon often comes in waves and may be associated with constipation, bloating, or changes in stool pattern. One common condition is diverticulitis, an inflammation and infection of small outpouchings in the colon wall called diverticula. These pockets can trap stool, leading to infection, localized pain—most often in the left lower quadrant—along with fever and tenderness. Without antibiotics, diverticulitis can worsen and even lead to perforation of the colon, which, again, is a surgical emergency.

What are the functions of the liver and gallbladder?

The liver, located in the upper right abdomen, is one of the body's most vital organs. It filters toxins from the blood, metabolizes drugs and alcohol, stores glucose in the form of glycogen, produces proteins needed for blood clotting, and generates bile to help digest fats. It also plays a role in hormone regulation and immune function. The gallbladder, a small sac tucked beneath the liver, stores and concentrates bile, releasing it into the small intestine after meals—especially those high in fat—to aid digestion.

When bile flow is blocked—typically by gallstones—pressure builds in the gallbladder, triggering sharp, cramping pain under the right ribs, often after eating fatty food. This is known as biliary colic. If the blockage persists, inflammation and bacterial infection can follow, resulting in cholecystitis. In severe cases, this may lead to perforation, abscess, or systemic infection requiring urgent evacuation. The liver itself can also be affected by disease processes, including viral hepatitis, alcohol damage, or drug toxicity—all of which can impair its ability to clear toxins and regulate metabolism.

What does the pancreas do, and why does it matter?

The pancreas sits deep in the upper abdomen, behind the stomach. It serves two key functions: It produces digestive enzymes that help break down food in the small intestine, and it regulates blood sugar by releasing insulin and glucagon. Because of its location and function, inflammation or injury to the pancreas can affect both digestion and metabolic stability.

Pancreatitis—an inflammation of the pancreas—can be triggered by heavy alcohol use, gallstones, certain medications, or trauma. It causes deep, constant pain in the upper abdomen, often radiating to the back, and may be accompanied by nausea, vomiting, or signs of shock in severe cases. In the wilderness setting, pancreatitis should be considered in anyone with persistent upper abdominal pain and no clear explanation, especially if they've consumed alcohol. Suspected cases require evacuation as there is no field treatment beyond hydration and supportive care.

What does the spleen do, and why is it important?

The spleen, tucked under the left ribs, filters blood, removes old or damaged red blood cells, and plays a critical role in immune defense by producing and storing white blood cells. It contains a dense network of blood vessels and lymphoid tissue, making it both highly vascular and immunologically active. The spleen also helps fight certain bacteria, particularly encapsulated organisms like *Streptococcus pneumoniae*, *Haemophilus influenzae*, and *Neisseria meningitidis*.

Although it's not a common source of abdominal pain on its own, the spleen is vulnerable to rupture from blunt trauma, such as a fall or impact to the left side. A ruptured spleen can cause life-threatening internal bleeding, often with referred pain to the left shoulder (Kehr's sign). Any left upper quadrant pain following trauma must be taken seriously and monitored closely, even if the injury seems minor at first.

What does the appendix do?

Truthfully, no one *really* knows. The appendix is a small, finger-like pouch off the colon in the lower right abdomen. It may help maintain healthy gut bacteria or serve an immunologic function, but its exact role remains unclear. What is clear is that when the appendix becomes blocked—typically by stool or, less commonly, by a tumor—it can become inflamed, leading to appendicitis.

Pain often starts near the belly button and shifts to the lower right side, progressively worsening. It may be accompanied by nausea, loss of appetite, or low-grade fever. A ruptured appendix can lead to widespread infection and is a life-threatening emergency requiring surgery. In the field, worsening abdominal pain with guarding or rebound in the lower right quadrant should raise immediate concern, antibiotics, and evacuation.

What does the bladder do, and how can it cause pain?

The bladder collects and stores urine, expanding as it fills and sending signals to the brain once it reaches around 250-300 mL. It sits low in the pelvis, just behind the pubic bone, and receives urine from the kidneys through two narrow tubes called ureters. When the bladder becomes irritated or inflamed—such as during a urinary tract infection—it can cause suprapubic pain, pressure, and symptoms like burning, urgency, or frequent urination. In older adults, retention becomes more common due to weaker bladder muscles, outlet obstruction (like from prostate enlargement), or certain medications, especially antihistamines, decongestants, and anticholinergics like diphenhydramine (Benadryl). This can lead to a chronically overfilled bladder, vague lower abdominal discomfort, and the sense of incomplete emptying. In the field, the presence of a firm, distended bladder or the inability to urinate despite discomfort should raise concern. If basic measures fail and drainage isn't possible, immediate evacuation is warranted.

What is a hernia, and is it dangerous?

A hernia occurs when part of the intestine or abdominal tissue pushes through a weak spot in the abdominal wall—commonly in the groin, around the navel, or near a surgical scar. It may present as a bulge that becomes more noticeable with coughing, straining, or lifting. Early signs include a sense of pressure, dull aching, or localized discomfort.

If the hernia is soft, painless, and easily reducible—meaning it can be gently pushed back in—it can typically be monitored in the field. But if it becomes firm, tender, irreducible, or the overlying skin turns red, dusky, or inflamed, it may be incarcerated (trapped) or strangulated (trapped with compromised blood flow). Strangulation can quickly lead to tissue death, bowel perforation, and sepsis. Persistent or worsening pain—especially in a hernia that was previously reducible—is a big red flag. In such cases, antibiotics should be given, and immediate evacuation is essential.

What is ovarian torsion, and how does it present?

Ovarian torsion occurs when the ovary twists around the ligaments and blood vessels that support it, cutting off its blood supply. This leads to sudden, severe lower abdominal pain, usually on one side (unilateral). The pain is often sharp and constant, and may be accompanied by nausea, vomiting, or a feeling of lightheadedness. It can occur with or without a known ovarian cyst, though a history of previous cysts and enlarged ovaries increase the risk. In the field, this diagnosis is difficult to confirm without imaging, but any sudden, unexplained lower abdominal pain in someone with ovaries should be taken seriously. If torsion is suspected, urgent evacuation is required, as delays in treatment can lead to loss of the ovary and permanent reproductive damage.

What is constipation, and how do I manage it in the wilderness?

Constipation, defined as infrequent or difficult bowel movements, is a common issue in the field. Dehydration reduces the water available in the colon, causing stool to become hard and dry. A low-fiber diet means less bulk to stimulate intestinal movement. Disrupted routines—such as changes in sleeping, eating, or bathroom timing—interfere with the body's natural rhythm. And stress shifts the nervous system into "fight or flight" mode, slowing digestion and reducing bowel motility. The result is delayed transit, harder stool, and increased straining.

Hydration, movement, and fiber-rich foods are key for prevention. Fruits like prunes, pears, and apricots are especially useful in the field because they combine insoluble fiber, which adds bulk, with sorbitol, a natural sugar alcohol that draws water into the bowel. Juices made from these fruits have a similar effect. Magnesium-based laxatives, such as milk of magnesia, work by the same principle—pulling water into the intestines to soften stool. Warm fluids like coffee may also help stimulate bowel activity.

If the patient is passing gas and appears otherwise stable, conservative measures are appropriate. But increasing pain, bloating, or the *absence* of gas suggests a more serious problem and warrants evacuation for further evaluation.

What causes nausea and vomiting in the wilderness, and what do I need to know?

First off, nausea and vomiting are *symptoms*, not diagnoses per se; and they can result from a wide range of physiological disturbances. Understanding the mechanism helps guide field assessment. Vomiting is coordinated by a region in the brainstem that receives signals from multiple sources: the digestive tract, the inner ear (which senses motion and balance), the cerebral cortex, and the chemoreceptor trigger zone (CTZ, a specialized area that detects toxins in the blood). This explains why vomiting can be triggered by everything from infection and injury to motion sickness or chemical exposures.

- *Head injury* can trigger vomiting through increased intracranial pressure or direct irritation of the brain's vomiting center. Blunt trauma—especially to the occiput—can cause nausea, vomiting, and altered mental status. In children, vomiting may be an early red flag in head trauma. In the wilderness, any vomiting associated with confusion, severe headache, or unsteady gait after a fall or impact should raise concern for brain injury, and prompt evacuation is warranted.
- *Small bowel obstruction* leads to a mechanical backup of intestinal contents. The stomach and small intestine continue to secrete fluid and digest food, but nothing moves downstream. Stretching of the intestinal wall and chemical signals from the gut stimulate the

vomiting reflex. Pain is typically crampy and episodic, often accompanied by abdominal distension and the absence of normal bowel movements. Vomiting tends to be bilious (green or yellow) and becomes feculent (smells like feces) in later stages. Bowel obstruction requires urgent evacuation.

- *Gastroenteritis*—inflammation of the GI tract from viral, bacterial, or parasitic infection—is one of the most common causes of nausea and vomiting in the field. Pathogens irritate the lining of the stomach and intestine, triggering both the CTZ and the gut-brain axis. Symptoms include vomiting, diarrhea, fever, and abdominal cramping. Though self-limited in most (not all) cases, dehydration is a major concern, especially in hot or remote environments. Oral rehydration, rest, and electrolyte replacement are key. If vomiting persists beyond 24 hours, or if the patient cannot keep fluids down, evacuation should be considered.
- *Severe constipation* (obstipation)—particularly in older adults or those on medications like opioids—can also cause nausea and vomiting. When the colon is severely backed up, pressure builds throughout the GI tract, and the stomach begins to empty in reverse. Vomiting may be preceded by bloating and a prolonged absence of bowel movements. This diagnosis can be missed if stool is still present in small amounts. Rehydration, movement, and gentle abdominal massage may help. If there's no improvement or if pain increases, the patient should be evacuated.
- *Seasickness* is a form of motion sickness caused by a mismatch between what the eyes see and what the inner ear detects. When the body senses motion through the vestibular system but the eyes don't confirm it—like on a rocking boat—the brain interprets it as a possible poisoning event and triggers the vomiting reflex. Symptoms include nausea, yawning, pallor, and cold sweat, often followed by vomiting. Seasickness is more likely when dehydrated, hungry, or overtired. It can be

managed with acupressure (notably on the P6 (Neiguan) point, located centrally, three finger-widths below the wrist crease on the inner forearm), ginger, hydration, and fresh air. Keeping the eyes fixed on the horizon can reduce sensory mismatch. Pharmacologic options like scopolamine or antihistamines (e.g., meclizine) may help but can cause drowsiness.

Nausea and vomiting should always be evaluated using a structured approach like OPQRST (Onset, Provocation, Quality, Region/Radiation, Severity, and Time) and a focused physical exam. Non-pharmacologic management includes placing a cool rag on the back of the neck or forehead, elevating the head and torso, applying pressure to the P6 acupressure point (remember this one), using shaded environments, avoiding strong odors, and encouraging slow sips of electrolyte-rich fluids. Keep in mind that nausea is not just a nuisance; it may be the first sign of a serious medical condition. In the field, assess for red flags: persistent vomiting, signs of dehydration (dry mucous membranes, sunken eyes, low urine output), altered mental status, abdominal rigidity, fever, or recent head trauma.

Evacuation is indicated for any suspected bowel obstruction, head injury, ongoing vomiting despite care, or inability to tolerate fluids.

What is an anal fissure?

An anal fissure is a small tear in the thin lining of the anal canal, usually caused by passing hard stool or repeated straining. Less commonly, it can result from prolonged diarrhea, which softens and inflames the tissue, making it more prone to tearing. The injury exposes the sensitive underlying layer (the anoderm), which is rich in nerve endings—causing sharp, cutting pain during or after bowel movements. In response, the internal anal sphincter—a ring of muscle that helps control bowel continence—often spasms. This muscle spasm restricts blood flow to the area, slows healing, and can trap the fissure in a cycle of pain and delayed recovery. Bleeding is usually minimal, often seen as bright red streaks on toilet paper or the stool surface.

In the field, the priority is softening the stool to avoid further trauma. The individual should avoid straining and clean the area gently using baby wipes or a clean, damp cloth—dry wiping can worsen the tear. Applying zinc oxide or a topical antibiotic ointment may reduce friction and promote healing. If available, topical lidocaine can help with pain, and nonsteroidal anti-inflammatory drugs (NSAIDs) may ease discomfort and reduce the internal sphincter spasm. Most anal fissures will heal within a few days if the stool remains soft and the area is kept clean.

What are hemorrhoids?

Hemorrhoids are swollen veins in the lower rectum or around the anus. They're grouped into two types based on location. Internal hemorrhoids form deeper inside the rectum, where there are fewer pain nerves—so they may bleed but usually don't hurt. External hemorrhoids form closer to the skin, where nerve endings are dense. These can become painful, especially if a blood clot forms inside (a thrombosed hemorrhoid), causing a firm, tender, often purple lump near the anal opening.

In the wilderness, several common factors contribute: dehydration, constipation, straining during bowel movements, and prolonged sitting—especially on hard, hot, or vibrating surfaces like saddles, rafts, or vehicle benches. These conditions increase pressure on the veins around the anus, leading to swelling and irritation.

Field care focuses on reducing pressure, easing pain, and keeping the area clean. Hydration is key to softening stool. NSAIDs help reduce swelling and pain. Cold compresses (ice, wet cloth, or a cool stream) can offer relief. Barrier creams like zinc oxide may help reduce friction. After bowel movements, gently clean with wipes or water instead of dry toilet paper.

If a thrombosed external hemorrhoid becomes so painful it limits walking or sitting, lancing may be considered—but only if you have sterile tools, basic wound care supplies, and the training to do it safely. The best time is 48–72 hours after it appears, when the clot is close to the surface and the skin is stretched thin.

Without the ability to irrigate, monitor, or manage bleeding, evacuation may still be the better call; but if the pain prohibits function or movement, you may have little choice.

What is a perianal abscess?

A perianal abscess is a localized bacterial infection near the anus, usually caused by bacteria entering through hair follicles, sweat glands, or minor abrasions. In wilderness settings, it's often the result of prolonged pressure, friction, and sweat—common in rafters, horseback riders, and anyone sitting for long periods in heat and grit. Saddle sores and raft rash frequently precede abscess formation. The infection develops into a painful, swollen, red mass that worsens over 24–72 hours. Pain increases with sitting, walking, or bowel movements. Fever may indicate systemic involvement.

Once the abscess becomes fluctuant, incision and drainage (I&D) is the appropriate treatment. Without drainage, the pain becomes disabling, the guest cannot continue participating in the trip, and the infection may progress to cellulitis or sepsis. Using sterile technique, make a controlled incision at the point of maximal fluctuance, express the pus, and irrigate the cavity with clean (treated or boiled) water. After drainage, the wound should be lightly packed with clean gauze or fabric to prevent the skin from closing prematurely and trapping residual infection. Packing material should be changed daily and the site kept open, clean, and as dry as possible.

Apply antibiotic ointment around the wound margin if available. Loosely cover the area with clean, breathable material to reduce contamination and friction. Avoid occlusive dressings or tight clothing. Wound care must be ongoing—monitor for signs of spreading infection, fever, or worsening symptoms. If any of these develop, or if proper care can't be continued, the guest should be evacuated.

What is diarrhea, and what are the basic principles of field management?

Diarrhea is defined as the passage of three or more loose or watery stools in a 24-hour period. It results from increased water content in the stool, often due to impaired absorption, increased secretion, or rapid transit through the intestines. In the wilderness, infections—viral, bacterial, or parasitic—are the most important causes to consider. While factors like contaminated food or water, sudden dietary changes, and stress can all contribute, the priority—in the wilderness setting—is identifying and managing infectious causes.

Treatment begins with aggressive oral hydration. Water alone is inadequate. Electrolytes and glucose are needed to facilitate fluid absorption in the small intestine. A simple oral rehydration solution (ORS) can be prepared with 1 liter of clean water, 1/2 teaspoon of salt, and 6 teaspoons of sugar. Commercial ORS packets or diluted fruit juices can also be used.

Avoid high-fat foods, dairy, and caffeine, which can worsen symptoms. If diarrhea is mild and the patient is otherwise well, they can continue activity with close monitoring. Evacuation is indicated for diarrhea when there is persistent fever, bloody stools, severe dehydration, worsening abdominal pain, or no improvement after 72 hours of supportive care.

How big of a problem is diarrhea, really?

Diarrhea remains one of the most common illnesses worldwide, responsible for an estimated 1.6 million deaths annually, primarily in children under five and individuals in low-resource settings. Globally, billions of cases occur each year, leading to significant morbidity, lost productivity, and medical complications—even in otherwise healthy adults. Because of its frequency, potential severity, and near-universal occurrence in remote and travel settings, diarrhea warrants focused attention in this book.

When should antibiotics be given for diarrhea?

Antibiotics are indicated when diarrhea is accompanied by systemic symptoms such as fever, bloody stools, abdominal pain, or worsening dehydration. In these situations, a bacterial infection is likely, and the benefits of treatment outweigh the risks. Azithromycin or ciprofloxacin are preferred first-line agents in most regions. If symptoms persist beyond 48 to 72 hours or systemic illness is evident, antibiotics should be started.

However, caution is warranted when there is bloody diarrhea and severe cramping *without* fever—especially in children. This pattern may signal infection with Shiga toxin-producing *E. coli* (e.g., *E. coli* O157:H7), where antibiotics can increase the risk of hemolytic uremic syndrome (HUS), a serious complication that can lead to kidney failure. In such cases, focus on hydration and arrange evacuation for monitoring and further care.

Even when the exact cause is unknown, field management should emphasize hydration, reserve antibiotics for appropriate cases, and recognize red flags that require evacuation.

Are there over-the-counter (OTC) medications to manage traveler's diarrhea?

There are. Pepto-Bismol (bismuth subsalicylate), also sold internationally under names like *Bismuth Subsalicylate Suspension* or *Gastro-Bismol* (Central/South America), *Gastro-Stop Plus* (Australia), and *Pepti-Calm* (parts of Africa and Europe), is an over-the-counter option that may help prevent traveler's diarrhea by coating the stomach lining, reducing inflammation, and exerting mild antibacterial effects. *Imodium* (loperamide hydrochloride), known in some regions as *Dimor*, *Fortasec*, or *Lopedium*, slows gut motility to reduce stool frequency and urgency. While both can be helpful in the short term, each has precautions: bismuth subsalicylate should be avoided in those with aspirin allergies, bleeding risks, or in children recovering from viral illness. Loperamide should not be used with fever or bloody stools, as it can trap harmful organisms and worsen illness. In higher-risk situations, especially in areas with poor sanitation, a healthcare provider may recommend prophylactic antibiotics such as azithromycin or ciprofloxacin. A pre-travel consultation is advised to tailor prevention strategies safely.

What's dysentery?

Dysentery is a more severe form of diarrhea marked by the presence of blood and/or mucus in the stool. It usually reflects invasive infection of the intestinal lining, most commonly from *Shigella*, *Entamoeba histolytica*, or certain toxin-producing strains of *E. coli*. Dysentery is often associated with fever, abdominal pain, and tenesmus—the sensation of needing to pass stool despite an empty rectum. While many cases of diarrhea resolve without intervention, dysentery carries a higher risk of dehydration, systemic illness, and complications. In wilderness or remote travel settings, recognizing the distinction is critical, as dysentery often requires antibiotics and may even warrant evacuation.

How do I prevent diarrhea while traveling or guiding in remote areas?

Preventing diarrhea in remote environments begins with strict attention to food and water hygiene. Water should always be boiled, bottled, filtered, or chemically treated before consumption. Ice should be avoided unless it is known to be made from safe, clean water—even rainwater works. Meals should be freshly cooked and served hot. Raw milk products and uncooked foods carry a higher risk and should be avoided. Fruits and vegetables should be peeled, and salads or other raw preparations should be considered high-risk due to potential microbial contamination.

Frequent handwashing with soap and water remains the most effective way to reduce transmission, particularly after bathroom use or contact with animals. While alcohol-based hand sanitizers may serve as a backup, they are less effective and should not be relied on as a substitute for proper hygiene.

By adhering to these practices, guides can reduce the risk of diarrheal illness and protect both themselves and their clients during remote expeditions.

Does drinking Coca-Cola prevent food poisoning?

No. While Coca-Cola contains phosphoric and carbonic acids that may have mild antibacterial properties, it is not nearly strong enough to neutralize harmful microbes in contaminated food or water. At best, it might slightly reduce bacterial activity in the stomach, not prevent infection or illness. Preventing foodborne disease depends on proper food handling, strict hygiene, and consuming only safe, treated water. Coca-Cola is not a substitute for any of these measures.

Red Flag Framework: Gastrointestinal Emergencies

What's an easy way to remember what signs and symptoms warrant evacuation using the Red Flag Framework?

For the gastrointestinal system: **GUTS**

- **G**eneralized or localized abdominal pain lasting more than six hours.
- **U**nable to pass stool or gas with associated pain (possible bowel obstruction)
- **T**hrowing up (persistently)
- **S**ignificant abdominal firmness or distention (possible internal injury or obstruction)

Any of these signs indicate a potentially serious condition, requiring immediate evaluation and possible evacuation. When in doubt, follow the Red Flag Framework: GUTS = Evacuate.

Chest Pain in the Wilderness

What should guides know about chest pain?

Chest pain should always be taken seriously, especially in remote environments. This section provides a general approach to thinking through chest pain in the field; more detailed explanations of specific conditions follow later in the book. The goal isn't to make the perfect diagnosis—it's to recognize when the pain might be dangerous and decide whether evacuation is needed.

Start with the basics:

- When did the pain begin?
- Where exactly is it located?
- What does it feel like—sharp, dull, burning, tight?
- Does it spread to the arm, jaw, neck, or back?
- What makes it better or worse?
- Has the patient ever had this pain before?

Also look for red flags like shortness of breath, sweating, lightheadedness, gray or pale skin, cough, fever, or weakness. These can help narrow down the possible causes and signal life-threatening illness.

Most chest pain falls into four main categories: musculoskeletal, pulmonary, cardiovascular, and gastrointestinal.

Musculoskeletal pain comes from the chest wall—muscles, bones, or joints. It's usually sharp, reproducible with movement or touch, and doesn't cause fever or shortness of breath. It often follows a fall, heavy lifting, or overuse. The pain arises from inflammation or irritation of local structures like the costochondral joints (where ribs meet cartilage). If the patient is otherwise stable, treat with rest, NSAIDs (nonsteroidal anti-inflammatory drugs), and warm compresses.

Pulmonary causes include pneumonia, pneumothorax, and pulmonary embolism.

- *Pneumonia* is a lung infection that causes inflammation and fluid buildup. This irritates the pleura—the thin lining around the lungs—leading to sharp pain that worsens with deep breaths (pleuritic pain), plus fever, chills, cough, and fatigue. Start antibiotics if available and evacuate if symptoms worsen.
- *Pneumothorax* occurs when air leaks into the space between the lung and chest wall (the pleural space), causing lung collapse. It often follows trauma but can also happen spontaneously in tall, thin individuals or those with lung disease. Symptoms include sudden one-sided chest pain and trouble breathing. Breath sounds may be reduced on the affected side. If air pressure builds and begins to compress the heart and lungs (tension pneumothorax), this is life-threatening and may require emergency needle decompression.
- *Pulmonary embolism* is a clot in the lung's blood vessels. It disrupts oxygen exchange and strains the heart. Look for sudden pain, shortness of breath, fast heart rate, and sometimes coughing blood. Risk goes up after long travel, surgery, immobility, or in people with clotting disorders. Immediate evacuation is required.

Cardiovascular causes can be the most dangerous.

- *Myocardial infarction* (heart attack) occurs when blood flow to part of the heart is blocked, causing tissue damage. Pain is often described as pressure or tightness in the center of the chest that may radiate to the jaw, arm, or back. Other signs include sweating, nausea, anxiety, and difficulty breathing. Not all people have classic symptoms—older adults, women, and people with diabetes may present with vague complaints. If suspected, keep the person at rest, give 160–325 mg of chewable aspirin, and assist with prescribed nitroglycerin if available. Evacuate immediately.
- *Angina* is similar but temporary. It reflects reduced blood flow to the heart and typically goes away with

rest in under 15 minutes. If it's new, worsening, or unrelieved, treat it like a heart attack.

- *Aortic rupture* is rare but catastrophic. It happens when the wall of the aorta (the body's main artery) tears, often from a failed aneurysm. Pain is sudden, severe, and tearing—usually in the chest or abdomen and radiating to the back. Shock follows quickly. Survival without immediate surgical care is extremely unlikely.

Gastrointestinal causes such as acid reflux, esophageal spasms, or ulcers can mimic heart pain due to overlapping nerve pathways.

- *Gastroesophageal reflux disease (GERD)* causes a burning feeling behind the breastbone, often after meals or when lying down.
- *Esophageal spasms* may feel like tightness or pressure and can improve with swallowing.
- *Peptic ulcers* can cause upper abdominal pain that radiates toward the chest, especially when the stomach is empty. These diagnoses are made only after serious cardiopulmonary causes are ruled out.

Chest pain in the wilderness demands a high index of suspicion. Supportive care, limiting exertion, and early recognition of red flags are critical. When in doubt, consider the most dangerous possibility and evacuate early.

What are palpitations?

Palpitations are the sensation of an unusually fast, strong, or irregular heartbeat. They are common and can be triggered by stress, dehydration, electrolyte imbalances, excessive alcohol or caffeine intake, or exertion. While often benign, palpitations can also indicate serious heart conditions, particularly in individuals with a history of cardiac disease or arrhythmias such as atrial fibrillation, which increases the risk of stroke. Persistent or worsening palpitations—especially when accompanied by dizziness, chest pain, or shortness of breath—warrant medical evaluation and even evacuation from a remote setting.

Can alcohol cause palpitations?

Excessive alcohol consumption, particularly binge drinking, can trigger "holiday heart syndrome," a condition where alcohol irritates the heart's electrical system, leading to abnormal heart rhythms, most commonly atrial fibrillation. This is especially concerning for individuals without preexisting heart conditions who suddenly experience palpitations after heavy drinking.

Alcohol also depletes electrolytes such as magnesium and potassium, both of which are essential for normal heart function. Dehydration, fluctuations in blood sugar, and increased epinephrine levels further contribute to palpitations. These effects can occur even after moderate drinking in susceptible individuals, making alcohol a common but often overlooked trigger for heart rhythm disturbances.

How can palpitations be managed in the wilderness?

Managing palpitations in the wilderness is challenging, as there are no diagnostic tools to determine whether the cause is benign or dangerous. The priority is rest and rehydration with electrolyte replacement, especially if dehydration, alcohol, or exertion are suspected triggers. Identifying and avoiding exacerbating factors such as caffeine, nicotine, alcohol, or missed medications is also crucial.

For stable-appearing individuals, vagal maneuvers (stimulating the vagus nerve) may help slow certain rapid heart rhythms. This includes the Valsalva maneuver (bearing down as if having a bowel movement) and cold-water facial immersion (splashing cold water on the face to trigger the mammalian dive reflex). These maneuvers should not delay evacuation if symptoms persist or worsen.

If palpitations persist; worsen; or are accompanied by chest pain, dizziness, or shortness of breath or if the individual has a history of heart disease or arrhythmias, emergent evacuation is necessary. In the wilderness, the inability to monitor heart rhythms means that erring on the side of caution is always going to be the best approach.

What is a panic attack, and how is it managed?

A panic attack is a sudden episode of intense fear or discomfort that triggers severe physical reactions without an apparent cause. Symptoms often include a racing heartbeat, shortness of breath, dizziness, trembling, and muscle tension. These episodes can be particularly challenging in wilderness settings, where immediate medical assistance may not be available. Recognizing that an individual is experiencing a panic attack is crucial, as it allows for proper management and prevents unnecessary escalation.

Encouraging slow, controlled breathing is a key intervention. During panic or acute stress, rapid breathing—hyperventilation—lowers carbon dioxide levels in the blood. This shift raises the blood pH, triggering symptoms like tingling in the lips and fingertips, dizziness, and lightheadedness. Slowing the breath helps restore CO_2 balance and calms these sensations.

Grounding techniques also help interrupt the panic loop—focusing on nearby objects, light movement, or simple tasks can shift attention away from fear and restore a sense of control.

Minimizing sensory overload by guiding the individual to a quieter environment can also help them regain that critical calm. If symptoms persist, worsen, or mimic a medical emergency such as a heart attack, evacuation may be necessary to rule out serious conditions. While panic attacks can usually be managed in the field with supportive care, their impact on decision-making and group safety should be considered when determining whether continued travel is appropriate.

Red Flag Framework: Cardiovascular Emergencies

What's an easy way to remember what signs and symptoms warrant evacuation using the Red Flag Framework?

The Red Flag Framework for Cardiovascular Emergencies is **PULSE**:

- **P**ersistent chest pain lasting more than 10 minutes, especially if it radiates to the neck, arm, or jaw.
- **U**nusual heart rhythm, including irregular, too fast, or too slow heartbeats.
- **L**ightheadedness or dizziness associated with chest pain.
- **S**hortness of breath at rest, unrelated to exertion.
- **E**pisodes of nausea and/or vomiting with chest pain.

Any of these signs indicate a potentially serious condition, requiring immediate evaluation and possible evacuation. When in doubt, follow the Red Flag Framework: PULSE = Evacuae.

Eye, Ear, Nose, & Throat Emergencies

Why is an understanding of eye emergencies important for wilderness guides?

Eye emergencies are often underestimated and can escalate rapidly, leading to permanent vision loss if improperly managed. Wilderness environments expose individuals to dust, debris, strong UV light, chemical irritants, and high-impact activities, all of which increase the risk of eye injuries.

Studies show that eye trauma accounts for a significant portion of wilderness-related injuries requiring evacuation, with chemical burns, corneal abrasions, and blunt trauma being among the more common causes. For guides, recognizing the severity of eye injuries, applying proper management techniques, and making timely evacuation decisions is critical—not only for the good of the patient, but also for mitigating legal exposure. Permanent vision impairment can lead to significant liability for guides or outfitters, especially if injuries are mishandled or underappreciated in the field.

In an environment where access to specialized care is limited, early recognition, proper management, and knowing when to evacuate are critical skills—especially when it comes to the eye.

What is the basic eye anatomy?

The eye is a specialized organ that detects light, forms images, and supports spatial awareness—key for our survival as a species. Because so many of its parts are exposed or delicate, it helps to understand the basic anatomy, especially in remote settings where even small injuries can affect mobility and decision-making.

The cornea is the clear, curved front surface of the eye. It provides most of the eye's focusing power by bending incoming light toward the back of the eye. Despite its thinness, it's packed with nerve endings, making it highly sensitive to scratches, foreign bodies, and ultraviolet (UV) damage—common risks in wilderness settings.

Just behind the cornea is the iris—the colored part of the eye. It's a circular muscle that expands or contracts to adjust the size of the pupil, controlling how much light enters the eye. In bright conditions, the pupil constricts; in darkness, it dilates.

Behind the pupil is the lens, which fine-tunes focus so that we can see both near and far. Together, the cornea and lens direct light to the retina, a thin, light-sensitive layer at the back of the eye.

The retina functions like film in a camera. It contains photoreceptor cells that convert light into electrical signals, which travel through the optic nerve to the brain, allowing us to "see". If the retina is damaged—from trauma, detachment, or impaired blood flow—vision can be permanently lost.

The sclera (the white of the eye) provides structural support, while the conjunctiva—a thin membrane lining the eyelids and covering the sclera—is prone to irritation from dust, pollen, or contaminated water.

Several glands help keep the eye moist and protected. The lacrimal gland produces tears to flush debris and prevent infection while the meibomian glands, located in the eyelids, secrete oils that stabilize the tear film. Blocked or irritated glands can lead to dryness, inflammation, and discomfort—all of which impair vision.

This finely tuned system supports vision, depth perception, and situational awareness—functions that are vital not just for survival in the backcountry, but for perceiving and navigating the world around us.

Surface Anatomy of the Eye

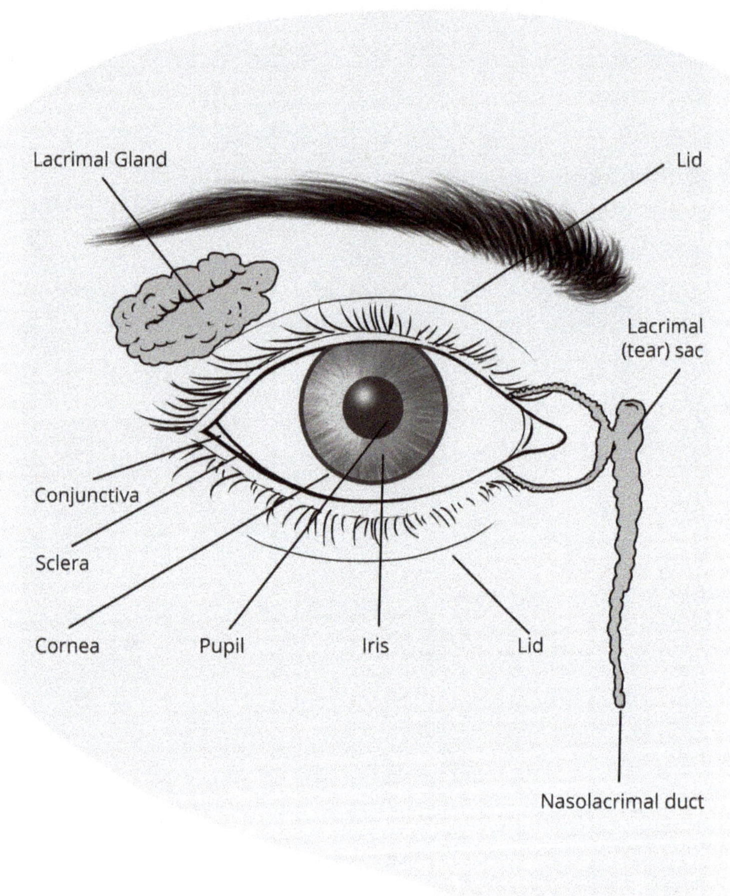

Is blood in the eye an emergency?

It depends. The key is distinguishing between a subconjunctival hemorrhage and a hyphema.

A subconjunctival hemorrhage occurs when blood collects beneath the conjunctiva—the clear membrane over the white of the eye (sclera). It appears as a sharply defined red patch that *doesn't cross into the colored part of the eye and doesn't affect vision.* It's typically painless and caused by minor trauma, coughing, or straining. Though it may look dramatic, it's harmless and resolves on its own within a week. No treatment is needed.

A hyphema, by contrast, is bleeding into the anterior chamber—the space between the cornea and the iris. It often follows trauma and *may partially or completely cover the iris and pupil*, causing pain, blurred vision, and light sensitivity. Hyphema can raise intraocular pressure and threatens permanent vision loss if not managed correctly.

In the wilderness, a hyphema is an emergency. Keep the patient upright to allow blood to settle, minimize activity, and avoid anything that increases eye pressure (bending, lifting, straining). Protect the eye without applying pressure and arrange urgent evacuation.

Knowing the difference between these two conditions ensures the right response and helps protect sight. This is one to get right.

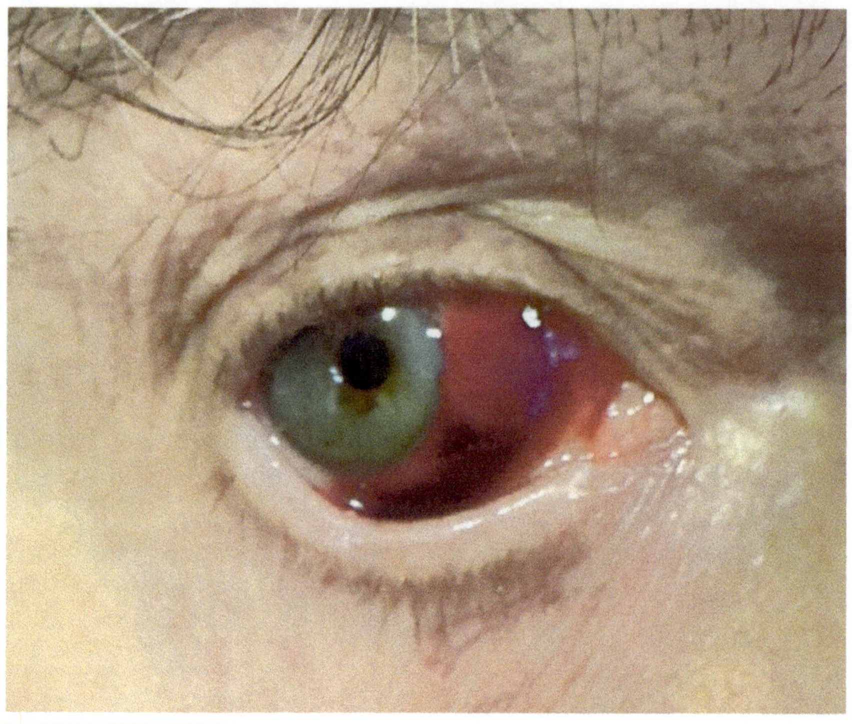

Subconjunctival hemorrhage. Not a vision-threatening emergency, but a striking presentation that often causes concern. The hemorrhage is limited to the conjunctival space and does not extend over the cornea or obscure the iris or pupil. Typically, painless and self-limited, resolving without treatment over one to two weeks. Image courtesy of the author.

What is the difference between preseptal and orbital cellulitis?

Both involve infection near the eye, but orbital cellulitis is significantly more dangerous than preseptal cellulitis and can lead to vision loss or life-threatening complications if not recognized and treated quickly.

Preseptal cellulitis is a superficial infection involving the eyelid and surrounding tissue, limited to structures in front of the orbital septum. It presents with redness, swelling, and tenderness of the eyelid but no pain with eye movement and no vision changes. It's often caused by minor trauma, insect bites, or local skin infections and typically responds to oral antibiotics.

Orbital cellulitis, in contrast, is a deep space infection within the orbit. It often starts as a sinus infection, trauma, or nearby bacterial spread. Key signs include proptosis (eye bulging), pain with eye movement and vision changes, fever, and a toxic appearance. If untreated, it can lead to abscess formation, optic nerve injury, or cavernous sinus thrombosis—a dangerous condition where infection spreads into the veins at the base of the brain, impairing blood drainage and risking stroke, brain infection, or even death.

In the field, distinguishing the two may be difficult. Any eye pain with movement, visual disturbance, or worsening swelling should be treated as orbital cellulitis until proven otherwise. Immediate oral antibiotics should be given if available, and urgent evacuation arranged. Delays in treatment dramatically increase the risk of permanent vision loss or neurological complications.

What should be done for sudden vision loss in the wilderness?

Sudden vision loss in the wilderness is a true emergency, even if it's painless. Several conditions can cause it, and many involve reduced blood flow or pressure changes affecting key parts of the eye. The retina—the thin, light-sensitive layer at the back of the eye—needs constant oxygen. When blood flow to the retina is blocked, vision can be lost quickly and painlessly. A central retinal *artery* occlusion is like a stroke in the eye—it cuts off oxygen to the retina, causing sudden, painless, and often permanent vision loss in the affected eye. A retinal *vein* occlusion, on the other hand, blocks the blood drainage from the retina, leading to swelling and blurred vision. Both are considered serious vascular events that require urgent medical attention, *even if the patient feels no discomfort*. Retinal detachment—when the retina pulls away from the back of the eye—is a painless but vision-threatening emergency. Because the retina has no pain receptors, the condition may progress without discomfort, despite the risk of permanent blindness. Warning signs include flashes of light, a sudden shower of floaters, or the sensation of a dark curtain sweeping across the visual field. Rapid loss of peripheral vision is a classic finding. Any of these symptoms require urgent evacuation, as early treatment greatly improves the chance of preserving sight.

Now, not all vision loss is retinal. Acute angle-closure glaucoma occurs when fluid (aqueous humor) inside the eye can't drain properly through its normal channel. This backup causes a rapid rise in intraocular pressure, which can compress the optic nerve and reduce blood flow to the retina. It often presents with severe pain, nausea, blurred vision, and a red or hard eye—but not always.

In the field, avoid putting pressure on the eye and limit exertion. Protect the eye from light and trauma. *Evacuation should be immediate*—even if symptoms seem to improve—as many causes of sudden vision loss can result in permanent damage within hours.

What is a corneal abrasion, and how is it managed in the field?

A corneal abrasion is a scratch on the cornea—the clear, dome-shaped surface that covers the iris and pupil. Despite being thin and transparent, the cornea is one of the most highly innervated tissues in the body, which makes even small injuries intensely painful. It has no blood vessels, allowing light to pass through without distortion. Instead, it relies on oxygen from the air and nutrients from the aqueous humor behind it. But this lack of blood supply also limits immune defenses, making it more prone to infection.

Injury often comes from sand, dust, contact lenses, or trauma. Symptoms include tearing, light sensitivity, redness, a gritty sensation, and sharp pain. Immediate irrigation with clean water or saline is the most important step—it helps flush out particles and prevent deeper damage. After flushing, antibiotic eye drops or ointment reduce the risk of infection. Lubricating drops may ease irritation, and NSAIDs can help with pain. The eye should be kept gently closed (but not patched tightly). If symptoms persist beyond 48 hours or if vision is affected, evacuation is warranted to rule out deeper injury or infection.

What should I know about contact lenses in the wilderness?

Contact lenses can be dangerous in the backcountry. They trap debris, restrict oxygen flow, and create a perfect environment for bacterial growth—especially from organisms like *Pseudomonas aeruginosa* and *Staphylococcus aureus*, which can cause rapid, vision-threatening infections. Risk increases with poor hygiene, extended wear, or exposure to contaminated water sources like lakes, rivers, or dirty lens cases.

Any eye symptoms—redness, irritation, pain, or blurred vision—warrant immediate removal and disposal of lenses. Leaving them in can trap bacteria, block tear flow, and delay healing. If infection is suspected, start broad-spectrum antibiotic drops, and don't resume lens use until fully recovered.

In remote environments, glasses are safer. Guides should urge clients to carry a backup pair and maintain strict hygiene if lenses are used. Clean water access and proper storage must be planned in advance. Untreated eye infections can escalate quickly and may require evacuation.

What is "pink eye," and how do I manage it?

Conjunctivitis, or pink eye, is inflammation of the conjunctiva—the thin, transparent membrane covering the sclera and inner eyelids. Because it is exposed and highly vascularized, the conjunctiva is especially vulnerable to irritation and infection.

There are three main types of conjunctivitis:

- Viral conjunctivitis is often associated with respiratory infections and causes watery discharge. It is highly contagious but usually self-limited.
- Bacterial conjunctivitis produces thicker discharge, eyelid crusting, and eye sticking, and often requires antibiotic eye drops.
- Allergic conjunctivitis is caused by environmental allergens such as pollen, dust, or animal dander. It leads to redness, tearing, and intense itching. It is not contagious and typically responds well to antihistamine drops and cold compresses.

While all types can cause discomfort, viral and bacterial conjunctivitis are contagious. Hand hygiene and avoiding eye contact or rubbing are essential to prevent spread. Contact lenses should not be worn during any form of eye irritation or infection, as they can trap bacteria, allergens, or debris against the cornea and worsen the condition.

If symptoms worsen or persist—especially if there are vision changes, severe pain, or progressive swelling—evacuation is warranted to rule out more serious conditions. Eye injuries and infections can progress rapidly in wilderness settings, where sanitation is limited, and environmental exposure increases risk. Any significant eye concern, particularly involving trauma or visual acuity changes, should be treated with a low threshold for evacuation.

What is a stye?

A hordeolum, commonly called a stye, is an acute localized infection of the eyelid, usually caused by Staphylococcus aureus. It involves either the sebaceous glands at the base of an eyelash (external hordeolum) or the meibomian glands within the eyelid (internal hordeolum). It presents as a painful, red, swollen bump near the lid margin, often with purulent drainage. Warm compresses are the first-line treatment to promote spontaneous drainage, though persistent cases may require antibiotics or even incision and drainage.

A chalazion is a chronic, noninfectious blockage of a meibomian gland, leading to a recurring inflammatory response. It appears as a firm, painless nodule within the eyelid, often away from the lash line. Chalazia may resolve on their own or with warm compresses, but persistent lesions may require steroid injections or even surgical excision.

The key difference is that a hordeolum is an acute bacterial infection that tends to be painful and may require antibiotics, while a chalazion is a sterile gland blockage that is typically painless, does not require antibiotics, and is longer-lasting.

The Ear

What is the relevant ear anatomy I need to know?

The ear is divided into three sections—outer, middle, and inner—each with distinct anatomy and clinical relevance.

The outer ear includes the pinna (the visible external portion) and the external auditory canal, which directs sound toward the tympanic membrane (eardrum). Conditions here, such as swimmer's ear (otitis externa), often result from moisture retention or trauma and present with localized pain, swelling, and drainage. Pain that worsens with movement of the outer ear or pressure on the tragus typically indicates an outer-ear source.

The middle ear begins at the tympanic membrane and contains the ossicles-three small bones (malleus, incus, stapes) that transmit sound vibrations. It connects to the nasopharynx via the eustachian tube, which equalizes pressure between the middle ear and the outside environment. Blockage of this tube-due to congestion, allergy, or infection-can cause pain, pressure, muffled hearing, or a sensation of fullness. Middle-ear infections (otitis media) occur behind the eardrum and often involve fluid accumulation; bacterial overgrowth; and symptoms such as pain, reduced hearing, and occasionally fever

The inner ear contains the cochlea, which converts mechanical sound waves into nerve signals, and the semicircular canals, which regulate balance and spatial orientation. Disorders affecting this region typically present with vertigo, imbalance, nausea, and hearing changes, but not localized ear pain.

Recognizing which part of the ear is involved can help distinguish between minor outer-ear irritation, treatable middle-ear infections, or more serious inner-ear dysfunction requiring further evaluation. Pain and drainage point toward the outer ear, pressure and hearing loss suggest middle-ear involvement, and dizziness or balance changes indicate inner-ear pathology.

Anatomy of the Ear

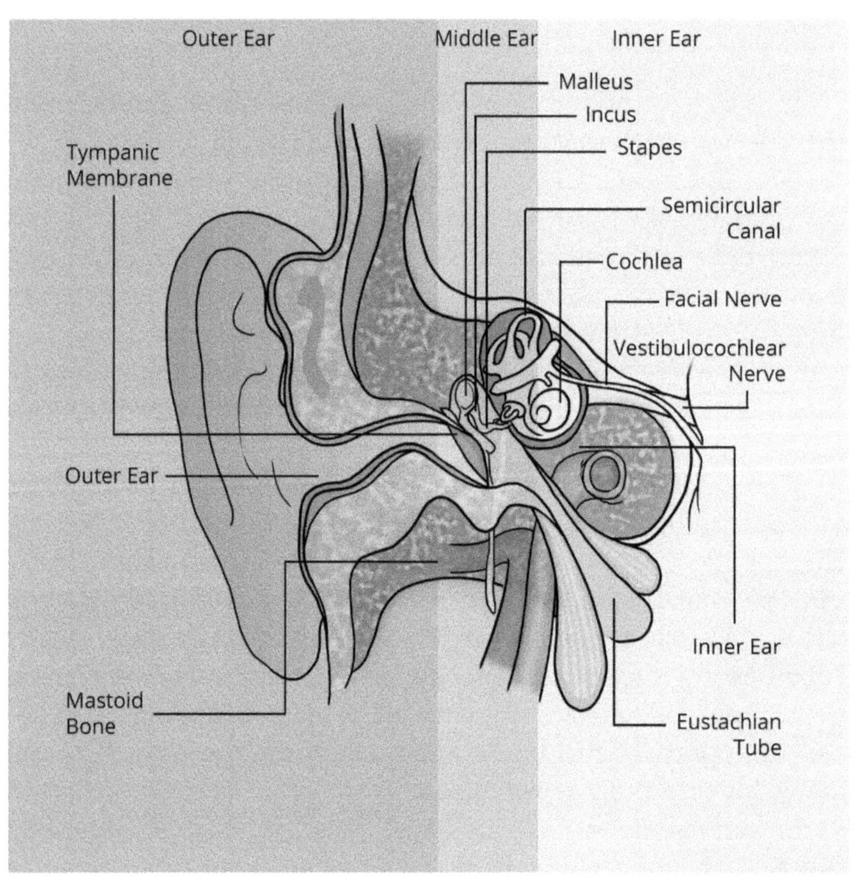

What is swimmer's ear, and how is it treated?

Swimmer's ear, or *otitis externa*, is an infection of the external auditory canal, most often caused by *Pseudomonas aeruginosa* or *Staphylococcus aureus*—bacteria that thrive in moist environments. Prolonged water exposure, especially in warm or dirty conditions, can break down the canal's protective barrier, allowing microbes to invade and trigger inflammation and infection.

Symptoms include pain (often worsened by pulling the ear or pressing the tragus), itching, redness, swelling, and possible drainage. In severe cases, the canal may swell shut, impair hearing and prevent ear drops from reaching the canal.

In susceptible individuals, prevention includes drying the ear after water exposure and maintaining a mildly acidic canal environment. A 1:1 mix of rubbing alcohol and white vinegar helps evaporate water and inhibit bacterial growth but should be avoided in anyone with a known eardrum perforation or ear tubes, as it may irritate the middle ear.

Mild cases can be treated with topical antibiotic drops—ideally combined with a corticosteroid to reduce inflammation. In a pinch, even antibiotic eye drops can be used in the ear (but *never* the other way around) and are often effective. If medicated drops aren't available, a 1:1 mix of rubbing alcohol and white vinegar can help: the alcohol dries the canal, and the vinegar lowers the pH to inhibit bacterial growth. If only one is available, either may offer some benefit, though the combination works best. Avoid use if there's concern for ear tubes or a ruptured eardrum. If swelling blocks the canal, a soft gauze wick can help deliver drops deeper. Over-the-counter pain relievers like ibuprofen and acetaminophen can ease discomfort.

If symptoms persist beyond 72 hours, worsen, or are accompanied by fever or swollen lymph nodes, oral antibiotics and evacuation should be considered.

What is otitis media?

Otitis media is a middle ear infection, most often caused by *Streptococcus pneumoniae* or *Haemophilus influenzae*. It typically follows a respiratory illness, when inflammation blocks the eustachian tube—the narrow channel that connects the middle ear to the back of the throat—trapping fluid behind the eardrum. Symptoms include deep ear pain, fullness, muffled hearing, and sometimes fever. Unlike swimmer's ear, which affects the *external* canal, eardrops are ineffective—oral antibiotics are usually required.

If untreated, otitis media can lead to serious complications such as mastoiditis (infection of the skull behind the ear) or meningitis (infection of the brain's protective layers). In wilderness settings, red flags include persistent fever, worsening pain, swelling or redness behind the ear, severe headache, or confusion—signs that warrant immediate evacuation. Early recognition is critical to preventing deterioration, especially in remote environments.

How should I manage insects or foreign objects in the ear?

They need to come out.

Insects: If an insect enters the ear and can't be safely grasped with forceps or tweezers, the first step is to immobilize or kill it to ease removal and reduce discomfort. A few drops of mineral oil, baby oil, or vegetable oil—warmed to body temperature—can be instilled into the canal to suffocate the insect. Cold fluid may trigger vertigo, so temperature matters. Once the insect is still, tilt the patient's head to allow it to drain out, or gently flush the ear with body-temperature water—only if there's no concern for a ruptured eardrum. Never use sharp instruments, which can damage the canal or eardrum and worsen the situation.

Foreign Objects: Nonliving foreign bodies in the ear require careful handling. If the object is clearly visible and easily grasped, it may be removed with tweezers. If not, further attempts should be avoided—pushing it deeper risks impaction or eardrum injury.

Evacuation is warranted if removal isn't straightforward; if pain, hearing loss, or signs of infection develop; or if there's any doubt about eardrum integrity. Sharp instruments should never be used in the ear canal. If symptoms worsen after attempted removal, oral antibiotics and evacuation are necessary to prevent complications.

The Nose

What is the relevant nose anatomy guides should know?

The nose is the body's primary entry point for air and plays a vital role in filtering, warming, and humidifying it before it reaches the lungs. Key anatomical components include the nares (nostrils), nasal cavity, septum, turbinates, sinuses, and olfactory receptors. The nasal cavity is lined with moist mucosa that traps airborne debris and pathogens while helping to maintain airway hydration.

The turbinates are curved bony projections covered in mucous membrane that extend into the nasal passages. They increase surface area, allowing for more efficient conditioning of incoming air—regulating temperature, humidity, and airflow direction.

The nasal septum, composed of cartilage and bone, divides the nasal cavity into two chambers. It contains two important vascular networks that are central to understanding nosebleeds:

- Kiesselbach's plexus, located on the anterior (front) part of the septum, is the most common source of nosebleeds. These anterior bleeds are typically visible, self-limited, and manageable with pressure and topical vasoconstrictors.
- Woodruff's plexus, located in the posterior nasal cavity, supplies deeper mucosal tissue. Posterior nosebleeds are less common but more serious due to their location

and higher-volume blood flow. These may require advanced medical intervention and can be difficult to control in the field.

The sinuses—frontal, maxillary, ethmoid, and sphenoid—are air-filled cavities that surround the nasal passages. They help reduce skull weight, enhance vocal resonance, and support immune defense by producing mucus to trap pathogens. When these cavities become inflamed or obstructed, sinusitis can develop, leading to facial pressure, congestion, and nasal discharge.

A basic understanding of nasal anatomy helps guides differentiate minor issues—like self-limited nosebleeds or congestion—from more serious conditions such as posterior epistaxis or severe sinus infections that may warrant antibiotics, intervention, or evacuation.

How should I manage nosebleeds in the wilderness?

Most nosebleeds originate from Kiesselbach's plexus, the highly vascular area at the front of the nasal septum. These anterior nosebleeds are common, typically self-limited, and respond well to direct pressure. The patient should sit upright, lean slightly forward, and firmly pinch the soft part of the nose just below the nasal bones for 10 to 20 minutes without interruption. Tilting the head forward prevents blood from draining into the throat, reducing the risk of nausea, vomiting, or aspiration. A cold compress applied to the bridge of the nose or back of the neck may help constrict vessels and slow bleeding.

If bleeding persists, inserting a nasal tampon (such as a Rhino Rocket®) or a rolled gauze soaked in saline can enhance clotting. The tampon or gauze applies pressure internally and can temporarily be left in place.

Posterior nosebleeds, arising from Woodruff's plexus deeper in the nasal cavity, are less common but more serious. These typically present with heavy bleeding that drains into the throat, causing coughing, choking, or vomiting of swallowed blood. Anterior pressure is usually ineffective. Field treatment may involve nasal packing with expandable tampons or an improvised balloon tamponade using a small balloon or even Foley catheter if available. Keep the patient seated, leaning forward, and allow blood to drain from the mouth to protect the airway.

Posterior bleeds require immediate evacuation. If bleeding continues or the patient shows signs of hypovolemia—pallor, dizziness, weakness, or a rapid pulse—treat as a medical emergency. In remote settings, early recognition and bleeding control are critical, as continued blood loss can lead to shock and airway compromise.

What should I know about sinus infections in the field?

Sinus infections (sinusitis) result from inflammation in the paranasal sinuses, often following prolonged congestion; allergies; or exposure to dry, dusty, or high-altitude environments. Symptoms include facial pressure, fever, headache, thick nasal discharge, and postnasal drip. In the wilderness, management includes hydration, nasal irrigation with *clean* water or saline, and decongestants if available. While the vast majority (98%) of sinus infections are viral, bacterial sinusitis should be suspected if fever, severe facial pain, swelling around the eyes, or persistent symptoms persist beyond a week. In these cases, antibiotics and evacuation may be required.

The Throat

What do I need to know about throat anatomy?

The throat, or pharynx, is a shared passageway for both air and food—responsible for breathing, swallowing, and vocalization. Because it performs multiple functions, the throat must carefully coordinate airflow to the lungs and food to the stomach to avoid choking.

At the top of the trachea sits the larynx (voice box), which houses the vocal cords that vibrate to produce sound. Just behind it runs the esophagus, which carries food and liquid to the stomach. In front, the trachea channels air toward the lungs.

To keep these systems separate, the body relies on the epiglottis—a leaf-shaped flap of cartilage that reflexively closes over the trachea during swallowing. If this mechanism fails, food or liquid may enter the airway, leading to choking or aspiration. This is why eating while talking is risky—both actions compete for the same passage and require precise coordination.

The throat also plays a key role in immune defense. It contains lymph nodes that help filter pathogens, and it is bordered by major blood vessels: the carotid arteries and jugular veins, which supply and drain the brain. Structural support comes from the thyroid and cricoid cartilage, which maintain the shape and openness of the airway.

Because the throat is involved in both breathing and swallowing, *any* injury, swelling, or obstruction can become life-threatening in seconds. Even a partial blockage can quickly progress to complete airway compromise, requiring immediate intervention.

What causes a sore throat, and how is it treated?

Most sore throats are a viral infection, caused by *rhinovirus, adenovirus, or influenza,* and resolve within a week. Supportive care—such as saltwater gargles, lozenges, honey, hydration, and over-the-counter pain relievers like ibuprofen—is usually sufficient. However, in a wilderness setting, bacterial infections such as strep throat (caused by *Streptococcus pyogenes*) require antibiotics to prevent complications. Left untreated, strep can lead to peritonsillar abscess, a deep-throat infection that can obstruct the airway, or rheumatic fever—an inflammatory disease that can cause long-term damage to the heart, joints, and nervous system.

Can a sore throat become life-threatening?

While most sore throats are mild and self-limited, severe infections can lead to airway obstruction or systemic complications. Ludwig's angina, a deep-neck infection often stemming from untreated dental or throat infections, can cause dangerous swelling that compromises the airway. Symptoms such as difficulty breathing, drooling, muffled voice, or swelling in the neck or floor of the mouth indicate a medical emergency requiring antibiotics and often immediate evacuation.

Red Flag Framework: Ear, Nose, & Throat Emergencies

What's an easy way to remember what signs and symptoms warrant evacuation using the Red Flag Framework?

For ears, nose, and throat: **HEAR**

- **H**ard-to-control nosebleeds (epistaxis), especially posterior or in anticoagulated patients
- **E**ar pain with fever, headache, or redness around the ear (e.g., mastoiditis)
- **A**irway swelling or worsening throat pain from infections (e.g., tonsillitis, abscess) with difficulty swallowing or fever
- **R**etained foreign object in the ear, nose, or throat

Any of these signs indicate a potentially serious condition, requiring immediate evaluation and possible evacuation. When in doubt, follow the Red Flag Framework: HEAR = Evacuate.

Can You Hear What I Hear?

Throw six guys on a mothership in the Maldives for a few weeks, and something's bound to happen. This trip was no exception.

We'd been running deep into the island chain, following the curve of atolls until we found a leeward lagoon tucked away from the southwest monsoon winds—the Hulhangu season, as the locals call it. For six days, life was simple. Sun, salt, surf, fishing, and the kind of camaraderie that only comes from long days on the water. Then, one evening at dinner, one of the boys showed up looking off.

Not tired. Not sunburned. Sick.

Where he should've been tan and salty, he was pale, shifting uncomfortably in his seat. Said his ear had been bothering him for a few days—happened now and then, but never like this. When I took a look, I knew why.

His left ear was swollen shut, hot to the touch, the skin stretched so tight it looked ready to split. Otitis externa. A nightmare case. The ear canal was the problem, but the swelling was so bad that even the eardrops we had onboard couldn't get through.

This wasn't something you just ride out. Although usually a mild infection, it can sometimes extend into the surrounding soft tissues, causing significant cellulitis.

He'd been dealing with discomfort for a couple days—some itching, irritation, and pressure. Like a lot of people, he'd tried using a cotton swab to relieve it, but that only rubbed the ear canal raw. The damaged skin made things worse by opening the door for infection—but it also gave us an opening.

I had a bottle of local anesthetic with epinephrine in my kit—normally used for wound care. Dripping it into his ear wasn't exactly textbook, but the risk was low, and the upside was real. The exposed tissue let the epinephrine shrink the surface blood vessels just enough to reduce the swelling and create a paper-thin gap in the canal. As a bonus, the anesthetic took the edge off the pain.

With that opening, we tucked in a tiny piece of gauze—a wick—to hold the space open and help the antibiotic drops reach the infection. That was all we could do for the night. We started him on oral antibiotics, pushed fluids, loaded him up on ibuprofen and Tylenol, and sent him to bed.

By morning, the swelling was down by half. The canal was finally open enough to let air and medication do their job. We stuck with the antibiotics—both oral and topical—and by the end of the day, he was pain-free, fever-free, and well on his way to recovery. Within forty-eight hours, he was back to himself. The rest of the trip, we had him rinse his ears after every session—a 50/50 mix of vinegar and alcohol straight from the galley.

Sometimes, the best tool in the kit isn't a tool at all. It's the ability to adapt. Improvisation isn't about having everything—it's about knowing what you have, what you can make work, and when to take a calculated risk.

Rashes, Blisters & the Skin

What should guides know about the skin?

The skin serves as the body's first line of defense—protecting against infection, injury, and environmental exposure. It regulates temperature, prevents water loss, and provides critical sensory input. Structurally, it consists of three layers: the epidermis, which acts as a waterproof barrier; the dermis, which houses blood vessels, nerves, and lymphatics; and the subcutaneous layer, which insulates, stores fat, and absorbs impact. In wilderness environments, maintaining skin integrity is essential. Even minor wounds can compromise fluid balance, temperature regulation, or immune defense. The skin also plays a key role in thermoregulation, adjusting blood flow and producing sweat to manage heat. Its nerve endings detect pressure, temperature, and pain—serving as an early warning system for injury or cold exposure. Friction, moisture, and extreme temperatures are common field stressors that can lead to blisters, maceration, frostbite, or sunburn—many of which are preventable with proper clothing and early care. Infections are a constant risk, particularly in hot, humid, or unsanitary conditions where even small cuts or insect bites may allow bacteria to enter and spread through deeper tissue. Allergic reactions and irritants—from plants, bites, or environmental exposure—can also trigger immune responses within the skin, leading to itching, rash, or swelling. Burns from fire, sun, or hot fluids further disrupt the skin's protective role and can quickly become serious. Recognizing early signs of damage or infection and taking basic precautions can prevent many minor skin issues from escalating into debilitating problems in the wilderness setting.

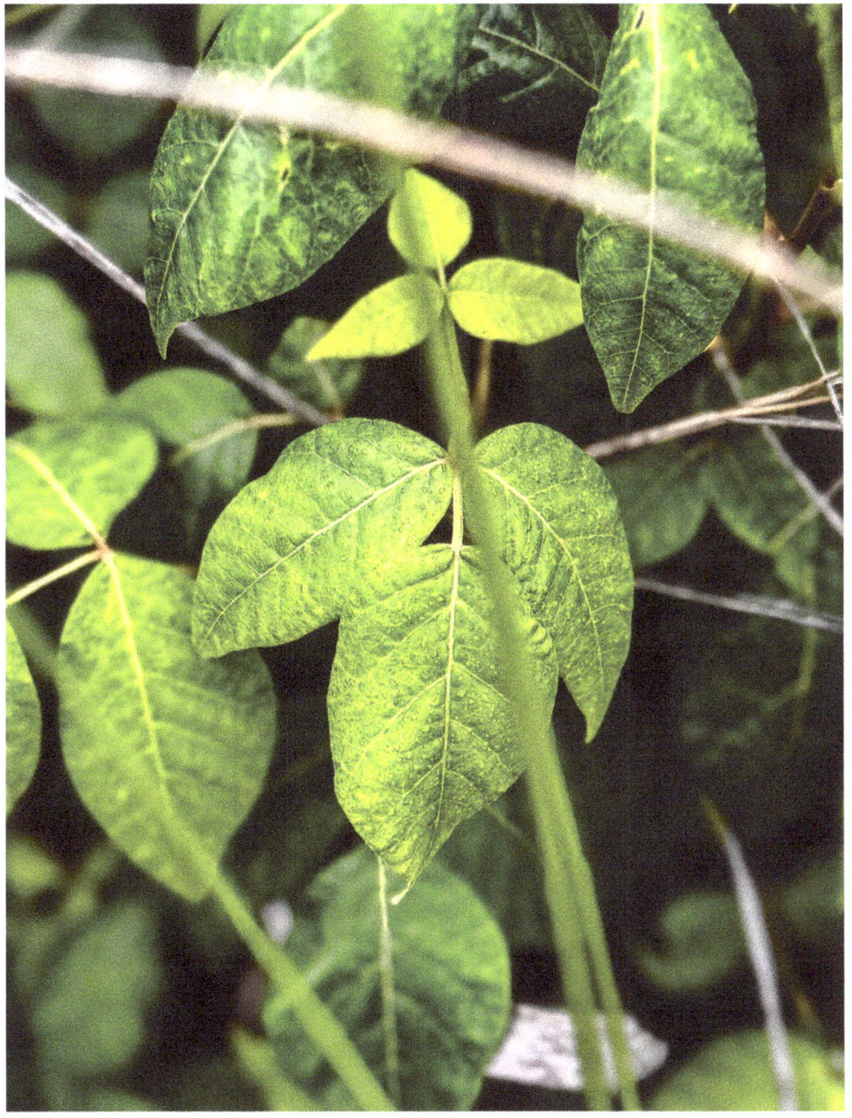

"Leaves of three, let them be." Poison ivy (Toxicodendron radicans) growing along the sand dunes of Brigantine Island, New Jersey. Photo courtesy of the author.

What is contact dermatitis, and how is it treated?

Contact dermatitis is a localized inflammatory reaction of the epidermis triggered by direct contact with an irritant or allergen. It typically presents as redness, itching, burning, swelling, and sometimes blistering or oozing. There are two main types: *irritant contact dermatitis*, caused by direct damage from substances like soaps, solvents, or plant oils; and *allergic contact dermatitis*, an immune response to triggers such as poison ivy or certain topical medications.

Symptoms usually appear within hours to a few days and usually remain limited to the area of contact. In the wilderness, common triggers include poison ivy or oak, insect repellent, sunscreen, resin-treated gear, or contaminated clothing. Commercial dish soap is particularly effective for removing urushiol—the toxic oil in poison ivy—as it's designed to dissolve grease. Early, thorough washing is critical. If exposure involves fine plant hairs (setae), toxic sap, or calcium oxalate crystals—as in nettles or Dieffenbachia—immediate cleansing helps prevent further irritation and absorption.

Once clean, cool compresses can reduce itching and inflammation. Topical corticosteroids, if available, are highly effective. Oral antihistamines like diphenhydramine may reduce itching and help prevent secondary infection from scratching.

More severe reactions—especially on the face, genitals, large surface areas, or accompanied by fever or malaise—may require oral corticosteroids and evacuation. Signs of secondary infection, such as spreading redness or drainage, warrant antibiotics and further care.

Prevention is key: wear protective clothing, use barrier creams, and wash exposed skin promptly after contact. Early field management can keep minor irritants from becoming disabling conditions.

What is cellulitis?

Cellulitis is a bacterial infection of the skin and soft tissue, most commonly caused by *Streptococcus pyogenes* or *Staphylococcus aureus*, including methicillin-resistant *S. aureus* (MRSA). In specific settings, other organisms—such as *Pasteurella* from animal bites or *Vibrio* from saltwater exposure—may be involved.

It occurs when bacteria enter through a break in the skin-such as a cut, scrape, blister, insect bite, or puncture wound—and begin spreading through the dermis and subcutaneous tissue.

The infection typically presents with localized redness, swelling, warmth, and pain, often with a distinct leading edge of spreading redness (erythema). The area may feel firm or tender to the touch, and skin may appear shiny or taut. As the infection progresses, systemic symptoms such as fever, chills, malaise, or swollen lymph nodes may develop. In some cases, blistering, skin breakdown, or purulent drainage may occur, indicating a more severe infection or developing abscess.

In wilderness settings, where hygiene and access to medical care are limited, cellulitis can rapidly progress. Delayed treatment increases the risk of deeper tissue involvement, abscess formation, necrotizing infection, or sepsis. *Any infection that continues to spread despite cleaning and wound care or is accompanied by systemic symptoms, requires oral antibiotic treatment.* If there are signs of rapid progression, tissue destruction, or systemic compromise like fever or malaise, evacuation is mandatory.

Wound prevention and early management are key to reducing cellulitis risk in the field. This includes thorough cleaning of all skin breaks; covering wounds with clean, dry dressings; and avoiding exposure to contaminated water sources. Minor skin infections should be monitored closely; and any signs of expanding redness, increasing pain, or systemic symptoms should be taken seriously. In remote environments, early intervention is the best chance to avoid serious complications and prevent the need for urgent evacuation.

What are shingles, and how should they be managed in the wilderness?

Shingles, or herpes zoster, is a reactivation of the *varicella-zoster virus*—the same virus that causes chickenpox. After the initial infection, the virus remains dormant in nerve roots and may reactivate later in life, especially during periods of stress, illness, or immune suppression. Once reactivated, it travels along the affected nerve, causing inflammation and a painful, localized rash.

Shingles typically presents with burning, tingling, or itching in a single dermatome—one side of the chest, abdomen, back, or face is most common—followed by red patches and grouped fluid-filled blisters. The rash usually *does not cross the midline* and often lasts two to four weeks. Pain can range from mild to severe, and some patients develop postherpetic neuralgia, a lingering nerve pain that can persist for months after the rash resolves.

In wilderness settings, the focus is on preventing secondary bacterial infection and managing pain. Keep the rash clean and dry. Avoid scratching or covering it with occlusive dressings. For pain, start with acetaminophen or ibuprofen. If pain is severe and opioid analgesics are available and appropriate, they may be used. Antiviral medications (acyclovir, valacyclovir, or famciclovir) are most effective if started within 72 hours of symptom onset and can shorten the course of illness and reduce complications. Evacuate if the rash involves the face, eyes, or ears—due to risk of vision or hearing loss—or if the patient has systemic symptoms like fever, fatigue, altered mental status or widespread involvement. Signs of bacterial superinfection—warmth, redness, swelling, or pus—also warrant antibiotics and evacuation for advanced care.

Vaccination significantly reduces the risk of shingles and its complications especially for older adults or those frequently in remote environments.

How should I manage blisters in the wilderness?

Blisters form when shear forces separate the epidermis from the dermis, allowing plasma to accumulate in the space created. This fluid-filled sac cushions the underlying tissue and protects it—what many refer to as nature's Band-Aid.

The blister roof is sterile and should be preserved whenever possible.

If the blister is small, intact, and not interfering with movement, leave it alone. Cover it with moleskin, tape, or padding to reduce friction. If it's tense, painful, or likely to rupture under pressure, drain it by puncturing at the edge with a sterile needle or blade. Never remove the skin roof unless it's torn. Once the roof is gone, the wound is exposed and should be treated like any open injury—with irrigation, dressing, and monitoring for infection.

Blisters that become macerated—meaning the skin is softened and weakened from prolonged moisture exposure—are more likely to tear or become infected. In high-risk environments like wet terrain, reused socks, or prolonged activity, keeping feet dry and rotating footwear is just as important as treatment.

How can I prevent and manage athlete's foot in the wilderness?

Athlete's foot, or *tinea pedis*, is a common fungal skin infection that thrives in warm, moist environments—conditions frequently created by prolonged wear of tight or damp footwear. It usually begins between the last three toes, where heat, friction, and trapped moisture allow fungi to flourish. Early signs include itching, redness, peeling, and cracking of the skin. If left untreated, the condition can lead to painful fissures or secondary bacterial infection.

Prevention starts with keeping the feet clean, dry, and well-ventilated. Moisture-wicking socks, rotating footwear to allow full drying, and avoiding barefoot exposure in communal areas all reduce risk. In remote settings, this means removing shoes during rest periods, drying feet thoroughly each night, and airing out boots or waders whenever possible.

Treatment begins with daily washing—especially between the last three toes—followed by careful drying. Over-the-counter antifungals like clotrimazole or terbinafine are effective when available although often not needed. A 50%

vinegar soak can lower skin pH enough to slow fungal growth. Cornstarch or baking soda may help absorb moisture throughout the day.

In austere environments, placing dry gauze or clean paper strips between the toes at night promotes airflow and keeps the interdigital spaces dry. Powdering between the toes before inserting spacers can further reduce moisture and fungal persistence. This low-tech, high-impact strategy works well when supplies are limited, and hygiene is hard to maintain.

Guides should watch for signs of secondary bacterial infection—worsening redness, swelling, warmth, pus, or systemic symptoms. In those cases, antibiotics and evacuation may be necessary.

What causes cracked heels, and how should they be managed in the wilderness?

Cracked heels are a common problem in the field, often resulting from prolonged standing, dehydration, and repeated exposure to alternating wet and dry conditions. These factors dry out the skin and create pressure points, especially on the heel's outer margin, leading to fissures, painful cracks in the thickened skin. Left untreated, deep fissures can become portals for infection, bleed with movement, hurt like hell, and significantly impair mobility.

Management begins with cleaning the affected area thoroughly using soap and water to remove dirt and reduce bacterial load. After drying, cyanoacrylate glue or medical tape can be applied to seal superficial cracks. This helps protect exposed tissue, reduce pain, and limit further tearing. Additionally, the glue creates a temporary barrier that also aids in hydration retention and wound closure.

At night, applying a thick emollient such as petroleum jelly can help soften the skin and promote healing. Covering the feet with clean socks after applying the ointment enhances absorption and protects the skin from friction. During the day, padded socks or insoles reduce shear stress and pressure on the heel, preventing new fissures and reducing pain while walking.

Daily inspection is essential. Guides should look for signs of infection, including increased redness, warmth, swelling, pus, or worsening pain. If these signs appear or if fissures deepen and become increasingly painful, more aggressive wound care or evacuation may be necessary. In the wilderness, cracked heels can quickly compromise function and expose the patient to mostly avoidable complications. Early management, moisture control, and pressure protection are key to keeping feet operational in harsh environments.

How do I recognize a serious skin condition?

Serious skin conditions can be your canary in the coal mine. Widespread, blistering, or rapidly progressing rashes often indicate more than just a local problem—they may reflect *systemic* infection, toxin exposure, or a severe drug reaction. When the skin begins to peel, split, or form bullae (large fluid-filled blisters), the body's barrier is compromised, raising the risk of infection, fluid loss, and thermoregulation failure. Systemic symptoms like fever, chills, vomiting, muscle aches, or confusion raise the stakes significantly. Rashes involving the eyes, lips, genitals, or mouth should be treated as medical emergencies, especially when paired with mucosal erosion or signs of skin peeling. While minor irritation can be managed in the field, anything that spreads rapidly, affects those critical areas, or comes with systemic illness warrants evacuation.

The Lungs: Cough, Asthma, & Pneumonia

What is a cough?

A cough is a protective reflex that clears the airways of mucus, irritants, or foreign particles. It is a common symptom of respiratory infections; allergies; or environmental exposure to dust, smoke, or cold air. In most cases, a cough is harmless and self-limited; but in the wilderness, it can indicate a more serious condition, such as pneumonia, bronchitis, asthma, or even a pulmonary embolism.

Persistent coughing can lead to dehydration, fatigue, and difficulty sleeping-all of which can impair decision-making and physical performance in remote environments. A worsening or prolonged cough—especially if accompanied by fever, shortness of breath, chest pain, or coughing up blood—requires careful assessment and likely warrants evacuation. Recognizing when a cough is minor versus when it signals a more serious problem is essential for effective wilderness management.

What is asthma and how should it be managed in the wilderness?

Asthma is a chronic airway disease defined by bronchospasm, airway swelling, and excess mucus production. During an attack, these combine to narrow the airways, making *exhalation* slow and inefficient. Air becomes trapped in the lungs, the chest hyperinflates, and the patient has to work harder with each breath. This increases fatigue, raises carbon dioxide levels in the blood, and can eventually lead to respiratory failure.

The first-line treatment is inhaled albuterol. It acts on beta-2 receptors in the airway smooth muscle, causing rapid bronchodilation. It works within minutes and treats the *spasm*, not the *inflammation*. Corticosteroids like prednisone suppress the immune response, reduce swelling, and blunt mucus production. In the field, a 5-day course of prednisone (e.g., 40 mg. daily) can help reduce the risk of rebound symptoms during evacuation.

Signs of a severe attack include cyanosis, altered mental status, a silent chest, or the inability to speak in full sentences. Epinephrine should be used in these cases, particularly if there's any concern for airway swelling or anaphylaxis.

Manual external chest compression (MECC) can be considered as a last resort when the chest is visibly overinflated, and the patient can't fully exhale. This involves applying firm, controlled pressure to the chest wall during *exhalation*—using a hand, forearm, or any safe method available—to help push trapped air out. It's a temporary maneuver to reduce hyperinflation and buy time when other measures aren't enough. Any moderate or severe attack in a remote setting requires aggressive intervention and evacuation.

What is COPD, and how is it managed in the wilderness?

Chronic obstructive pulmonary disease (COPD) is a progressive, *irreversible* condition marked by airflow limitation from chronic bronchitis, emphysema, or both. Chronic bronchitis causes airway inflammation and mucus overproduction; emphysema destroys alveolar walls, reducing gas exchange and trapping air; and both lead to poor exhalation, breathlessness, and inefficient oxygen uptake.

Symptoms include chronic cough, wheezing, fatigue, and difficulty breathing that worsens with cold air, altitude, smoke, or respiratory infections. In the field, even mild exertion can cause severe distress during an exacerbation.

Wilderness management focuses on stabilization and trigger avoidance. Patients should carry their maintenance inhalers—typically a long-acting and a short-acting beta-agonist like albuterol.

Exacerbations—marked by increased cough, sputum, wheezing, or breathlessness—warrant immediate albuterol use. A 5–7-day course of oral prednisone (e.g., 40 mg. daily) may reduce inflammation. If there's fever, dark sputum, or signs of infection, antibiotics are indicated and always evacuate for worsening respiratory distress, altered mental status, or failure to improve with treatment. Unlike asthma, COPD damage is permanent, and decompensation in remote settings carries high risk.

What is pneumonia, and how is it managed in the wilderness?

Pneumonia is a lung infection that causes inflammation and fluid buildup in the alveoli, the tiny air sacs responsible for gas exchange. Normally, these sacs stay air-filled, allowing oxygen to enter the bloodstream and carbon dioxide to be removed. In pneumonia, the alveoli fill with fluid, pus, and immune cells, which limits oxygen absorption and leads to cough, shortness of breath, fever, and fatigue. Chest pain that worsens with breathing or coughing (pleuritic pain) may occur when inflamed lung tissue irritates the chest wall lining.

In the wilderness, pneumonia can limit physical capacity quickly, especially with exertion, altitude, or cold air. It often begins with a productive cough, fever, and chills, then progresses to rapid breathing (tachypnea), low oxygen levels, or confusion—especially in older adults where sudden fatigue or altered mental status may be the only early signs.

Field management includes rest, hydration, and early antibiotics if available. Azithromycin or doxycycline are reasonable empiric choices depending on availability and allergy history. NSAIDs like ibuprofen can reduce pleuritic pain and support deeper breathing while positional changes and active coughing help clear secretions.

Evacuate for respiratory distress, persistent fever, altered mental status, or inability to tolerate fluids or oral medications. Without treatment, pneumonia can progress to respiratory failure, or sepsis—especially when evacuation is delayed.

Red Flag Framework: Respiratory Emergencies

What's an easy way to remember what signs and symptoms warrant evacuation using the Red Flag Framework?

For the Respiratory Emergencies: **AIR**

- **A**udible wheezing, stridor, or difficulty breathing OR

- **I**ncreased respiratory effort (gasping, labored breathing) OR
- **R**apid breathing or signs of hypoxia (low oxygen) (blue lips or extremities)

Any of these signs indicate a potentially serious condition, requiring immediate evaluation and possible evacuation. When in doubt, follow the Red Flag Framework: AIR = Evacuate.

Acute Psychotic Episodes

What is an acute psychotic episode, and why is it significant in the wilderness?

An acute psychotic episode is a sudden break from reality, marked by hallucinations, delusions, disorganized thinking, paranoia, or agitation. Triggers can include preexisting mental illness, substance abuse or withdrawal, dehydration, hypoglycemia, infections, medication noncompliance, or extreme stress. In the wilderness, the lack of medical resources, social support, and the addition of environmental stressors can quickly escalate the situation, making early recognition and intervention critical. Individuals experiencing psychosis may become disoriented, unresponsive to reason, or unpredictable, creating potential safety risks for both them and the group.

How do I handle a psychotic episode?

Managing a psychotic episode in the wilderness requires a focus on safety, de-escalation, and evacuation. Remove potential weapons—sharp objects, shoelaces, or anything that could be used for self-harm—and avoid leaving the person alone if they appear confused, paranoid, or agitated. Speak calmly, using simple, direct language without challenging delusions or hallucinations. Avoid sudden movements or confrontational posture, which can escalate distress. If the person is confused but cooperative, allow them space to rest while monitoring for changes.

Basic needs come first. Hydration, food, and sleep can reduce, or even reverse symptoms caused by dehydration, hypoglycemia, or exhaustion. If psychiatric medications are part of the patient's routine and available, help them take their usual dose. For severe agitation, benzodiazepines such as diazepam, lorazepam, or alprazolam (if on hand) may provide short-term relief but should not delay evacuation.

Evacuation is required unless symptoms resolve fully and rapidly. Persistent paranoia, disorientation, or unsafe behavior—either to self or others—warrants immediate removal. Keep in mind that aeromedical crews may be reluctant to transport a behaviorally unstable patient in a confined aircraft. Sedation, physical restraint, or ground-based alternatives may be necessary. While awaiting transport; maintain close observation; protect the group; and document symptoms, history, medications, triggers, and any actions taken.

What is alcohol withdrawal?

While alcohol withdrawal can mimic psychosis, it's a substance-induced medical emergency—not a primary psychiatric condition. In remote environments, it's unpredictable and potentially fatal.

Alcohol acts as a central nervous system depressant. It enhances gamma-aminobutyric acid (GABA)—the brain's primary *inhibitory* neurotransmitter—slowing neural activity and producing a calming effect, while simultaneously suppressing glutamate, the main *excitatory* neurotransmitter. With chronic use, the brain is constantly bathed in alcohol. To maintain function, it adapts by downregulating GABA and ramping up excitatory systems just to stay balanced. When alcohol is suddenly removed, that governor effect disappears, and the primed glutamate system hits overdrive. The result is nervous system chaos: tremors, agitation, hallucinations, and, in severe cases, seizures.

Withdrawal typically starts 6–24 hours after the last drink with tremors, sweating, nausea, headache, anxiety, and insomnia. It can then progress to hypertension, agitation, hallucinations, and confusion. Delirium tremens (DTs)—the most severe form—usually hits at 48–96 hours and involves disorientation, seizures, and unstable vitals. Untreated, mortality can reach 40%.

In the wilderness, there's no real treatment—only evacuation. At the first signs of agitation or anxiety in any heavy drinker, get them out. If benzodiazepines aren't available, a short-term fallback is small, controlled doses of alcohol—not as treatment, but to buy time. The goal is seizure prevention, not sedation.

Hydration and electrolytes are also critical. Withdrawal worsens deficits in sodium, potassium, magnesium, and glucose—raising seizure and cardiac risk. Start oral fluids if possible.

Once hallucinations, confusion, or seizures appear, there's no safe field option. Early recognition and prompt evacuation are essential.

Sepsis

What is sepsis, and why is it a serious concern in the wilderness?

Sepsis is a systemic response to infection that disrupts circulation, oxygen delivery, and organ function. It often begins when a localized infection—such as a wound, pneumonia, or GI illness—triggers a widespread inflammatory cascade. Blood vessels dilate, become leaky, and lose their vascular tone. As fluid shifts out of the bloodstream, circulating volume drops, leading to impaired tissue perfusion.

As perfusion declines, oxygen delivery drops. Cells switch from aerobic metabolism (which uses oxygen efficiently) to anaerobic metabolism, a less effective backup that produces lactic acid as waste. This leads to metabolic acidosis and early organ dysfunction. The lungs, kidneys, and brain—organs with high oxygen needs—are often the first to fail.

Sepsis can evolve from routine infections and remains a major cause of death worldwide. In wilderness settings, where delays are common and resources are limited, it's a high-risk condition. Signs include fever or hypothermia, tachycardia, fast breathing, altered mental status, pallor, low urine output, or a known infection that's worsening despite care.

Empiric oral antibiotics should be initiated, along with oral rehydration and preparation for evacuation. There is no role for watchful waiting in sepsis. Early recognition and timely transfer to definitive care are the only interventions likely to improve the outcome.

Shock: The Most Important Concept in Medicine

Why is understanding shock so important?

Because shock is the common pathway to death in all cases of critical illness or injury, making it essential to understand in wilderness medicine. At its core, shock is a state of inadequate tissue perfusion—meaning the body's organs aren't receiving the oxygenated blood they need to survive. This happens when the circulatory system can no longer maintain sufficient blood *pressure* to the organs. The causes vary: in hypovolemic shock—such as from bleeding or severe fluid loss through vomiting or diarrhea—there simply isn't enough circulating volume. In distributive shock, including anaphylaxis and sepsis, the blood vessels dilate and become leaky, causing pressure to fall sharply. In neurogenic shock, like after spinal cord injury, the vessels lose their normal muscle tone and can't constrict to maintain adequate blood pressure. And in cardiogenic shock, the heart itself fails to pump effectively—whether from trauma, arrhythmia, or infarction (heart attack). Though the mechanisms may differ, the end result is the same: blood pressure drops below a critical threshold, tissues are starved of oxygen, and organ failure begins.

In wilderness settings, early recognition is critical. Delays are expected and resources limited. Guides who understand the underlying physiology can spot red flags early, support perfusion, and trigger evacuation before the *brief* window to act closes.

What are the types of shock and their field management?

There are four main types of shock: hypovolemic, distributive, cardiogenic, and obstructive. While their causes differ, all lead to inadequate tissue perfusion and progressive organ dysfunction. Field management starts with recognizing the likely category and supporting circulation until evacuation.

Hypovolemic shock is caused by fluid loss—most often from bleeding, diarrhea, vomiting, or dehydration. Circulating volume drops, blood pressure falls, and oxygen delivery to organs declines. This is the most common form seen in trauma and wilderness settings. Treatment includes controlling external bleeding, starting oral rehydration with electrolytes if tolerated, and elevating the legs to support blood flow. Evacuation is time-sensitive.

Distributive shock includes sepsis, anaphylaxis, and neurogenic shock. In these cases, blood vessels lose tone and dilate, making even normal blood volume inadequate for circulation. Early signs may include flushed or warm skin that later turns cool or mottled as perfusion drops. Rehydration is still the priority. Epinephrine should be administered immediately for suspected anaphylaxis, and oral antibiotics started for suspected sepsis. Urgent evacuation is required in all forms.

Cardiogenic shock results from pump failure—usually due to a heart attack, arrhythmia, or longstanding heart disease. It's uncommon in wilderness settings but can occur in older adults or anyone with known cardiac conditions. Patients may appear pale, short of breath, cold to the touch, or extremely fatigued. Oral fluids may worsen symptoms, as the heart is already struggling to pump and added volume only increases the workload. The patient should be kept upright and resting.

Aggressive rehydration should be avoided unless the patient is clearly volume-depleted. Evacuation is immediate.

Obstructive shock occurs when something physically blocks blood flow. In the wilderness, this might include:

- Tension pneumothorax: Air becomes trapped in the chest, collapsing a lung and shifting pressure onto the heart and remaining lung—usually after blunt or penetrating chest trauma. May present with severe shortness of breath, uneven chest rise, absent breath sounds on one side, or tracheal deviation (if visible). Rapid recognition and intervention are critical.
- Cardiac tamponade: A life-threatening buildup of fluid around the heart, often following chest trauma. Without equipment, field clues may include worsening shortness of breath, weak or fading pulses, confusion, or visible neck vein distention.
- Pulmonary embolism: A blood clot blocks arteries in the lungs, often without any trauma. May present as sudden shortness of breath, sharp chest pain (especially with breathing), rapid heart rate, and sometimes unexplained anxiety or a sense of impending doom. Signs may appear abruptly in otherwise stable individuals, especially after prolonged travel, immobilization, or recent illness.

In all forms of shock, definitive treatment is limited in the field. Rapid recognition and prompt evacuation remain the most effective interventions. Early signs often include confusion, weak pulses, rapid breathing, delayed capillary refill, and reduced urine output. Rehydration is appropriate in most cases—except in cardiogenic shock. Keep the patient warm, calm, and under close observation until evacuation.

Men's Health in The Wilderness

What is testicular torsion?

Testicular torsion occurs when the testicle twists on its blood supply, cutting off circulation. It's one of the few true urologic emergencies in wilderness medicine as once blood flow stops, the testicle begins to die. Damage can begin within six hours, and after twelve, the chances of saving it drop dramatically.

The testicle is a dense, coiled marvel of male biology—essential, delicate, and proudly on display. It hangs from the spermatic cord like an ornate chandelier, suspended by arteries, veins, nerves, lymphatics, and the sperm-carrying vas deferens. Normally, the testicle is anchored within the scrotum, preventing it from rotating. But in some males—especially adolescents and young adults—a variation called the "bell clapper deformity" leaves the testicle more mobile. This allows it to twist, first blocking venous return, then arterial flow, cutting off circulation and causing severe pain.

The left testicle is more commonly affected, likely because it hangs slightly lower and has a longer spermatic cord—both of which increase its vulnerability to torsion.

Because the testicles share nerve roots with the lower abdomen, the pain often radiates upward and is frequently accompanied by nausea and vomiting. In some cases, abdominal pain is more prominent than scrotal pain early on, which can delay diagnosis.

Torsion usually strikes without trauma. The affected testicle will ride high, feel firm, and lie at an unusual angle. Pain worsens with movement, and the scrotum may appear red or swollen.

If the story fits—sudden, one-sided testicular pain with or without abdominal pain or vomiting—treat it as torsion. Some trained providers may attempt manual detorsion by rotating the testicle outward—*like opening a book*: clockwise for the patient's left testicle, counterclockwise for the right, as viewed from the provider's perspective below. This maneuver must be done correctly as twisting the wrong direction can worsen the torsion. Relief is usually immediate if successful, but surgical fixation is still required.

Regardless of field intervention or outcome, evacuation is mandatory. This is not a condition that allows for observation as delay can result in permanent loss and lasting consequences.

Any other causes of testicular pain besides torsion I should know?

Yep. If testicular pain comes on slowly, worsens with movement, and is paired with swelling or aching that builds over time, it may be epididymitis (inflammation of the sperm duct) or orchitis (inflammation of the testicle). These often happen together.

While urinary tract infections and sexually transmitted infections are common triggers, viral infections (like mumps) can inflame the testicle as well. Other cases are mechanical; and at least as likely in the wilderness setting, long periods of sitting on a bike or saddle, trauma, or pressure can all cause irritation and swelling even *without* infection.

In the field, the testicle will usually feel sore and heavy. Walking makes it worse. The scrotum may look red or feel warm, and the pain may improve a bit when the scrotum is elevated, reducing the pull of gravity on inflamed structures.

Treatment includes rest, ice, NSAIDs, and scrotal support. While oral broad-spectrum antibiotics like levofloxacin (or even ciprofloxacin) and doxycycline can be started in the field if available, they are *not* to be considered definitive therapy. Proper care still requires clinical management, and if a sexually transmitted infection is suspected, any recent sexual partners should also be treated.

Always think about testicular torsion first. If the pain came on suddenly, the testicle is riding high, or the diagnosis isn't clear, open the book, start antibiotics, evacuate, and treat it like torsion. The risk of missing a dying testicle outweighs the risk of over-triage.

What is a penile fracture?

Penile fracture isn't just slang; it's a real tear of the tunica albuginea, the thick outer sheath that surrounds the blood-filled erectile bodies of the penis. During a full erection, internal pressure is high, and if the penis bends sharply—during sex or a direct blow—that sheath can rupture. The result: an audible "pop," sudden pain, rapid loss of erection, and swelling or bruising. Sometimes the penis will visibly curve or twist to one side.

This is a surgical problem, but not a life-threatening emergency. Most fractures need repair within 24 to 72 hours to avoid long-term complications like scarring, chronic pain, or erectile dysfunction. It doesn't need a helicopter per se, but it does need timely evacuation.

In the field, avoid aspirin or NSAIDs (like ibuprofen) since they can worsen bleeding. Use acetaminophen for pain. Don't attempt to manipulate or "straighten" the penis. Support it gently, apply cool compresses, and keep the patient calm. Evacuation should happen as soon as feasible even if the patient minimizes it or is embarrassed to bring it up. This is not something that heals well on its own.

Women's Health in the Wilderness

Why is women's health important in wilderness settings?

More women are participating in wilderness travel and remote expeditions than ever before, bringing essential skills, leadership, and perspective to these environments. As this involvement grows, it's increasingly important for guides and responders to recognize and prepare for medical conditions that may uniquely affect women in the field. Common concerns include urinary tract infections, vaginal infections, and pregnancy-related complications. Management relies on prevention, early identification, and practical intervention using the resources at hand. Addressing these issues directly not only supports safety and group function—it also reflects good planning and reinforces inclusive, competent expedition leadership.

What unique health issues should guides be aware of for women in the wilderness?

Women in the wilderness encounter unique health challenges, including urinary tract infections (UTIs), vaginal infections, and pregnancy-related complications. The demands of the wilderness environment, such as dehydration, limited hygiene options, and restricted access to medical care, can heighten the risk and severity of these conditions. Guides should prepare their medical kits to address the needs of female participants, including items such as antifungal creams, antibiotics, pregnancy tests, and menstrual supplies. Emphasizing hygiene and hydration is critical to prevention, especially for UTIs, which are often triggered by dehydration or limited opportunities to urinate. Open communication between guides and participants can help identify concerns early and guide proper management. Guys, talk to the ladies.

Are there additional risks for pregnant women in the wilderness?

Of course. Pregnancy introduces distinct challenges in wilderness settings, particularly when medical care or evacuation is delayed. The second trimester is generally considered the safest period for extended outdoor activities, as the risks of miscarriage and preterm labor are lower, and physical endurance is often better than during the first or third trimesters. However, guides must remain vigilant for serious complications that can escalate rapidly, such as an ectopic pregnancy or miscarriage.

Ectopic pregnancy, occurring in about 1-2% of pregnancies, presents a significant risk in remote settings. An ectopic pregnancy involves the implantation of a fertilized egg outside the uterus, most commonly in a fallopian tube, and can cause life-threatening bleeding if ruptured. Symptoms include sharp abdominal or pelvic pain, vaginal spotting, dizziness, and signs of shock. These signs in a woman of child-bearing age demand immediate evaluation and evacuation.

Miscarriage, or pregnancy loss before 20 weeks, occurs in roughly 10-20% of known pregnancies, with many happening before the woman is even aware she is pregnant. In the wilderness, symptoms of a miscarriage such as heavy bleeding, severe cramping, or the passage of tissue require prompt evacuation to manage complications like excessive blood loss or infection.

Guides should also be aware that pregnant women face a higher risk of dehydration and infections, which can complicate both their health and that of the fetus. Foodborne illnesses or exposure to mosquito borne diseases like malaria and Zika can pose serious risks, particularly in tropical or subtropical regions. Providing access to clean water, maintaining proper nutrition, and minimizing environmental hazards are critical steps to supporting the health of a pregnant participant.

Gynecological Infections

What causes a urinary tract infection?

A urinary tract infection (UTI) occurs when bacteria, most commonly *Escherichia coli* (*E. coli*), enter the urinary system—leading to infection of the urethra, bladder, or kidneys. In the wilderness, limited access to medical care can allow a minor UTI to progress into serious complications such as pyelonephritis (kidney infection) or sepsis (a life-threatening systemic infection). Due to anatomical differences, UTIs are more common in females, as their shorter urethra and its proximity to the anus provide a more direct route for bacteria to reach the bladder. Recognizing early symptoms—burning with urination, frequent urges to urinate, and lower abdominal discomfort—is essential to prevent complications in remote settings.

What is pyelonephritis?

Pyelonephritis is a bacterial infection of the *kidneys* that typically starts as a lower urinary tract infection and *ascends* to the upper urinary system. It causes significant inflammation and can lead to significant complications if untreated. Symptoms include fever, chills, *flank pain*, nausea, and vomiting. Unlike bladder infections, pyelonephritis often presents with systemic signs of illness, indicating a more severe infection that can lead to kidney damage, abscess formation, or sepsis.

In wilderness settings, prompt management is critical. Encourage aggressive oral hydration if tolerated, as dehydration worsens kidney stress and impairs recovery. If antibiotics are available, they should be started immediately. Pain can be managed with acetaminophen, but NSAIDs should generally be avoided due to their potential to impair kidney function. Close monitoring for worsening symptoms, such as persistent vomiting, confusion, or signs of sepsis, is essential. Any suspected case of pyelonephritis require urgent evacuation as progression without treatment can lead to permanent kidney damage or life-threatening systemic infection.

How can UTIs and their complications be prevented in the wilderness?

Preventing UTIs in remote environments relies on proper hydration, hygiene, and early intervention. Staying well hydrated encourages regular urination, which helps flush bacteria from the urinary tract before they can cause infection. Basic hygiene practices, such as wiping front to back, urinating after sexual activity, and avoiding prolonged holding of urine, reduce bacterial migration into the urethra. Wearing loose, breathable clothing and changing out of wet or damp garments can prevent bacterial overgrowth in the perineal area.

In communal wilderness settings, regular handwashing, especially before eating or handling personal hygiene items helps limit bacterial exposure. If access to clean water is limited, alcohol-based hand sanitizers can be an effective alternative. Recognizing early signs of infection—such as urinary urgency, burning, or lower abdominal discomfort—allows for prompt management with hydration and, if available, antibiotics. By implementing these preventive measures, wilderness guides can help reduce the risk of UTIs and minimize the likelihood of complications requiring evacuation.

How can I tell the difference between vaginal irritation and infection?

Vaginal irritation is usually caused by external factors such as friction, moisture, prolonged damp conditions, or exposure to irritants like scented soaps, tight clothing, or synthetic fabrics. It typically presents with localized redness, mild swelling, itching, or a general sense of discomfort. There is often no abnormal discharge, odor, or internal pain. Managing irritation in the field involves identifying and removing the cause—switching to breathable, moisture-wicking clothing, improving hygiene, avoiding wipes or soaps with fragrance, and keeping the area dry. Symptoms often improve within 24 to 48 hours once the irritant is eliminated.

Vaginal infections, however, involve an overgrowth of normal flora or introduction of new bacteria and usually cause more specific symptoms. Unlike irritation, infections often involve changes in discharge and odor, and the discomfort is more persistent and internal—infections often require medical management.

What are the signs and treatment of a yeast infection?

Yeast infections occur when *Candida albicans*—a fungus normally present in the vaginal microbiome—grows unchecked. Under typical conditions, beneficial bacteria help keep *Candida* in balance, but factors like antibiotic use, prolonged moisture, hormonal shifts, or immune suppression can tip the scale toward overgrowth. Symptoms include intense itching, redness, irritation, and a thick, white, clumpy discharge—burning with urination or intercourse may also occur.

In standard settings, treatment involves antifungal medications such as clotrimazole or miconazole, often available over the counter in topical or suppository form. Recovery is supported by keeping the area dry, avoiding irritants like scented soaps or synthetic underwear, and wearing breathable clothing.

In the wilderness, where antifungals may not be available, moisture control becomes the priority. Changing into dry clothing regularly, avoiding prolonged dampness, and allowing airflow to the area can slow fungal growth. Probiotic-rich foods like yogurt—or oral probiotics—may help restore the natural bacterial balance. Yeast infections *generally* do not cause systemic illness, and evacuation is rarely necessary unless symptoms are severe, persistent, or interfere with movement or daily function.

What is bacterial vaginosis, and how is it treated?

Bacterial vaginosis (BV) occurs when the normal balance of vaginal bacteria is disrupted, allowing anaerobic organisms—most commonly *Gardnerella vaginalis*—to overgrow. Long considered a simple imbalance, BV is now recognized as a sexually transmitted infection (STI). Male partners contribute to reinfection and treating both partners improves cure rates.

The strongest risk factor is recent unprotected intercourse. BV typically presents with a thin, gray-white discharge and a strong fishy odor, often more noticeable after sex. Unlike yeast infections, it rarely causes itching or redness. Left untreated, BV increases the risk of secondary infections and complications, including pelvic inflammatory disease (PID), which can lead to sepsis and long-term reproductive issues. Any patient with pelvic pain, fever, or worsening symptoms requires antibiotics and evacuation.

Definitive treatment includes antibiotics—most commonly metronidazole or clindamycin. In wilderness settings where these may not be available, management focuses on prevention and symptom control. Avoiding douching, maintaining hygiene, and staying hydrated may help support recovery. Probiotics containing *Lactobacillus* may be beneficial, but evidence is mixed.

Early recognition matters. Patients with mild symptoms may not need immediate evacuation, but worsening symptoms or systemic signs demand treatment. With BV now classified as an STI, partner treatment should be addressed to prevent recurrence. In remote environments, education on risk factors and prevention is critical.

What is a Bartholin's abscess, and how is it managed in the wilderness?

The Bartholin's glands, located on either side of the vaginal opening, produce mucus to lubricate the area—primarily during sexual activity. A Bartholin's cyst forms when one of these glands becomes blocked, leading to fluid buildup. Small, painless cysts may resolve on their own or with warm compresses. However, if infected, the cyst can form a Bartholin's abscess—marked by pain, redness, swelling, and impaired mobility.

Like most abscesses, antibiotics alone are not sufficient—drainage is required. In the wilderness, recognizing when incision and drainage (I&D) is needed is critical to prevent abscess progression or systemic illness.

If the abscess is soft and fluctuant, a small incision should be made at the softest—most swollen point using a clean blade. Pus should be expressed; and the cavity irrigated with clean water, hydrogen peroxide, or a diluted povidone-iodine solution. The wound must remain open and loosely packed with gauze to allow continued drainage as closure increases the risk of recurrence.

Pain relief is usually immediate. Adjunct antibiotics—such as doxycycline or trimethoprim-sulfamethoxazole

(Bactrim)—are appropriate if fever or surrounding cellulitis is present. NSAIDs or acetaminophen can help manage discomfort, and dressings should be changed daily.

Evacuate if the abscess worsens despite drainage, systemic symptoms develop, *the patient has diabetes* or cannot function due to pain or illness. Close monitoring is essential.

When is evacuation necessary for vaginal infections?

Most cases of vaginal irritation can be managed in the field without evacuation. Improving hygiene, keeping the area dry, and avoiding irritants like scented soaps or synthetic fabrics are often sufficient. Yeast infections, while uncomfortable, typically respond to antifungal treatments such as fluconazole or topical clotrimazole. If treated early, symptoms usually improve within a few days. Evacuation is rarely needed unless symptoms are severe, persistent, or limit mobility.

Bacterial infections are more concerning, especially in prolonged or remote settings. If abnormal discharge, strong odor, or irritation persists for several days without improvement—and no treatment is available—evacuation should be considered. Untreated infections may progress upward into the reproductive tract, leading to pelvic inflammatory disease (PID)—a serious ascending infection involving the uterus, fallopian tubes, or ovaries. Immediate evacuation is warranted if abdominal or pelvic pain, fever, or uterine tenderness develops, as PID requires antibiotics and definitive care.

Early recognition of worsening symptoms is essential. Delays in treatment increase the risk of complications especially in remote environments.

Red Flag Framework: Genitourinary Emergencies

What's an easy way to remember what signs and symptoms warrant evacuation using the Red Flag Framework?

For Genitourinary Emergencies: **BURN**

- **B**urning, painful, or blood with urination, fever, pelvic pain
- **U**nable to urinate despite urgency (urinary retention)
- **R**adiating flank pain (possible kidney infection/stone)
- **N**asty discharge (foul-smelling, discolored)

Any of these signs indicate a potentially serious condition, requiring immediate evaluation and possible evacuation to prevent permanent damage. When in doubt, follow the Red Flag Framework: BURN= Evacuate.

Emergency Childbirth in the Wilderness

Why is childbirth included in this book?

Childbirth is a natural process that has unfolded safely for millennia, even in remote and resource-limited environments. In most cases, labor progresses without the need for significant intervention, as the body is remarkably equipped to manage childbirth. Globally, most births happen uneventfully, and this remains true even in a wilderness setting.

So why include it? Because you never know. Most guides and guests will never have to assist in a birth, but the more you travel, the more unexpected situations arise. Wilderness guides are often the most capable person present in an emergency, and while childbirth is rare in the field—having a basic understanding of the process is valuable.

The reality is that childbirth is not a medical crisis unless something goes wrong. In most cases, the best thing a guide can offer is a calm, prepared approach. The goal is to support the natural process while ensuring the safety of both the mother and baby. With a steady demeanor, basic preparation, and a willingness to assist, a guide can help ensure a safe and natural delivery, even in a challenging environment.

Okay, so how do I assist with childbirth in the wilderness?

- *Check your own pulse first*, slow your breathing, and relax—you got this.
- *Prepare the area:* Create a clean, warm, and private space. Use sterile or clean supplies, including gloves, towels, and any antiseptics available. Position the mother semi reclined, with knees bent and feet supported, for comfort and access.
- *Recognize the stages of labor:* Delivery is imminent when contractions occur every 2-3 minutes and last for about a minute. Crowning, when the baby's head becomes visible at the vaginal opening, is a clear sign that birth is near.
- *Guide the delivery*: As the baby's head emerges, gently support it with your hands—avoiding any pulling. If the umbilical cord is wrapped around the neck, gently try to slip it over the baby's head. If that's not possible, clamp the cord in two places and cut between the clamps. After the head is delivered, the shoulders will follow—typically one at a time. Gently guide the head downward to help deliver the upper (anterior) shoulder, then slightly upward to assist with the lower (posterior) shoulder. Once the shoulders are clear, the rest of the body usually follows easily. Babies are slippery, so maintain a firm but controlled hold to prevent dropping.
- *Provide postpartum care for the baby*: Immediately dry the baby with clean towels to prevent heat loss and encourage skin-to-skin contact with the mother to keep warm. Clear the baby's nose and mouth of fluids if necessary. Tie (tightly) or clamp the umbilical cord in two places—first about 4 inches from the baby's belly and

the second about 2 inches further toward the placenta. Using a clean, sharp tool, cut the cord between the two clamps and *do not remove* the clamps or ties.

- *Deliver the placenta:* The placenta should be delivered naturally within 30 minutes. Do not pull on the umbilical cord. Place the placenta in a clean bag for medical evaluation if reasonable.

What are the postpartum priorities in the wilderness?

The main priorities after childbirth in remote settings are controlling bleeding, preventing infection, and supporting recovery. Once the placenta is delivered, the uterus must contract down tightly to compress the blood vessels that supplied it during pregnancy. This muscular contraction is the body's primary method of controlling bleeding. If the uterus stays soft, bleeding can continue unchecked. Gently massaging the lower abdomen—just above the pubic bone—can help stimulate contraction. If bleeding remains heavy—soaking more than one pad per hour or passing large clots—this may signal a serious complication, and evacuation should be arranged.

Infection is rarely an immediate concern but can develop over several days. Watch for rising fever, chills, increasing abdominal pain, or foul-smelling discharge starting around postpartum day 3 to 5. If a tear or episiotomy occurred during delivery, monitor the area daily for redness, swelling, or pus. If the wound is large and the patient is stable, it's acceptable to suture the laceration using clean technique and basic supplies—even if the sutures are temporary. A loosely approximated closure is better than leaving the tissue open, both for comfort and infection control. Clean gently with warm water only; avoid wipes, soaps, or antiseptics that may irritate healing tissue.

Additional considerations include hydration, warmth, calorie intake, and rest. Postpartum women lose a significant amount of fluid during delivery and are at higher risk for dizziness, fatigue, and hypothermia—especially in cold or high-altitude environments. Encourage frequent fluid intake and calorie-dense snacks to support healing and lactation. Protect from exposure, provide physical support when moving, and encourage short walks as tolerated to prevent blood clot formation in the legs. Pain is best managed with acetaminophen, as ibuprofen may increase bleeding risk in the immediate postpartum window.

Evacuation is necessary if bleeding does not slow after an hour, if infection is suspected, or if the mother shows signs of worsening weakness, confusion, or is unable to care for herself or the infant. When in doubt, support early and maintain a low threshold to evacuate.

Traumatic Injuries in Wilderness Settings

Overview

Why is there so much focus on traumatic injuries in the wilderness?

While wilderness medicine covers a broad range of clinical challenges, trauma remains one of the most common and consequential issues in remote settings. Unlike medical conditions that often develop gradually, injuries often occur without warning and demand rapid assessment, clear decision-making, and timely intervention—especially when definitive care may be hours or even days away.

Data from wilderness expeditions and backcountry rescue research show that soft tissue injuries, sprains, strains, and lower extremity fractures are among the most frequent problems encountered in the backcountry. Falls, slips, and overuse injuries top the list of mechanisms, especially during hiking, climbing, or backpacking. In mountainous or alpine regions, altitude illness, hypothermia, and dehydration often complicate otherwise manageable injuries. The combination of environmental exposure, varied terrain, and prolonged evacuation times means even minor trauma can quickly escalate to life-threatening if not managed correctly.

While this book isn't solely about trauma, injury management in remote settings is a core skill. Guides and responders must act decisively, improvise with limited resources, and know when to initiate evacuation. These decisions are trip, career and even life defining. In the moment, there may be no protocol, no second opinion, and no outside support. The ability to act—calmly, competently, and with limited resources—defines not just the outcome for the patient but the reputation and credibility of the responder.

Why is scene safety a priority?

Ensuring scene safety protects responders, patients, and bystanders. Wilderness settings pose unique hazards, including unstable terrain, extreme weather, and wildlife threats. Approaching an injured person without assessing the risks can turn one casualty into multiple, further complicating rescue efforts. A bad situation becomes much, much worse when an unaware rescuer becomes the next patient.

What is body substance isolation, and why does it matter in the wilderness?

Body substance isolation (BSI) is a critical infection-control practice that prevents exposure to blood, saliva, or other bodily fluids that may carry diseases like hepatitis B, hepatitis C, or HIV. With an estimated 300 million people living with hepatitis B and nearly 40 million with HIV, exposure risks in medical aid situations are very real considerations.

In wilderness settings, limited clean water, prolonged patient contact, and unpredictable emergency settings increase contamination risks. Gloves, CPR barrier devices, and alcohol-based sanitizers are essential. Masks protect against respiratory droplets in cases of coughing, bleeding, or suspected infections. While wilderness care often requires improvisation, body substance isolation (BSI) is a critical intervention ensuring both responder and patient safety and a higher standard of care.

What is the "golden hour," and does it apply in the wilderness?

The golden hour refers to the critical first 60 minutes after a traumatic injury, historically believed to be the window in which rapid intervention significantly improves survival outcomes. While modern research has challenged the strict time-dependent nature of this principle, studies continue to emphasize that early stabilization plays a crucial role in patient survival.

In wilderness medicine, where definitive care is often hours or even days away, the underlying concept of the golden hour remains highly relevant. Unlike urban settings with rapid Emergency Medical Services (EMS) transport and waiting trauma centers, wilderness guides must act as the first and often only responders for an extended period of time. In these scenarios, early interventions—controlling bleeding, stabilizing fractures, and preventing hypothermia—are critical to preventing the rapid deterioration of a patient. Even when evacuation is delayed, addressing immediate life threats within the first hour can significantly improve the chances of survival by slowing shock progression and preserving organ function until higher-level care is reached.

What is the "lethal triad" in trauma, and why does it matter?

The "lethal triad" describes a dangerous cycle involving *hypothermia*, *acidosis*, and *impaired blood clotting*—three factors that can rapidly worsen traumatic injuries and increase the risk of death. It all starts with major blood loss, which reduces circulating volume in the body and limits oxygen delivery to vital tissues. In response, cells shift to anaerobic metabolism, which produces lactic acid and lowers the body's pH. This acidotic state weakens heart function, impairs circulation, and disrupts enzymes needed for vital processes—including coagulation. As circulation declines, oxygen delivery falls even further, clotting becomes increasingly impaired, and bleeding accelerates—continuing the spiral.

Simultaneously, blood loss and environmental exposure drive down core body temperature. Hypothermia reduces platelet function and slows the enzymatic reactions of the coagulation cascade—as clotting fails, bleeding continues. This leads to further volume loss, worsening perfusion, and progressive shock.

The cycle is self-sustaining: tissue hypoxia drives acidosis, acidosis and hypothermia impair clotting, and this coagulopathy causes more bleeding. Once established, this physiologic spiral is difficult to reverse without blood products, warming measures, and advanced care.

In the wilderness, prevention is the only effective strategy. Stop the bleeding early, insulate aggressively to prevent heat loss, and support perfusion through fluid resuscitation and patient positioning. Recognizing the early signs and acting before this triad takes hold is ultimately going to be the difference between survival and collapse.

Why all this? Can't I just evacuate?

You could—but without immediate access to a helicopter and a trauma team, and with evacuation often delayed or logistically complex, you shouldn't. Wilderness trauma isn't the same as urban trauma. There's no imaging, no surgery, and no definitive care on standby. Delay, exposure, and limited resources are guaranteed.

Here's the reality: the situation won't be perfect. Often, it won't even be good. You won't always know if you're right. That's exactly why preparation, training, and a working understanding of the why behind your decisions matter. You're not just guiding evacuation—you're treating, stabilizing, and deciding how to move forward in real time.

Rapid Trauma Assessment: The Primary & Secondary Survey

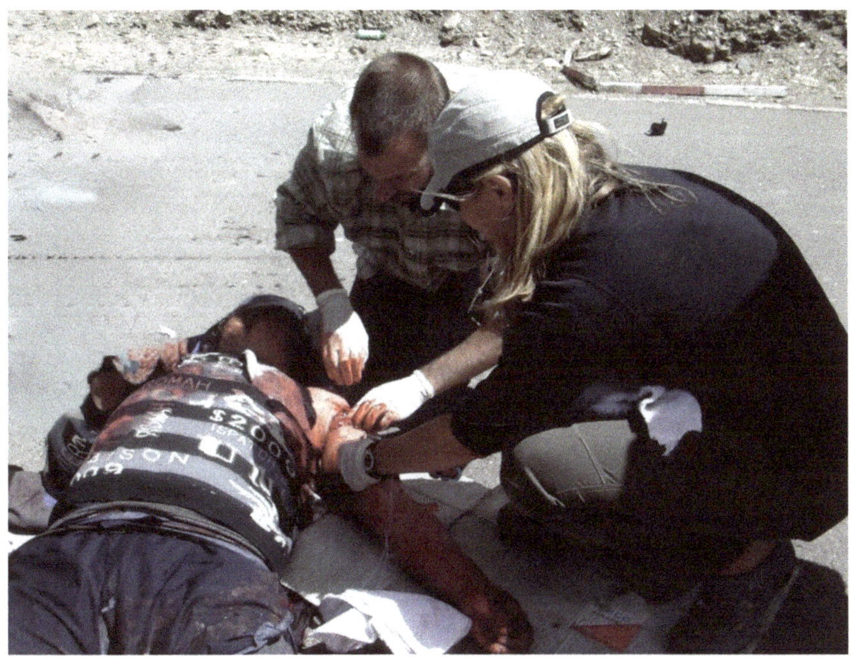

The author and expedition members rendering care to a motorcyclist who was thrown beneath a truck en route to the headwaters during the Yangtze River expedition. Massive extremity and head trauma required immediate hemorrhage control and field stabilization. Image courtesy of the author.

How are trauma assessments done?

From head-to-toe, the same way every time. The assessment is about *systematically* identifying injuries that require immediate stabilization or evacuation. The *primary* survey focuses on life-threatening issues: airway, breathing, circulation, disability (neurological status), and exposure. The *secondary* survey is a more detailed evaluation, looking for injuries that might have been missed initially.

Trauma patients in the wilderness aren't just dealing with their injuries. Environmental conditions, dehydration, exhaustion, and the stress of remote care all affect their ability to function—and yours. Understanding how the injury *fits* into the broader situation—terrain, weather, time, and resources—is often just as important as identifying the injury itself.

How should I perform the primary survey?

The goal of the primary survey is to *rapidly* identify and address immediate life threats. The components of the primary trauma survey include airway, breathing, circulation, disability (neurologic status), and exposure. Each component is assessed quickly, in order, and without interruption. This sequence is designed to catch the most serious problems first and guide immediate interventions—*especially* when resources are limited:

- *Airway and cervical spine*

  Ensure the airway is open. If the patient is unconscious or injured above the shoulders, assume a spinal injury until proven otherwise. Use manual stabilization while opening the airway. If the patient can talk clearly, the airway is intact. If not, assess for obstruction, facial trauma, or swelling. Inspect the mouth and jaw for deformity or bleeding. Stabilize the cervical spine if there's midline tenderness, altered mental status, or distracting injuries.
- *Breathing*

  Expose the chest and inspect for obvious deformity, bruising, or paradoxical motion. Listen for breath sounds—decreased or absent sounds may suggest pneumothorax or hemothorax. Palpate for tenderness or crepitus. If respiratory distress is worsening, initiate evacuation immediately.
- *Circulation*

  Check for signs of major bleeding. Control external hemorrhage with pressure and tourniquets as needed. Assess for skin color, temperature, and capillary refill—these give early clues about perfusion. Feel for radial pulses. Weak or absent pulses suggest hypovolemia or shock. A rising heart rate with cool, clammy skin is a warning sign.

- *Disability* (Neurologic Status)

  Use the *AVPU* scale to assess mental status: *Al*ert, responds to *V*erbal, responds to *P*ain, *U*nresponsive. Any decline from baseline, or new confusion, agitation, or unresponsiveness, should raise concern for head injury, shock, or low oxygenation.
- *Exposure/Environmental Control*

  Expose the patient fully to assess for hidden injuries, then immediately protect them from cold, wind, or wet conditions. Even mild hypothermia can worsen bleeding and shock.

Note: While the traditional sequence for the primary survey is ABCD—airway, breathing, circulation, disability—there are situations, particularly in the setting of massive hemorrhage, where circulation must take priority. In those cases, CAB may be the appropriate order to control life-threatening bleeding *before* managing airway and breathing.

What is the role of the secondary survey?

Once life-threatening issues have been addressed, the secondary survey provides a systematic head-to-toe assessment to identify additional injuries that may not have been apparent during the primary evaluation. This step ensures that potentially serious conditions are not missed and helps guide further stabilization and decision-making. In remote settings where evacuation is delayed, ongoing reassessment are critical. Early recognition of deterioration can make the difference between a manageable injury and a crisis.

During the secondary survey, the head and neck are examined for bleeding, deformities, or signs of skull or facial fractures. Pupil size and reactivity are checked, and cervical spine precautions are maintained. The chest is evaluated for tenderness, bruising, or asymmetrical movement, which could signal internal injury, rib fractures, a flail chest, or a pneumothorax. The abdomen is palpated for tenderness, rigidity, or distension—findings that raise concern for internal bleeding and organ injury. The pelvis is assessed for stability and signs of trauma, such as bruising or blood at the urethra.

Extremities are inspected for deformity, swelling, open wounds, and checked for circulation, sensation, and movement. Suspected fractures or dislocations should be reduced and stabilized and wounds managed. Neurologic function should be reassessed frequently, as changes in mental status, speech, or limb function may indicate evolving brain or spinal cord injury.

The secondary survey refines the treatment plan, helping to prioritize injuries, guides evacuation decisions, and improve patient outcomes—especially in prolonged wilderness care scenarios, where early recognition of evolving conditions is critical.

Further discussion regarding anatomy, physiology, and management considerations for each anatomical region are addressed in the following sections.

When is evacuation necessary for trauma patients?

Usually. Evacuation is necessary when a patient's condition exceeds the capacity of field care or when delaying definitive treatment increases the risk of serious complications or death. Life-threatening conditions—including airway compromise, uncontrollable hemorrhage, shock, altered mental status, head injuries, or environmental threats—require immediate evacuation, as they often demand advanced medical interventions that cannot be safely or effectively performed in a remote setting.

When determining the need for evacuation, consider the patient's overall trajectory, recognizing that an initially stable injury can deteriorate due to infection, worsening of the condition, or environmental challenges. If there is any uncertainty about the ability to manage the patient effectively in the field, evacuation should always be prioritized.

On the Edge of the Yangtze

The smoke—it's probably just burning trash, but it always gets me. It takes me back to remote places, the smell of it heavy in the air, pungent…now familiar.

We were traveling through the highlands of China, en route to explore the headwaters of the Yangtze. The road cut through windswept plateaus, where paved roads gave way to gravel paths, and then back again, as we passed through sparse towns. Brightly colored shops lined the streets, offering a sharp contrast to the rugged landscape. The sun hung high, its light harsh and unfamiliar compared to home—now a lifetime away. The air was thin, and the mountainous landscape stretched forever, jagged peaks towering over us like silent sentinels.

It was during this stretch that the truck came to a sudden stop, jerking everyone awake from their momentary daze. Stepping out into the dusty air, the scene unfolded before us: a man lay in the middle of the road, his motorcycle a twisted wreck beside him. He'd tried to overtake a large truck, clipped the mirror, and was thrown beneath the wheels

The injuries were severe. A large head laceration—nearly a scalping—exposed skull. His humerus was broken near the shoulder, glistening bone out in the sun. But the worst was his left leg—a near-complete traumatic amputation below the knee, with blood pulsing out with every beat of his heart, pooling on the oily tarmac.

Acting quickly, with an ER nurse and a couple of guides making up our medical team, a strap was turned into a makeshift tourniquet and applied a few inches above the knee. The bleeding stopped like a faucet shut off. His olive skin had gone gray—shock was washing over him.

A bystander's umbrella became an impromptu splint. The aged, hand-smoothed wooden umbrella handle was positioned in his armpit, and his wrist was secured to it, realigning the broken humerus, immediately slowing the bleeding.

The scalp tissue was repositioned as best as possible and wrapped tight under a pressure dressing. A blanket from the back of a passing mechanic truck went around him, preserving his valuable body heat.

We loaded him into that same truck and asked the driver to transport him to the nearest town.

Three weeks later, after completing the expedition, we got word: he made it. The leg was amputated in the hospital. But he lived.

This case highlights the critical importance of sticking to the basics—a thorough primary survey, hemorrhage control, fracture stabilization, and hypothermia prevention.

In this case, the basics of trauma care worked out for our patient, even far from home.

Head Injuries

Why are head injuries a significant concern in wilderness settings?

Head injuries present unique challenges in the wilderness due to the lack of diagnostic imaging, advanced monitoring, and critical interventions. Clinical evaluation and your knowledge are the only tools available to assess severity, making the recognition of worsening symptoms critical. Falls, climbing accidents, and high-impact activities can result in head trauma ranging from minor concussions to life-threatening brain injuries. The variability in how head injuries present across individuals further complicates assessment, as some patients may initially appear stable before deteriorating rapidly.

Complications such as swelling, bleeding, or increased intracranial pressure (ICP) can develop gradually or suddenly. Symptoms like persistent headache, nausea, vomiting, confusion, or changes in consciousness signal a worsening condition that requires immediate attention. In remote environments, where evacuation is often delayed, these complications can become life-threatening.

What should I know about the anatomy of the head?

The head is made up of the scalp, skull, and brain—each with a distinct role in protection and function. The scalp is highly vascular and helps absorb impact, but even minor cuts can bleed significantly. Beneath it, the skull forms a rigid barrier around the brain. It has only one major exit—the foramen magnum at the base of the occipital bone—where the brainstem connects to the spinal cord.

Inside the skull, the brain is surrounded by three protective layers called meninges and suspended in cerebrospinal fluid (CSF). This fluid cushions against impact, delivers nutrients, and clears waste. The brain controls everything from movement, thought, and coordination to breathing and heart rate. Because it's confined within a closed space, any swelling or bleeding can raise intracranial pressure—something that can become life-threatening, *especially in remote settings*.

Bones of the Skull

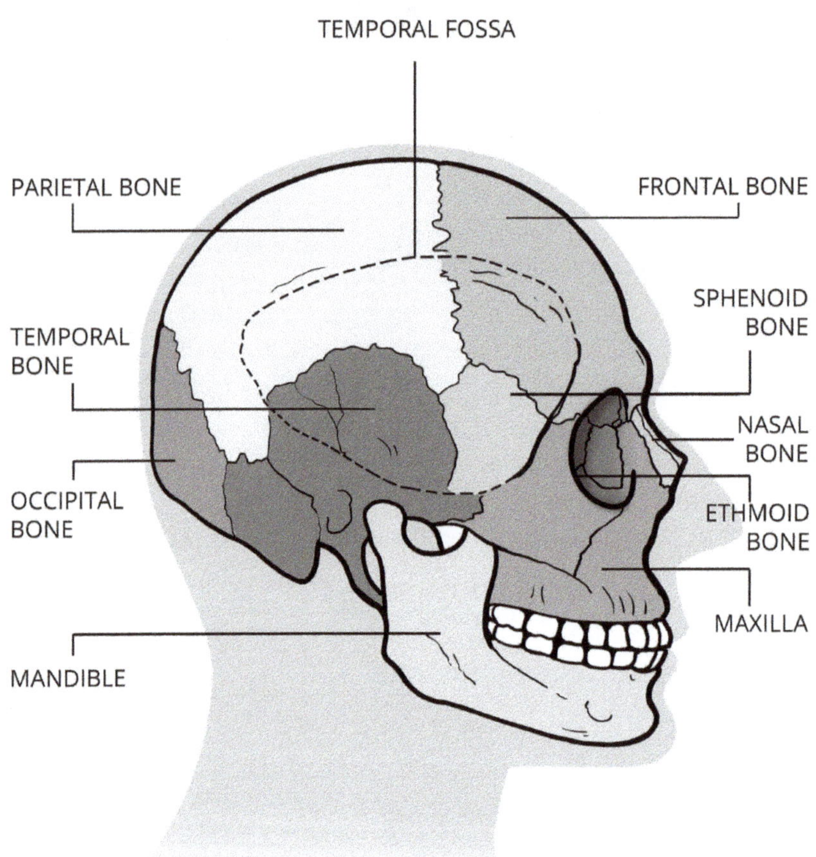

What is the Monro-Kellie Doctrine?

The Monro-Kellie Doctrine describes the skull as a closed, fixed space containing three main components: brain tissue, blood, and cerebrospinal fluid (CSF). Because the skull can't expand, any increase in one component must be offset by a decrease in another to keep intracranial pressure (ICP) stable. When bleeding, swelling, or fluid buildup occurs, pressure rises. With nowhere else to go, the brain is forced downward toward the only opening in the skull—the foramen magnum at the base of the occipital bone.

This process, called brain herniation, compresses the brainstem—the area responsible for breathing, heart rate, and blood pressure. If pressure continues to rise, the brainstem fails. Breathing stops. Circulation collapses. Death follows.

In the wilderness, there's no imaging, no surgical relief, and no way to control intracranial bleeding. Once herniation starts, reversal is unlikely. Early signs—worsening headache, persistent vomiting, confusion, unequal pupils, and declining mental status—require urgent evacuation. Any delay increases the risk of permanent injury or death.

This Monroe-Kellie Doctrine is not to be confused with the Monroe Doctrine of 1823—a U.S. foreign policy warning European powers to stay out of the Americas—the Monro-Kellie Doctrine deals with anatomy and the consequences of swelling in a confined space.

How is intracranial hemorrhage managed in the wilderness?

It isn't. Intracranial hemorrhage (ICH) is a life-threatening emergency that requires surgical intervention. There is no definitive treatment in the field beyond stabilization and immediate evacuation. Patients on anticoagulants are at significantly higher risk, even from minor trauma, due to impaired clotting and uncontrolled bleeding—conditions that cannot be managed in a remote setting.

Field care focuses on minimizing secondary injury. The patient's head should be elevated to approximately 30° to help reduce intracranial pressure. NSAIDs and aspirin should be avoided; acetaminophen is the preferred option for pain control. Neurologic status should be monitored using the AVPU scale (alert, verbal, pain, unresponsive), with close observation for any signs of deterioration. Oxygen should be administered if available. Hypothermia must be prevented, and hydration should be maintained without excessive fluid intake, which can worsen cerebral swelling.

Evacuation is mandatory for any suspected ICH or worsening head injury symptoms. Prolonged unconsciousness, repeated vomiting, slurred speech, seizures, or signs of rising ICP—such as confusion, unequal pupils, or declining mental status—require immediate transport. In the most severe cases, abnormal "posturing" may develop. This occurs when rising intracranial pressure causes compression of motor pathways in the brain. There are two main patterns:

- *Decorticate* posturing appears when the arms bend toward the chest ("to the core"), the legs extend, and the fists clench. It typically signals a brain injury above the brainstem, usually involving the cerebral hemispheres. This posturing happens when higher brain centers lose control but the midbrain remains partially functional, allowing some reflex pathways to remain active.
- *Decerebrate* posturing presents as full extension and inward rotation of the arms, straightened legs, and sometimes arching of the neck and back. It reflects a more severe brain injury involving the brainstem, where even midbrain control is lost. With higher centers no longer regulating movement, lower brainstem pathways dominate, producing an unopposed extensor response throughout the body.

Both patterns are late signs of catastrophic brain injury and should be considered premorbid findings in the wilderness setting. They are useful for recognizing the severity of damage but do not change field management. If you're seeing posturing, the chance of meaningful neurologic recovery is extremely low.

Because deterioration can occur without warning and intracranial pressure cannot be monitored in the field, early evacuation remains the safest and only viable option. Prompt recognition, stabilization, and transport give the patient the best chance of survival.

What is a concussion, and how should it be managed?

A concussion is a mild traumatic brain injury (mTBI) caused by a blow to the head or rapid acceleration–deceleration forces that disrupt normal brain function. The sudden movement of the brain within the skull stretches and shears neurons, triggering a cascade of metabolic changes that temporarily impair the brain's ability to regulate function. Following the injury, the brain enters a period of altered metabolism where it demands *more* energy for recovery, but experiences *reduced* blood flow, contributing to symptoms such as headache, dizziness, nausea, and cognitive fog.

In the wilderness, rest and symptom monitoring are the priorities. Physical and cognitive exertion should be minimized to allow the brain to recover. Acetaminophen can be used for headache relief, but NSAIDs like ibuprofen or aspirin should be avoided initially due to the risk of bleeding. If symptoms worsen, new neurological deficits appear, or there is any decline in mental status, immediate evacuation is required. Concussions are common in high-impact outdoor activities such as climbing, biking, skiing, and whitewater sports; and without proper management, symptoms can persist, worsening recovery time and increasing the risk of long-term complications.

When should a concussed patient be evacuated, and when can they return to activity?

Evacuation is mandatory for any patient with deteriorating mental status, repeated vomiting, worsening headache, difficulty waking, unequal pupils, or seizures. Even if symptoms seem mild, delayed complications like post-concussion syndrome or intracranial bleeding remain possible, especially in remote settings where early warning signs may go unnoticed. If there is any doubt about the severity of the injury, erring on the side of evacuation is always the safest option.

Returning to activity should be a gradual process, with light exertion reintroduced slowly. Any increase in symptoms-such as headaches, dizziness, nausea, or cognitive difficulties-indicates that the brain is still healing and requires more rest. Pushing through symptoms prolongs recovery and increases the risk of post-concussion syndrome, where symptoms persist for weeks or months, significantly impairing function in remote environments. Activities with a high risk of head impact, such as climbing, skiing, or rafting, must be strictly avoided until full recovery is confirmed. Sustaining a second head injury before healing is complete can result in severe swelling, long-term neurologic damage, or in extreme cases, fatal complications. In the wilderness, reinjury can be devastating, making a cautious approach to recovery essential before resuming any physically demanding or high-risk tasks. If symptoms persist longer than expected or worsen over time, evacuation should be considered to rule out more serious complications.

How do I identify and manage a skull fracture in the wilderness?

Managing a skull fracture in the wilderness requires caution and prompt action to prevent further injury or complications. A fracture should be suspected with significant head trauma, visible deformity, deep scalp lacerations, or signs of a basilar skull fracture—such as bruising around the eyes (raccoon eyes), bruising behind the ears (Battle's sign), or clear fluid leaking from the nose or ears, which may indicate cerebrospinal fluid (CSF) leakage.

Direct pressure should not be applied to the injury, especially if the skull is depressed or the wound is open. Instead, cover the area lightly with a sterile, noncompressive dressing to limit contamination without increasing pressure. If CSF is leaking, keeping the wound clean is critical to reducing the risk of infection (meningitis). If available, oral antibiotics should be given to help prevent infection, and the head should be elevated to approximately 30° to help lower intracranial pressure.

Evacuation is mandatory. Skull fractures often require imaging to assess for swelling, bleeding, or infection. Neurological status should be monitored closely, including level of consciousness, pupil response, and motor function. Even minor-appearing injuries can conceal serious underlying brain trauma, making early transport to definitive care essential.

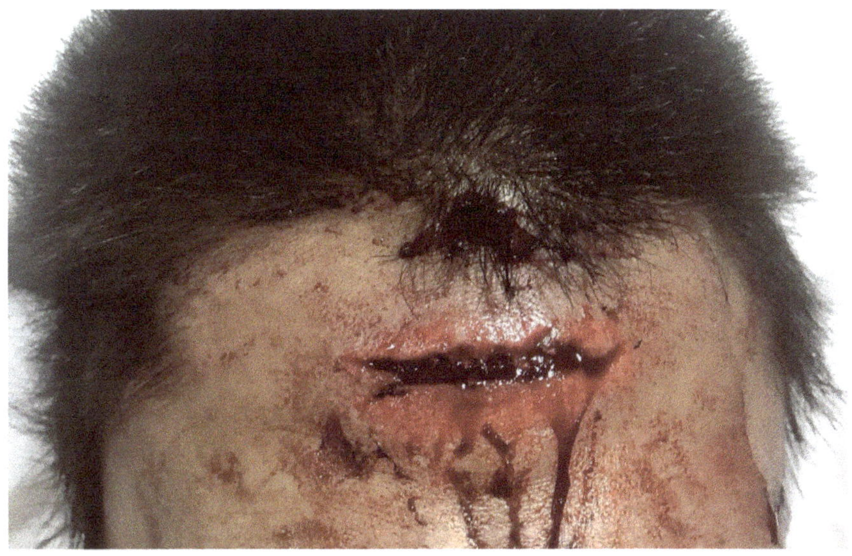

Scalp laceration with underlying skull fracture. Blunt-force trauma to an (unhelmeted) forehead from an oar strike while whitewater rafting, with obvious soft tissue injury and instability of the underlying skull. Managed in the field with cervical precautions, hemorrhage control, and prompt evacuation. Image courtesy of the author.

What should I do for scalp lacerations?

Scalp lacerations often bleed heavily due to the scalp's dense vascular supply. Bleeding is typically controlled with firm, direct pressure using a clean dressing or cloth. Pressure may need to be held for several minutes to allow clot formation. If bleeding persists, a hemostatic dressing or compressive bandage may help. Once bleeding is controlled, the wound should be gently rinsed with clean water or saline to remove debris. Excessive probing should be avoided, especially if a skull fracture is suspected.

Minor, superficial lacerations can be closed with sutures, staples, or adhesive strips. In remote settings, tying adjacent hair strands across the wound can help approximate the edges when no formal closure tools are available. A sterile, nonstick dressing should be applied to protect the wound, with ongoing monitoring for infection–redness, swelling, or discharge. If signs of infection develop, antibiotics should be started and evacuation considered.

Tetanus vaccination status must be verified. If the wound is heavily contaminated or if closure is delayed, empiric antibiotics should be considered to reduce the risk of infection. Evacuation is necessary if the wound exposes bone, continues bleeding despite proper pressure, or shows signs of infection. If there is visible deformity, palpable step-off, or associated neurologic symptoms suggesting a skull fracture, immediate evacuation is required.

Head High

A decade back, me and the boys were in El Salvador, chasing waves and shaking off the frigid Colorado winter. Mornings were slow, afternoons thick with heat, and the ocean was everything we needed. We'd been taking a panga up the coast to a reef break—nothing but warm-water, empty waves, and a boat captain half-asleep in the sun.

That morning, the setup was perfect. Head high, light offshores with an easy takeoff, finishing with a little barrel section over the edge of the rock reef. No crowds, no noise—just smiles.

I dropped in—easy, clean entry—everything lining up. But as the wave hit the deep channel and lost its speed, and I kicked into the deep water, something went wrong. Maybe my foot slipped, maybe the board caught wind—whatever it was, I came down hard—my skull slamming into the bottom of the board.

That was one of those moments where you inherently know the difference between being hurt and being injured.

I knew I hit hard, but it didn't seem like that big of a big deal. At least, that's what I thought—until the boys paddled over, asking what the hell I was doing floating around in the impact zone. I didn't have an answer.

By the time we got back to the boat, my head was pounding. By the time we hit the cabanas, I was in a bad way. The headache was relentless—deep, brutal—different. My roommate, an orthopedic surgeon, and I—both with extensive experience in trauma care—took one look at each other and knew what the real concern was. Brain bleed. Not a diagnosis—yet—but something we couldn't ignore. And we were stuck. No flights out, no real options. Not much in the way of choices.

Around the 30-hour mark, I could finally sit up, but even a sip of water came right back up. Turns out, when the brain takes a hit like that, it needs the only fuel source it can handle—sugar. I don't drink soda. Don't touch refined sugars. But in that moment, there wasn't enough Coca-Cola and white bread in the country for me.

I finally got a CT scan when we made it back to Colorado. This one turned out not to be a bleed—thankfully, a concussion. Appropriately, we avoided ibuprofen or aspirin, stuck with Tylenol and rest, because, frankly, that was the best we could manage at the time.

Looking back, I keep thinking, what if this had happened to someone else? If I'd been the one taking care of them? Or worse, if I did have a bleed, far from help in El Salvador?

The mechanism wasn't all that dramatic, but it doesn't need to be to end a trip—or worse.

Traumatic Eye Injuries

How should eyelid lacerations be managed in the wilderness?

Eyelid lacerations require careful assessment to rule out globe injury before addressing the wound itself. Signs of serious ocular involvement—such as an irregular pupil, decreased visual acuity, or visible foreign material—must be identified early. Missed globe injuries can result in permanent vision loss.

For superficial lacerations that do not involve the eyelid margin or deeper structures, the wound should be irrigated thoroughly with clean or sterile water to remove debris. Temporary closure can often be achieved using adhesive strips (e.g., Steri-Strips) to approximate wound edges with minimal trauma. A topical antibiotic ointment can reduce infection risk, and the wound should be monitored for signs of infection, including increasing redness, swelling, or discharge.

More complex lacerations require additional caution. Deep or full-thickness wounds, or those involving the eyelid margin or tear drainage system (the nasolacrimal duct), should not be manipulated in the field. The nasolacrimal duct helps drain tears from the eye into the nose, and damage can lead to chronic tearing or infection. After gentle cleaning to reduce contamination, the area should be covered with a nonadhesive sterile dressing. If the globe is intact, it should be protected with a rigid shield (e.g., a clean cup) to prevent further trauma. In cases of delayed evacuation, oral antibiotics are recommended, especially for contaminated or high-risk wounds.

Evacuation is required for any full-thickness laceration, involvement of the eyelid margin or tear ducts, or injuries with significant tissue loss. These wounds typically require surgical repair to preserve eyelid function and protect the eye.

What is an orbital fracture, and how is it managed in the wilderness?

An orbital fracture occurs when one or more bones of the eye socket break due to blunt trauma, such as a fall, punch, or impact from an object. The orbit is a thin, complex bony structure that supports the globe and houses muscles, nerves, and vessels. The floor and medial wall are particularly fragile and prone to fracture when intraorbital pressure increases suddenly during trauma.

Depending on location and severity, an orbital fracture can impair vision, restrict eye movement, or damage nearby structures. Blowout fractures of the orbital floor may allow fat and the inferior rectus muscle to herniate into the maxillary sinus, leading to entrapment. This often presents as restricted upward gaze and double vision (diplopia). Air from the sinuses may enter the orbit through fracture lines, resulting in *orbital emphysema*, with swelling, and limited eye movement. A retrobulbar hemorrhage, or bleeding behind the globe, is a vision-threatening emergency. Rapid accumulation of blood increases intraorbital pressure, compresses the optic nerve and central retinal artery, and may cause permanent vision loss.

Common signs of orbital fracture include:

- Periorbital swelling and bruising (black eye)
- Restricted or painful eye movement, especially upward
- Double vision in specific directions
- A sunken (enophthalmic) or bulging (exophthalmic) eye
- Numbness in the cheek or upper lip (infraorbital nerve involvement)
- Sudden vision changes or signs of orbital pressure

Field management begins with stabilizing the patient and protecting the injured eye. No pressure should be applied to the orbit. A rigid eye shield, such as a clean cup, should be used to prevent further trauma. The patient should avoid blowing the nose or sneezing, as this can force air into the orbit and worsen emphysema or swelling.

Eye movement should be assessed. Inability to look upward or worsening diplopia (double vision) suggests muscle entrapment and requires urgent evacuation. Progressive swelling, vision loss, or signs of optic nerve compression suggest retrobulbar hemorrhage, a surgical emergency.

Pain may be treated with acetaminophen. If evacuation is delayed, oral antibiotics should be considered to reduce the risk of sinus-related infection. All suspected orbital fractures require evacuation for imaging and definitive care to prevent long-term complications, including persistent diplopia, infection, or vision loss.

What is orbital compartment syndrome, and how is it managed in the wilderness?

Orbital compartment syndrome is a vision-threatening emergency caused by a rapid rise in pressure within the eye itself. This is most often due to a retrobulbar hematoma—bleeding behind the eye that accumulates within the confined bony socket. As pressure builds, it compresses the optic nerve and retinal blood vessels, eventually cutting off blood flow. If not recognized and treated quickly, permanent vision loss can occur within hours.

In wilderness settings, orbital compartment syndrome can result from blunt facial trauma, orbital fractures, penetrating injuries, burns, and infections. The orbit is a fixed space, and even a small amount of bleeding or swelling can critically increase intraorbital pressure. Key findings include a bulging eye (proptosis), marked orbital swelling, pain with eye movement, blurred or double vision, and a dilated, *nonreactive* pupil—a red flag for optic nerve compromise. Patients often describe a deep pressure or tightness behind the eye. These signs should be considered an emergency requiring immediate action.

Definitive treatment is surgical decompression, typically a lateral canthotomy, which is rarely possible in the field. Management focuses on protecting the eye and arranging rapid evacuation. The affected eye should be shielded using a rigid, noncompressive barrier such as a clean cup or improvised shield. Pressure must never be applied to the eye or orbit. Elevating the patient's head can help reduce intraorbital pressure. Pain should be treated with acetaminophen rather than NSAIDs, as nonsteroidal agents may worsen bleeding. If evacuation will be delayed or there is concern for open fracture or penetrating injury, oral antibiotics should be given to reduce infection risk. *Gentle* cold compresses may help reduce swelling, but they are not a substitute for definitive care.

Evacuation is mandatory. Orbital compartment syndrome is a time-sensitive emergency. Field stabilization may buy time, but vision can only be preserved with prompt surgical intervention.

What is an open globe injury, and how is it managed?

An open globe injury is a full-thickness rupture or laceration of the eye, typically caused by penetrating trauma or severe blunt force. It compromises the structural integrity of the globe, exposing internal contents and creating a high risk of infection and permanent vision loss. Key signs include a soft or sunken eye, an irregular or teardrop-shaped pupil, visible extrusion of intraocular contents, and hyphema (blood pooling in the anterior chamber). Patients may report sudden vision loss, severe pain, or a sensation that part of the eye is missing. Any penetrating or high-impact eye trauma should be treated as an open globe injury until proven otherwise.

Management in the field centers on protection and preventing further damage. No pressure should be applied to the eye. The globe should be shielded with a rigid barrier, such as a clean cup, to avoid contact or contamination. The eye should *not* be irrigated or manipulated. Oral antibiotics should be started if available, especially when evacuation is delayed.

The patient should remain calm and avoid straining, bending over, or movement that increases intraocular pressure. Pain may be managed with acetaminophen. NSAIDs should be avoided due to bleeding risk. If possible, the head should be kept elevated roughly 30°. Evacuation is mandatory. Open globe injuries require surgical repair and carry a high risk of vision loss if not addressed quickly.

How should chemical eye injuries be managed?

Chemical eye injuries require immediate and sustained irrigation to remove the harmful substance and limit tissue damage. The cleanest available water—bottled, previously boiled, or filtered—should be used to flush the eye continuously for at least 20 minutes. The patient's head should be positioned so the affected eye is lower than the uninjured one to prevent cross-contamination. Flushing should continue until symptoms such as burning or irritation begin to subside. After irrigation, ophthalmic antibiotics should be applied if available to reduce the risk of infection. Pain may be managed with acetaminophen or ibuprofen.

Evacuation is necessary for any chemical exposure that results in severe pain, vision changes, or persistent irritation despite adequate flushing. Alkaline burns—from substances like lye, ammonia, or cement dust—are especially dangerous, as they penetrate deeper and continue causing damage long after contact. Acidic burns are usually more superficial but can still result in serious corneal injury.

If pain, redness, or blurred vision persists after 30 minutes of continuous irrigation, urgent evacuation is required. Delayed complications—such as corneal scarring, ulceration, or secondary infection—can occur even after minor exposure. Any worsening discomfort increased light sensitivity, difficulty keeping the eye open, or changes in vision should prompt immediate evacuation to prevent permanent damage.

Red Flag Framework: Ocular Emergencies

What's an easy way to remember what signs and symptoms warrant evacuation using the Red Flag Framework?

For Ocular Emergencies: **SEE**

- **S**udden vision changes or loss
- **E**ye pain, redness, or swelling in or around the eye
- **E**xternal trauma or globe penetration

Any of these signs indicate a potentially serious condition, requiring immediate evaluation and possible evacuation. When in doubt, follow the Red Flag Framework: SEE = Evacuate.

Neck & Cervical Spine Injuries

How common are cervical spine injuries in wilderness settings?

Overall, cervical spine injuries are present in an estimated 2–5% of trauma patients with higher rates observed in those with blunt head trauma, altered mental status, or focal neurologic findings. These injuries are particularly concerning in wilderness settings, where limited diagnostics, prolonged extrication, and the risk of secondary spinal cord injury demand a cautious approach to assessment and stabilization.

What is the anatomy of the cervical spine, and why is it important?

The cervical spine consists of the first seven vertebrae (C1–C7). It supports the skull, allows head movement, and protects the spinal cord as it exits the brainstem. The upper vertebrae—the atlas (C1) and axis (C2)—control rotation and nodding and are especially prone to injury due to their mobility.

The spinal cord travels through the vertebral canal and paired spinal nerve roots exit between each vertebra to supply motor and sensory function to the upper body. Damage at any level can affect the corresponding nerve roots, leading to weakness, numbness, or paralysis. High cervical injuries (C1–C4) can impair breathing by disrupting input to the phrenic nerve, which controls the diaphragm. Lower injuries (C5–C7) often affect arm and shoulder function while sparing respiration.

Cervical spine injuries typically result from sudden acceleration or deceleration, hyperflexion, hyperextension, or axial loading—such as diving into shallow water and striking the bottom. These forces can cause fractures, dislocations, or ligament disruption. When the spinal cord or nerve roots are involved, the consequences may be permanent.

How do I assess and manage cervical spine injuries?

Cervical spine evaluation in wilderness settings relies entirely on clinical assessment. The goal is to identify injuries that may threaten the spinal cord while avoiding unnecessary immobilization, which can complicate transport and delay care.

The following criteria are adapted from two of the most widely used decision tools in emergency medicine: the NEXUS Criteria and the Canadian C-Spine Rule. While this combined approach hasn't been formally validated for wilderness use, it remains a practical field reference to help guides and responders recognize red flags. It's an educational tool—not a clinical directive—and should always be applied with judgment.

This framework is intended for patients who are alert, stable, under the age of 65, and without high-risk features. The decision to immobilize or evacuate must be based on the mechanism of injury, the patient's presentation, and the responder's training.

Cervical spine injury should be assumed if any of the following are present:

- Midline cervical spine tenderness
- Intoxication or altered mental status

- Neurologic symptoms (e.g., weakness, numbness, or loss of coordination)
- A distracting or significant secondary injury
- A high-risk mechanism (e.g., fall from height or direct axial load to the head)
- Pain with neck flexion, extension, or rotation

If any of these features are present, spinal precautions should be maintained and evacuation prioritized. *Even when all criteria are met, a subtle injury may still be present.* This tool is a guide—not a guarantee. In remote settings, early stabilization and motion control are critical, as spinal cord compromise is often irreversible.

What are the risks of unnecessary immobilization in wilderness settings?

Unnecessary immobilization can worsen hypothermia, increase discomfort, and complicate evacuation. Rigid collars and spinal precautions can restrict natural movement, making transport far more difficult through rough terrain. In remote environments, balancing the *risks* of injury with the *realities* of evacuation is crucial, and cervical spine immobilization should not be applied indiscriminately.

What makes penetrating neck trauma so dangerous?

It's a hot mess. The neck is compact and unforgiving: Major arteries, veins, airway structures, the spinal cord, and key nerve pathways all run within centimeters of one another. Penetrating trauma here can rapidly compromise multiple systems at once. Airway involvement may present as hoarseness, stridor, gurgling respirations, or subcutaneous emphysema from air leaking into soft tissue. Tracheal injury can cause bubbling at the wound site. Vascular injury is suggested by pulsatile bleeding or an expanding hematoma. Neurologic signs like weakness, numbness, or altered mental status signal spinal cord or nerve root damage. Difficulty speaking or swallowing can indicate esophageal violation. Bleeding in this region is often brisk and difficult to control due to the high-pressure arterial system and lack of available space for compression.

Initial field treatment is rapid hemorrhage control and airway protection. If direct pressure fails and the wound is deep, balloon tamponade is a viable field intervention. A Foley catheter or any long, narrow balloon can be carefully inserted to the *base of the wound*. Even if done blind, the goal is to advance fully to the *bottom* of the wound tract before inflation. Inflate slowly while monitoring for bleeding control—this may be the only way to tamponade bleeding from deep arterial or venous structures in the neck when surgical control is not available. Once the bleeding stops, secure the catheter in place and leave it during evacuation.

The Rest of the Spine

Why is spinal trauma a critical concern in the wilderness?

The spine is both a structural support and a protective channel for the spinal cord, which transmits signals between the brain and body. It consists of 33 vertebrae, divided into cervical (7), thoracic (12), lumbar (5), sacral (5, fused), and coccygeal (4, fused) regions. Intervertebral discs between most vertebrae act as shock absorbers and allow flexibility. Paired spinal nerve roots exit between each vertebra, carrying motor and sensory signals to specific regions of the body.

Spinal trauma—including fractures, dislocations, or ligament injuries—can compromise the spinal cord or its nerve roots, leading to temporary or permanent neurologic deficits. In wilderness settings, common causes include falls, blunt trauma, and high-energy impacts. The higher the injury, the more severe the functional loss. Cervical spine injuries are especially dangerous due to the risk of respiratory compromise. In the field, spinal cord injury is potentially life-altering, and early recognition with careful handling is critical to preventing further harm.

What are the key signs and symptoms of spinal trauma?

Spinal injuries may present with pain, tenderness, swelling, or visible deformity along the spine, but the most concerning signs are neurological. Numbness, tingling, weakness, or paralysis below the injury level suggest spinal cord involvement. Loss of bowel or bladder control, difficulty breathing, or signs of spinal shock(such as a slow heart rate and low blood pressure)indicate a severe injury requiring immediate attention.

Each region of the spine plays a distinct role in movement, sensation, and autonomic function and injuries at different levels result in different deficits:

- Cervical spine (C1-C7): Injuries at or above C3 can impair breathing due to phrenic nerve dysfunction, which controls the diaphragm. Damage at these levels can result in quadriplegia (loss of function in all four limbs) and, in severe cases, complete respiratory failure.
- Thoracic spine (T1-T12): Injuries can affect the ribcage and autonomic nervous system, leading to issues with temperature regulation, blood pressure control, and loss of sensation on the chest and abdomen. Loss of motor function at the thoracic level typically affects the lower body, while arm and hand function may remain intact.
- Lumbar spine (L1-L5): Injuries may impair leg strength and coordination, potentially leading to weakness, paralysis, or difficulty walking. In severe cases, lumbar injuries can cause cauda equina syndrome, a condition where nerve compression disrupts bowel and bladder function, "saddle" sensation, and lower limb control. This is a surgical emergency even in hospital settings and requires urgent evacuation from remote environments.
- Sacral spine (S1-S5): Damage at this level can interfere with pelvic control, bowel and bladder function, and lower limb movement. While sacral injuries are less

common, they can still cause debilitating effects on mobility and sensation.

Any high-force mechanism of injury, particularly if the patient is unconscious, disoriented, or has associated head trauma, warrants a high suspicion of spinal injury, even in the absence of obvious symptoms on physical exam. Any uncertainty should favor immobilization and evacuation, as missing an unstable spine injury can result in permanent disability.

How should spinal trauma be managed?

The priority in managing suspected spinal injury is to prevent further harm by minimizing movement. Keep the patient still and stabilize the head and neck in a neutral position. If a cervical collar is available, apply it. If not, use rolled clothing or soft padding secured with tape or straps to limit motion.

Assessment begins with careful palpation of the midline spine for tenderness, deformity, or step-offs—any of which may indicate fracture or ligament injury. A basic neurological exam should include motor strength and sensation in all four limbs. If there is midline tenderness, neurologic deficit, or an unreliable exam, assume spinal injury and immobilize.

Rigid immobilization is ideal but not always practical during prolonged evacuations, where it may contribute to hypothermia, pressure injuries, airway complications, or responder fatigue. If spinal injury cannot be confidently ruled out, immobilization should still be maintained.

Immediate evacuation is required for any neurologic findings—weakness, numbness, paralysis, difficulty breathing—or severe, persistent spinal pain. Even in stable patients, evacuation should be considered if spinal injury remains a possibility. Without imaging, wilderness responders must rely entirely on clinical judgment to guide care and transport decisions.

Headfirst

It was the kind of Colorado morning that makes you grateful to be on the mountain—crisp air, bright sun, and fresh corduroy laid out like a blank canvas. I was a paramedic and now ski patroller, sipping coffee after running through the morning equipment checks, when the call came in—skier down.

The lifts had barely started spinning. Too early for wrecks. We grabbed our gear and headed out.

When we arrived, a man in his sixties lay motionless in the snow. Conscious, breathing, but something was off. He tried to explain—said he'd caught an edge, gone forward, and slammed the crown of his head against the hardpack. But it seemed like he couldn't take a deep enough breath to get the words out.

That stopped me cold.

No blood, no chest pain or shortness of breath, no obvious fractures, nothing. But then we noticed his upper extremities were spastic. It was subtle. As we rolled him over, keeping firm in-line immobilization of his cervical spine, gravity took over and his body slid slightly down the corduroy. My hands stayed fixed on his head, but that shift created just enough traction to gently stretch the cervical spine—and I felt a subtle realignment of the bones beneath my fingers.

Then something happened I wasn't expecting. The moment that gentle traction took effect, his breathing improved. His voice steadied. He could move his arms—slightly, but with intention. It wasn't much, but it was enough to tell us what we were likely dealing with: unstable fractures high up in the cervical spine—and when left to their own accord— were compressing his spinal cord.

A cervical collar alone wasn't going to fix this. We had to maintain our in-line traction of his cervical spine to keep him breathing.

Now came the challenge: getting him off the mountain. Protocols called for full spinal immobilization but locking him down for the sled ride would have very likely undone the traction that was keeping the delicate spinal cord decompressed and allowing him to breathe. We didn't have a backboard that could fine-tune cervical traction, and the last thing any of us wanted was to strip away the one thing that was helping.

We talked it through and decided the best approach was to maintain the gentle, manual traction all the way down. I positioned myself at the head of the toboggan for the descent, keeping him as stable as possible. It certainly wasn't by the book, but it was what was needed.

With this careful approach, his airway stayed open, his voice stayed strong, and he could even use his arm slightly, grasping the heavy blankets covering him during the evacuation. At the helicopter landing zone, we briefed the flight crew, and after a discussion, they agreed—manual traction would be maintained all the way to the trauma center.

His injuries were as severe as we had feared—unstable fractures from C3 through C5. Injuries that often don't come with second chances.

But six months later, he walked into ski patrol headquarters, smiling, leaning on a cane. He shook our hands and told us he'd been given a second chance. His neurosurgeon later confirmed—the sequence of events that day had been as unusual as they were lifesaving.

Wilderness care rarely hands you clean solutions. Sometimes, you read the situation and make the best call with what you have.

It's not about perfect choices—it's about the right one in the moment.

Facial Trauma

What unique challenges does the wilderness present in managing facial trauma?

Facial trauma in the wilderness presents unique challenges due to dense vascularity, proximity to critical structures, and high risk of airway compromise and infection. Even minor injuries can bleed heavily, making hemorrhage control a priority when resources are limited. Trauma to the nose, mouth, eyes, or jaw can interfere with breathing, vision, or hydration, complicating care in remote settings.

The primary concern is airway obstruction. Swelling, jaw fractures, displaced teeth, or pooled blood can rapidly impair breathing. Blood in the stomach may induce vomiting and raise the risk of aspiration. Patients should be kept upright or in the recovery position whenever possible to protect the airway. Significant swelling, uncontrolled bleeding, or any signs of airway compromise require urgent hemorrhage control and evacuation.

Nasal injuries often bleed heavily and can obstruct airflow. Manage nosebleeds with direct pressure, nasal packing (see "Nosebleeds"), and a forward-leaning posture to reduce aspiration risk. Dental trauma—including broken, displaced, or missing teeth—should prompt concern for aspiration. Loose teeth may be stabilized; avulsed teeth should be stored in saline, milk, or the patient's saliva for transport.

Cervical spine injury should be assumed in any patient with significant facial trauma. High-force impact, altered mental status, or swelling or bruising along the neck warrant spinal motion restriction until cleared. Infection risk is high with open fractures, deep lacerations, or dirty wounds. Irrigate thoroughly with clean water or saline. If evacuation is delayed, start oral antibiotics for contaminated or high-risk wounds, particularly those involving the mouth or sinuses. Pills can be crushed and mixed with clean water if swallowing is difficult.

Pain management, hydration, and airway monitoring are critical during extended field care. Use acetaminophen or ibuprofen as available. Patients with jaw injuries may need a soft or liquid diet to maintain nutrition. Evacuation is mandatory for any facial trauma that impairs breathing, causes persistent bleeding, or threatens the airway. In remote settings, facial injuries can escalate rapidly into life-threatening emergencies. Early recognition and decisive intervention are essential.

Why is facial anatomy important to know?

The face is a complex structure of bones, soft tissues, nerves, and blood vessels, all essential for breathing, eating, speaking, expression, and sensory function. The mandible (lower jaw), maxilla (upper jaw), nasal bones, zygomatic bones (cheekbones), and orbital structures form the facial skeleton, providing both structural support and protection for critical areas like the airway, sinuses, and eyes. Facial injuries often bleed heavily due to dense vascularity, though this same circulation promotes rapid healing.

The facial nerve (cranial nerve VII) controls muscle movement, including facial expression, eyelid closure, and lip function. The trigeminal nerve (cranial nerve V) provides sensation to the face. Damage to these nerves can result in facial asymmetry, weakness, or numbness and should prompt a focused neurological assessment. Fractures or swelling in certain regions can obstruct the airway, making early recognition and intervention critical in remote settings.

In wilderness environments, understanding facial anatomy helps guides recognize injury patterns, anticipate complications, and make informed evacuation decisions. High-force facial trauma is rarely isolated—cervical spine, head, or neck injuries should always be suspected. Spinal precautions and ongoing reassessment are essential throughout field care.

Facial Bones

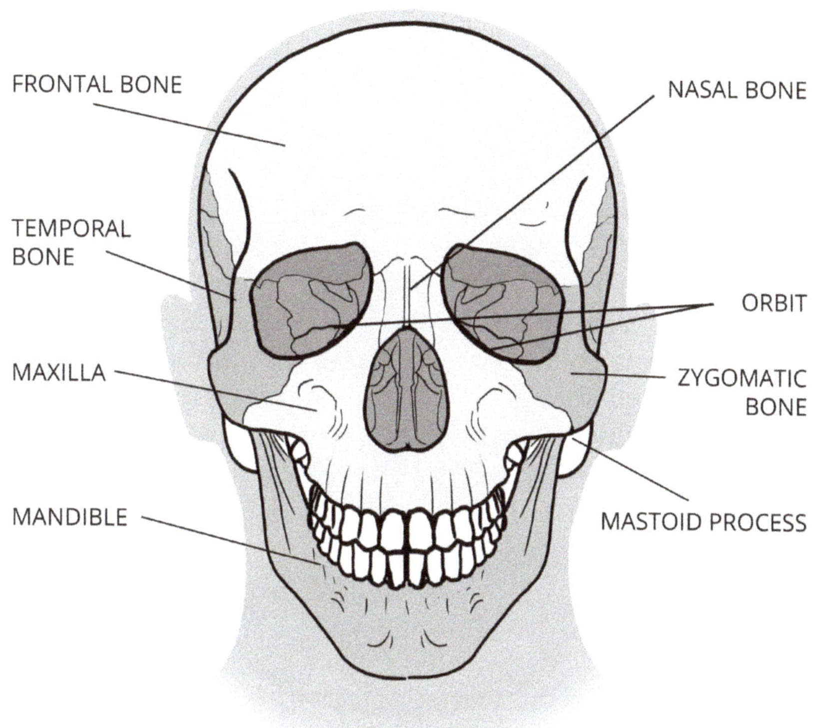

What are Le Fort fractures, and why are they important to understand?

Le Fort fractures are a classification system for midface fractures involving the maxilla, the central bone that anchors the upper teeth and supports the orbits and nasal, structures. They are divided into three types based on the pattern and extent of the fracture:

- Le Fort I: A horizontal fracture separating the upper jaw (maxilla) from the rest of the face—essentially a detachment of the upper teeth from the face.

- Le Fort II: A pyramidal fracture that extends from the *nasal* bridge through the orbital floors down through the maxilla, separating the midface from the skull base.
- Le Fort III: A complete craniofacial dissociation or "floating face," where the facial skeleton is separated from the skull. This is the most severe form and involves the orbits, zygomas, and nasal structures.

These injuries usually result from high-energy blunt trauma to the face, such as vehicle collisions, falls, or direct blows. They're relevant in wilderness medicine because they can compromise the airway, cause significant bleeding, damage the eyes or brain, and indicate high-force mechanisms often associated with cervical spine or brain injury. If facial instability, malocclusion, nasal flattening, or signs of CSF leak (clear fluid from nose) are present after blunt trauma, suspect a midface fracture and prioritize spinal precautions and evacuation.

How is a mandible dislocation managed in the field?

A jaw (mandible) dislocation occurs when the lower jawbone pops out of its socket at the temporomandibular joint (TMJ)—the hinge just in front of each ear that allows the mouth to open and close. Dislocation can happen from yawning, excessive mouth opening, trauma, or a direct hit to the jaw. It results in severe pain, visible jaw misalignment, difficulty speaking, and an inability to close the mouth.

If no other injuries prevent it, the jaw can sometimes be reduced (put back in place) in the field. Position the patient upright or semi-reclined and encourage calm breathing. Wearing gloves, place your thumbs on the lower back teeth (molars) inside the mouth while wrapping the rest of your fingers under the jawline on either side. Apply steady downward pressure to ease the jaw out of its locked position, then gently guide it back and upward into place. Once reduced, the patient should keep their mouth closed as much as possible to prevent it from slipping out again.

After reduction, check that the jaw opens and closes normally and that the teeth line up properly. If available, use a soft band or cloth tied under the chin and over the top of the head (Barton's bandage) to support the jaw and limit movement. The patient should avoid wide mouth opening, tough foods, or excessive talking for at least 24 hours. Evacuate if reduction is unsuccessful, if the injury recurs, or if a fracture is suspected.

Thoracic Trauma

What is the basic anatomy of the thorax?

The thorax, or chest cavity, stretches from the base of the neck to the diaphragm and houses vital organs for breathing, circulation, and digestion. It contains the heart, lungs, esophagus, and major blood vessels—including the aorta, vena cava, and subclavian arteries and veins. These great vessels lie just in front of the spine and beneath the sternum, making them vulnerable in both penetrating and high-impact injuries. The esophagus runs behind the heart and trachea, along the front of the spine, carrying food from the mouth to the stomach.

The ribcage provides structural support and protection for these internal organs. It's made up of 12 pairs of ribs, the sternum (breastbone), and the thoracic spine. The upper part of the sternum is called the manubrium, and it connects with the clavicles (collarbones) and the first ribs. The first seven ribs connect directly to the sternum through cartilage. Ribs 8 through 10 attach to the cartilage of the rib above—not directly to the sternum. Ribs 11 and 12 are called floating ribs because they have no front attachment; they connect only to the thoracic spine in the back. The flexible costochondral cartilage between the ribs and sternum allows for chest expansion during breathing. Above the first ribs lie the subclavian arteries and veins, which supply blood to the arms and can be damaged by clavicle or upper rib fractures.

The lungs are large, spongy organs responsible for gas exchange—bringing oxygen into the blood and removing carbon dioxide. The right lung has three lobes, while the left has two to accommodate the space taken up by the heart. Each lung is encased in a thin membrane called the pleura, which also lines the inside of the chest wall. The narrow space between these layers—the pleural cavity—creates the pressure conditions necessary for lung expansion. When this space is disrupted by trauma, normal breathing can be severely impaired.

At the base of the thorax lies the diaphragm, a dome-shaped muscle critical to respiration. When it contracts, it flattens downward, expanding the chest cavity and drawing air into the lungs. The heart sits just left of center, protected by the sternum and upper ribs. It is enclosed in the pericardium, a fibrous sac that can become dangerously compressed if blood or fluid accumulates inside it.

Understanding this anatomy is essential for recognizing and managing thoracic injuries in wilderness environments. Whether caused by blunt trauma, falls, or penetrating injury, damage to the structures of the chest can quickly become life-threatening without early recognition and proper intervention.

Bony Anatomy of the Thorax

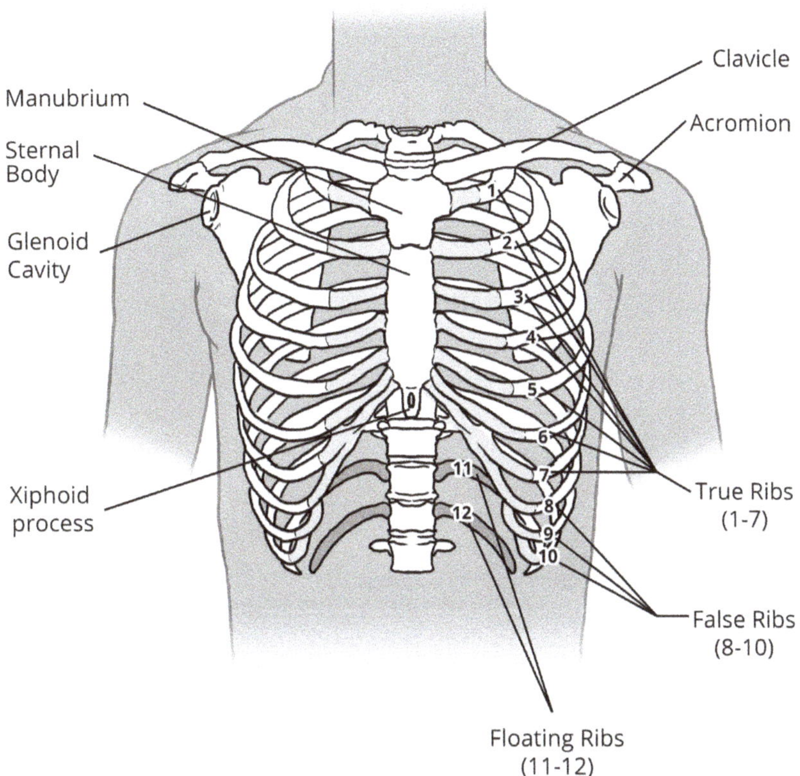

Is breathing just "sucking" in air?

No. One of the foundational tenets of our fragile, human existence is more complex than most realize. Breathing is *not* about sucking air in—it's about creating space. Let me explain.

When we expand the chest, we *decrease* the pressure inside the thorax compared to the atmospheric pressure around us, creating a pressure gradient. According to basic gas laws, air will move from areas of *higher* pressure to *lower* pressure. It's this gradient—not suction—that drives ventilation.

Here's how the system works, in sequence:

1. *Neurological Control and CO2 Detection*

Receptors in the brainstem monitor carbon dioxide levels in the blood. A rise in CO2–*not low oxygen*–is the primary trigger for respiration. The brainstem responds by sending signals through the phrenic nerves to contract the diaphragm. Intercostal muscles also receive input to help expand and stabilize the rib cage.

2. *Diaphragm Contraction Expands the Chest*

   The diaphragm contracts and flattens, increasing the vertical dimensions of the chest. This decreases intrathoracic pressure and reinforces the pressure gradient needed for airflow.

3. *Intercostal Muscles Support Chest Expansion*

   The external intercostals lift the ribs and sternum, increasing thoracic volume and helping maintain the pressure gradient during inhalation.

4. *Air Moves Along the Pressure Gradient*

   Because alveolar pressure (inside) is now lower than atmospheric pressure (outside), air flows *into* the lungs. It moves passively along the gradient *from high to low pressure*–no active sucking of air involved.

5. *Gas Exchange at the Alveolar Level*

   In the alveoli, oxygen diffuses into surrounding capillaries while carbon dioxide diffuses out. This exchange–oxygen in, CO2 out–is the reason we ventilate.

6. *Exhalation is Passive*

   When the diaphragm and intercostals relax, the thoracic cavity recoils and the available chest volume contracts. Pressure inside the lungs now *rises* above atmospheric pressure, and air flows back out along the now reversed pressure gradient.

7. *Ventilation Rate Matches CO_2 Load*

   The brainstem continuously adjusts rate and depth of breathing to maintain stable CO_2 levels. *Under normal conditions, carbon dioxide—not oxygen—is what drives the respiratory rate.*

A failure of any single component in this system leads to immediate respiratory distress. Ventilation breaks down, carbon dioxide builds up, and oxygen delivery to tissues drops. The result is a rapid cascade of compensatory responses—rapid breathing, increased work of breathing, and ultimately respiratory failure if uncorrected. Airway obstruction, chest trauma, diaphragm paralysis, or impaired neurological input can all interrupt the chain.

How do I recognize and manage rib fractures?

Rib fractures are common in outdoor settings, usually caused by blunt trauma. The ribs play two key roles: They protect underlying organs and provide the rigid casing needed to support the pressure-based mechanics of breathing. Surrounding each rib is a layer of intercostal muscle that expands and contracts with ventilation. Along the underside of each rib run small arteries, veins, and nerves, all of which can be damaged by displaced bone.

When ribs break, sharp bone edges can cut into nearby muscle, cause bleeding, or, if displaced inward, puncture the lung and lead to a collapsed lung (pneumothorax).

Rib injuries usually present with sharp, localized pain that worsens with deep breaths, coughing, or movement. Many patients instinctively take shallow breaths to avoid the pain. On exam, there may be tenderness or a crackling sensation of bony fragments rubbing against each other known as crepitus.

Pain control is the primary focus of treatment. NSAIDs like ibuprofen, coupled with acetaminophen, allow patients to take fuller breaths, which is essential to prevent complications. If breathing stays shallow, the smallest air sacs in the lungs, called alveoli, can collapse and begin to fill with fluid. This is known as atelectasis and sets the stage for pneumonia.

While rib belts or compression wraps can provide short-term relief during movement, they should not be used continuously. They restrict chest wall motion and make it harder to breathe deeply. Patients should be encouraged to sit or stand upright, breathe slowly and deeply, and allow gravity to assist diaphragm movement. This improves lung inflation and helps clear fluid.

In the field, rib fractures are often managed with supportive care, but they need to be watched closely. Evacuate if the patient has multiple fractures, fractures bilaterally (both sides of the chest), worsening shortness of breath, signs of poor oxygenation, fever, or a new productive cough that may indicate pneumonia or lung injury.

What is a flail chest, and how is it managed?

Flail chest occurs when multiple, sequential ribs break in *more* than one place, leaving a section of the chest wall detached from the rest of the ribcage. This segment moves in the *opposite* direction from the rest of the chest during breathing—pulled *inward* during inhalation and pushed *outward* during exhalation. That abnormal motion, called paradoxical movement, interferes with normal ventilation and greatly increases the risk of respiratory failure.

Anatomically, the instability prevents the chest wall from maintaining the pressure gradient needed for proper airflow. The lungs can't expand normally, and oxygen exchange becomes impaired. Pain from the injury often leads to shallow breathing, raising the risk of atelectasis and pneumonia.

In wilderness settings, the goal is to stabilize the flail segment and preserve ventilation. A rolled T-shirt, towel, or other soft item can be gently secured over the area to reduce movement. This should support the segment without restricting overall chest expansion. Tightly wrapping the chest should be avoided as it can significantly worsen ventilation.

Pain control is essential to allow for deeper breaths. NSAIDs and acetaminophen can help in mild cases, but more significant injuries often require stronger medications and supplemental oxygen—both of which are typically unavailable in the field.

Evacuation is mandatory. Flail chest often requires hospital-level care, including oxygen support, advanced pain management, close monitoring, and even surgical fixation.

In remote environments, early stabilization and prompt evacuation are critical to prevent decompensation.

What is a pneumothorax?

A pneumothorax occurs when air escapes *from* a hole in the lung *into* the chest, causing partial or full lung collapse. It impairs normal lung expansion and leads to respiratory distress. Most cases result from trauma, such as a rib fracture puncturing the lung, but spontaneous cases can occur in tall, thin individuals or those with underlying lung disease, forceful coughing, or sudden pressure changes.

Suspect pneumothorax when shortness of breath exceeds what pain alone would explain. Key signs include rapid, shallow breathing, pain, and decreased or even absent breath sounds on the affected side. Mild pneumothorax may be subtle. Worsening shortness of breath, cyanosis, or air hunger are red flags.

Subcutaneous emphysema occurs when air (that has escaped from the lung) dissects into the soft tissue beneath the skin, usually around the chest or neck. It's a sign that air has leaked from the lung into surrounding tissue planes. On palpation, it feels like bubble wrap under the skin: soft, crackling, and distinct.

In wilderness settings, consider pneumothorax in any chest trauma patient with worsening respiratory symptoms, asymmetrical breath sounds, cyanosis, or soft tissue air. Stable cases may allow for monitored evacuation, but any progression or signs of tension pneumothorax require immediate action and priority evacuation.

Can a pneumothorax be managed in the field?

Essentially, no. A presumed simple pneumothorax can often be managed with limited exertion, controlled breathing, and evacuation before it worsens. However, even minor lung collapses can deteriorate over time, particularly if air continues to leak from the lung and collect in the pleural cavity, further impairing lung expansion and oxygen exchange. Any suspected pneumothorax requires evacuation, as there is no way to predict whether it will remain stable or progress to a tension scenario

What is a tension pneumothorax?

Tension pneumothorax is the most grave acute complication of a pneumothorax. It occurs when each breath escapes the lung and stays trapped in the chest. The lung functions like a one-way valve—air enters the pleural space but cannot escape, and pressure builds rapidly with each breath.

As this pressure increases, it pushes the injured lung further inward and begins to shift the mediastinum—the space containing the heart, trachea, and major vessels. This shift compresses the opposite lung, squeezes venous blood return to the heart, and collapses circulatory function.

Tension Pneumothorax

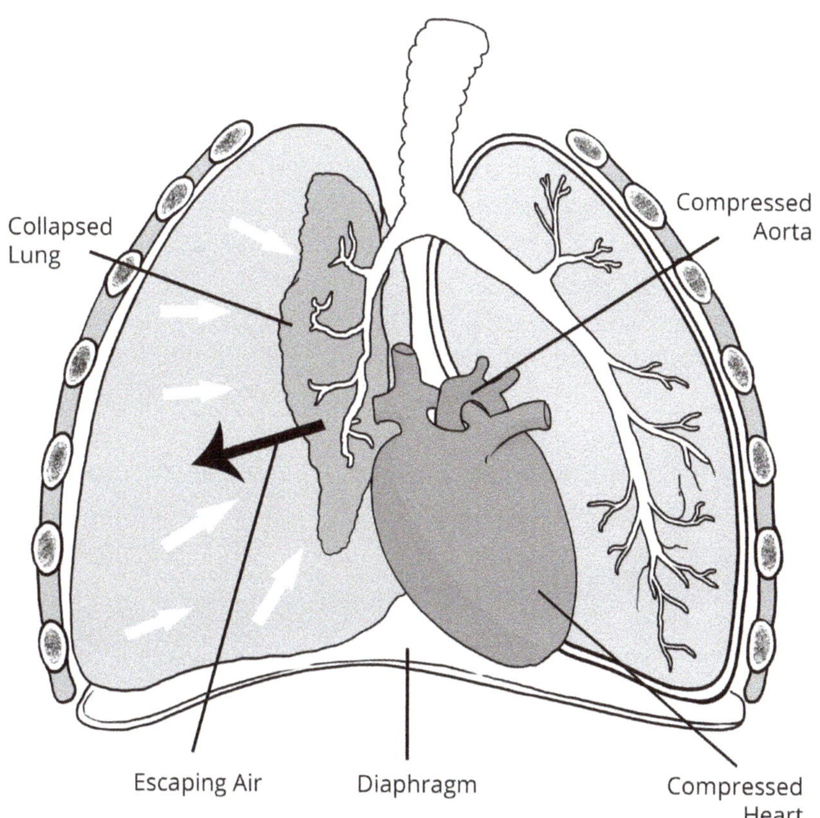

What is the field priority?

Early recognition is critical. Provide supplemental oxygen if available and keep the patient upright, or in the most tolerable position. Monitor closely for signs of progressive decompensation: absent breath sounds on one side, visible respiratory distress, worsening "air hunger," pallor, and altered mental status. These are indicators that the simple pneumothorax has progressed to tension physiology. If evacuation is delayed and the patient is *actively* deteriorating, the trapped air must be released, as without decompression, this condition is uniformly fatal.

A quick note before going further:

This is the part of the book where in-depth conversations around advanced procedures are unavoidable. It's also where protocols, medical direction, and advanced training become critical. While there are plenty of ways to skin this cat, I wanted to lay out the basics—to give guides and responders a working understanding of what's actually going on. None of this is meant as a how-to guide, or to encourage anyone to attempt advanced procedures without the right education, training, experience, and medical oversight. This section is provided for educational context only and is not a substitute for formal medical training. I'm not advocating for these interventions by guides, responders, or laypersons—but I believe understanding them matters. Leaving them out would feel like a glaring hole in any real discussion of trauma care.

Okay, so how do we decompress the chest with a needle?

Needle decompression is one of the first interventions taught to relieve a tension pneumothorax. The goal is to vent air trapped in the chest—air that's collapsing the lung, shifting the mediastinum, and restricting blood return to the heart. Relieving that pressure will allow the heart to fill, restore circulation, and buy time.

The classic site for needle placement is between the second and third ribs—on the affected side—at the midclavicular line (a vertical line down from the midpoint of the clavicle). An alternate is the fifth intercostal space at the anterior axillary line, also on the affected side. Regardless of location, the needle should pass just above the rib to avoid the neurovascular bundle beneath. Prep the skin with antiseptic if available. When inserted, the needle should go in perpendicular to the chest wall to improve the chances of cleanly reaching the pleural space.

The catheter should be large-bore (ideally 14-gauge) and at least 8 cm (3.25 inches) long. While relieving the pressure can buy time, it's rarely a perfect fix. Commercial angiocatheters often fall short—they kink easily, especially as the chest wall shifts with breathing or movement. Traditional teaching removes the needle and leaves the plastic catheter in place, but that tube can clog or collapse without warning. Leaving the needle in avoids kinking—but risks injuring vessels or deeper structures. Either way, it's temporizing at best—and your mind should already be on Plan B.

In the hospital, needle decompression is followed by a chest tube. In the field, the catheter may need to be replaced—or the whole approach escalated if pressure builds again. If no commercial catheter is available, improvisation may be necessary using whatever is on hand—but the goal doesn't change: create and maintain an open path for trapped air to escape.

Any time there's a hole in the chest, start antibiotics, monitor closely, and evacuate as soon as possible. Just to reiterate—this isn't something to attempt without proper training, education, and experience.

What would I do if needle decompression wasn't an option—or had already failed?

I include this question not as instruction or protocol, but because it comes up—almost every time chest trauma is discussed in a teaching setting. This isn't advice or a recommendation, and it's certainly not something I'm suggesting anyone should attempt. But the question gets asked for a reason, and because the stakes in this scenario are often life-or-death, it's worth addressing.

This kind of decision demands advanced training and the willingness to act when no other options remain. It's a low-frequency, high-acuity, last-resort maneuver—and once you make it, there's no walking it back.

This is for a patient in *extremis*—on the verge of death—from a tension pneumothorax, when no help is coming. I'd base that call on clinical findings: absent breath sounds, pallor, altered mental status, distended neck veins, *and* a clear mechanism for major chest trauma. The following describes a finger thoracostomy, which can be performed with limited supplies—even in a wilderness setting. This is a last-resort procedure, done only when the patient is dying, no help is in sight, and there's no other way to keep them alive.

And away we go:

1. Landmarks come first. Like any procedure, it starts with anatomy. I'd go to the fifth intercostal space at the midaxillary line—nipple level in men, inframammary (under the breast) fold in women. That's where to start.
2. Incision next. A 2–3 cm (about 0.8 to 1.2 inch) horizontal incision directly over the superior edge of the rib. If lidocaine is on hand, I'll use it—but in an imminent death scenario, I'm not delaying for anesthesia.
3. Then I go through the layers. Scalpel through skin, subcutaneous tissue, and intercostal muscle—tight to the top of the rib to stay clear of the neurovascular bundle beneath.
4. Finger follows. After palpating the rib, I push through the parietal pleura with a gloved finger applying steady, controlled pressure until I'm in—cautious of broken bone fragments from rib fractures as I push.
5. Pressure tells the story. A sudden rush of air and a hollow release confirms entry into the pleural space. I leave my finger in place to hold it open.
6. Then I watch. Signs of success are immediate—less work of breathing, better color, clearer mentation. If those don't come, something more is needed—and we're in for a long-er day ahead.
7. Last step: Stabilization, antibiotics, and evacuation. If decompression works, it's continuous monitoring and execution of the evacuation plan. And assuming there's no chest tube on hand, I'd either improvise a tube or stay ready to reinsert a finger if air reaccumulates and signs of tension return.

To reiterate, this is not advice or instruction—it's an inside look at how I might manage a patient who's otherwise going to die in the field. It's shared solely to deepen understanding in a worst-case, no-other-options scenario—not as a directive, recommendation, or endorsement of action. This is a procedure that should only be performed under the direction of licensed medical control.

What is a sucking chest wound?

A sucking chest wound is an open chest injury that pulls air into the pleural space with each breath–essentially a pneumothorax from the outside. Instead of leaking from the lung, air enters through the chest wall as the pressure gradient in the chest changes. The result is progressive lung collapse, impaired ventilation, and rapid deterioration if not managed. Common causes include gunshots, stabbings, or impalements.

The hallmark is a sucking or bubbling sound with breathing, often with frothy blood, chest pain, worsening shortness of breath, and visible respiratory distress. Left untreated, this can progress to a tension pneumothorax, where trapped air builds pressure, compressing the lungs, heart, and great vessels–leading to circulatory collapse and death (see above).

In a hospital, chest tubes and surgery follow. In the field, the goal is to stop more air from entering *while allowing trapped air to escape*. Use clean, nonporous material–plastic, sterile packaging, a clean food storage bag, or a chest seal–secured on *three* sides to create a flutter valve. This allows air to vent *out* on exhalation but blocks further entry on inhalation.

That's the principle. In practice, if the patient worsens–rising distress, distended neck veins, altered mental status–they may be developing a tension pneumothorax. Peel back the seal to vent it. If that fails, and you patient is decompensating, stick a gloved finger into the chest to clear the path and release the air.

Evacuation and antibiotics are mandatory. Without definitive treatment, the risk of further deterioration remains high, especially in remote settings.

Abdominal Trauma

What is the relevant anatomy of the abdomen?

The abdomen houses solid and hollow organs, major blood vessels, and key structural components—all vulnerable in trauma. Unlike the ribcage-protected chest, it lacks a rigid barrier, making it especially exposed. Internal bleeding or contamination here can be deadly—and can't be definitively managed in a wilderness setting.

Structurally, the abdominal cavity is lined by a thin, sensitive membrane called the peritoneum. Organs inside this lining—like the stomach, liver, spleen, and intestines—are referred to as peritoneal. Injuries here typically trigger early warning signs like sharp pain, guarding, or abdominal rigidity. In contrast, some organs—including the kidneys, pancreas, and major blood vessels—sit behind this lining in what's called the retroperitoneal space. Trauma in this space often progresses silently. There's no irritation of the peritoneum, so signs like pain or guarding may be absent. The first clue may be shock without obvious cause.

Solid organs—the liver, spleen, kidneys, pancreas, and adrenals—are highly vascular and bleed heavily when injured. The liver (right upper quadrant) and spleen (left upper quadrant) are especially prone to rupture. Retroperitoneal bleeding, especially from the kidneys or great vessels, may not present until blood loss is severe.

Hollow organs—like the stomach, intestines, gallbladder, and bladder—can spill their contents if perforated. This leads to peritonitis, a dangerous infection caused by contamination of the abdominal cavity. It often progresses quickly and can be fatal without surgical care.

Major vessels—the abdominal aorta and inferior vena cava—run deep and centrally. Injury to either causes massive internal bleeding and is almost always fatal without immediate intervention. The diaphragm, which separates chest from abdomen, can rupture from high-energy trauma, allowing abdominal organs to herniate into the chest and impair breathing and circulation.

In the wilderness, where imaging and surgery are unavailable, abdominal trauma must be taken seriously. Pain, rigidity, or signs of shock—especially without external bleeding—should raise immediate concern. Any suspicion of internal abdominal injury in a remote setting should trigger immediate plans for evacuation, as there's little that can be done in the field to change the outcome.

How should blunt abdominal trauma be assessed in the field?

Assessment begins with visual inspection. Look for bruising, swelling, deformity, or open wounds. Certain bruising patterns suggest internal injury—flank bruising (Grey-Turner's sign) or periumbilical bruising (Cullen's sign) indicate intra-abdominal or retroperitoneal bleeding. Bruising over the lower ribs raises concern for trauma to the liver or spleen.

Gently palpate the abdomen, watching for tenderness, rigidity, or guarding. Guarding—an involuntary tightening of the abdominal muscles—suggests peritoneal irritation or internal bleeding. Pain that worsens with movement, deep breaths, or coughing may signal diaphragm or peritoneal involvement. Diffuse tenderness raises concern for bowel injury. Avoid deep palpation if there is severe pain or rigidity, as this may worsen bleeding or organ damage.

Mechanism matters. Falls, blunt impacts, rockslides, or animal kicks can cause solid organ or bowel injury. High-energy mechanisms should heighten suspicion for multiple organ involvement, even when early symptoms seem mild.

Be alert for referred pain. Spleen injuries can cause left shoulder pain (Kehr's sign), which may be mistaken for an orthopedic injury. Liver injuries can cause right shoulder pain. Misinterpreting these signs can delay recognition of internal bleeding.

Monitor closely for signs of internal blood loss and early shock. Tachycardia, pallor, cold extremities, or unexplained fatigue may signal ongoing hemorrhage, even without obvious external trauma. A restless or anxious patient may be compensating; once decompensation begins, deterioration is often rapid.

Serial assessments are critical. Injuries that seem minor at first can become life-threatening. Any suspicion of internal bleeding, peritonitis, or shock mandates immediate evacuation. In wilderness settings, delays sharply narrow the window for survival.

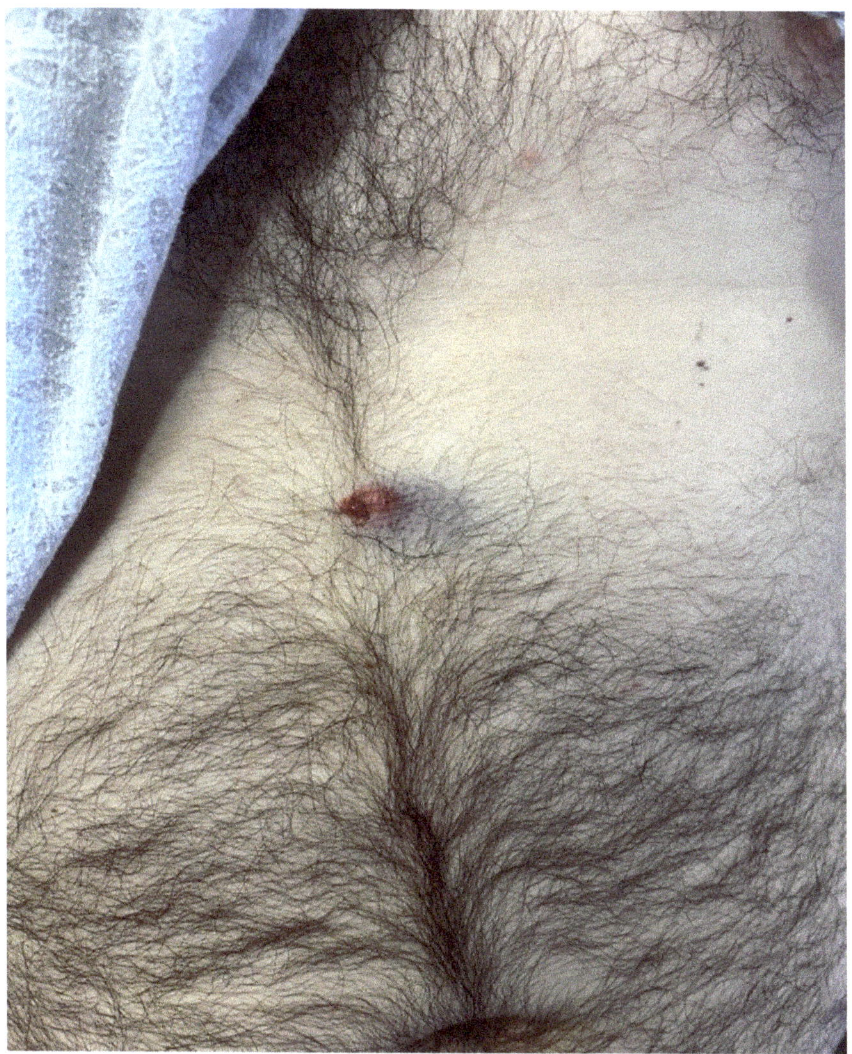

Abdominal gunshot wound from a .22 caliber round in a 53-year-old male. The injury was accidental. He traveled overnight by horseback to reach help, then underwent exploratory surgery and recovered without complication. Image courtesy of the author.

How is penetrating abdominal trauma managed in the wilderness?

Overall, not well. Penetrating injuries—gunshots, stabbings, and impalements—pose a major challenge in remote settings. Unlike blunt trauma, which distributes force, penetrating trauma creates deep, direct paths that can damage multiple organs, vessels, and bowel segments.

Impaled objects should not be removed in the field unless they obstruct the airway or prevent evacuation. Removal may disrupt clotting or worsen internal injury. Instead, stabilize the object with padding and secure it in place to limit movement during transport.

Control external bleeding with direct pressure. Avoid deep compression over the wound, which can worsen internal damage.

All penetrating abdominal injuries require immediate evacuation, regardless of initial appearance. Internal bleeding and contamination may progress silently. Intestinal perforation increases the risk of peritonitis and sepsis. Oral antibiotics should be started early in all suspected cases.

Penetrating injuries are progressive. What seems manageable at first may deteriorate rapidly. Increasing pain, abdominal distension, or any signs of shock must be treated as life-threatening.

In remote environments without imaging, surgery, or blood products, the window for meaningful intervention is narrow. Waiting too long may remove any realistic chance of survival.

What should be done if abdominal organs are exposed?

Evisceration—exposed bowel outside the abdominal wall—looks dramatic, but unless major vessels are involved, it isn't uniformly fatal. It usually doesn't compromise breathing or circulation. The real danger comes from drying, infection, and mechanical damage to the tissue.

These injuries can result from crashes, impalement, falls onto sharp objects, or even animal horns. Whatever the cause, the priorities are the same.

Cover the bowel immediately with a moist, sterile dressing—or the cleanest cloth available—to keep it protected.

If evacuation is imminent, leave the bowel in place—don't try to push it back in.

If evacuation is delayed—and the patient is stable, cooperative, and the tissue isn't badly swollen or contaminated—gentle reduction may be reasonable. Clean your hands, irrigate with clean water, and slowly guide the bowel back in, starting at the exit site using minimal pressure. Once reduced, loosely cover with a moist dressing and evacuate.

If reduction isn't possible, keep the tissue moist, shield it from further injury, and get the patient out as soon as possible.

Pelvic Trauma

Why are pelvic fractures so dangerous?

The pelvis is a critical load-bearing structure and protective ring for vital organs and major blood vessels. It's composed of the sacrum, coccyx, and paired ilium, ischium, and pubis bones—connecting at the sacroiliac joints in the back and the pubic symphysis in the front. When intact, it distributes force and provides structural stability. When fractured, that stability is lost, often resulting in severe bleeding and internal organ damage.

The pelvic cavity contains the bladder, urethra, reproductive organs, and segments of the intestines. These structures are vulnerable when the pelvic ring is disrupted. The rectum, located posteriorly, may be injured in open fractures, where sharp bone fragments tear into soft tissue.

The pelvis is one of the most vascular regions in the body. The common iliac arteries branch into external and internal iliac arteries, supplying the legs and pelvic organs. Venous structures, including the iliac veins and presacral venous plexus, lack muscular walls and are prone to continuous bleeding when injured. Venous bleeding here may not be externally visible but can still be life-threatening.

Disruption of the pelvic ring—from fractures, ligament damage, or dislocation—can shear blood vessels, resulting in uncontrolled hemorrhage. Movement of an unstable pelvis worsens bleeding and soft tissue injury. Stabilization in the field is essential. Minimizing motion and applying a pelvic binder are key to reducing further blood loss.

Pelvic fractures are high-risk injuries in any setting, but especially in remote environments without surgical care. Early recognition, immobilization, and evacuation are critical to survival.

Bony Anatomy of the Pelvis

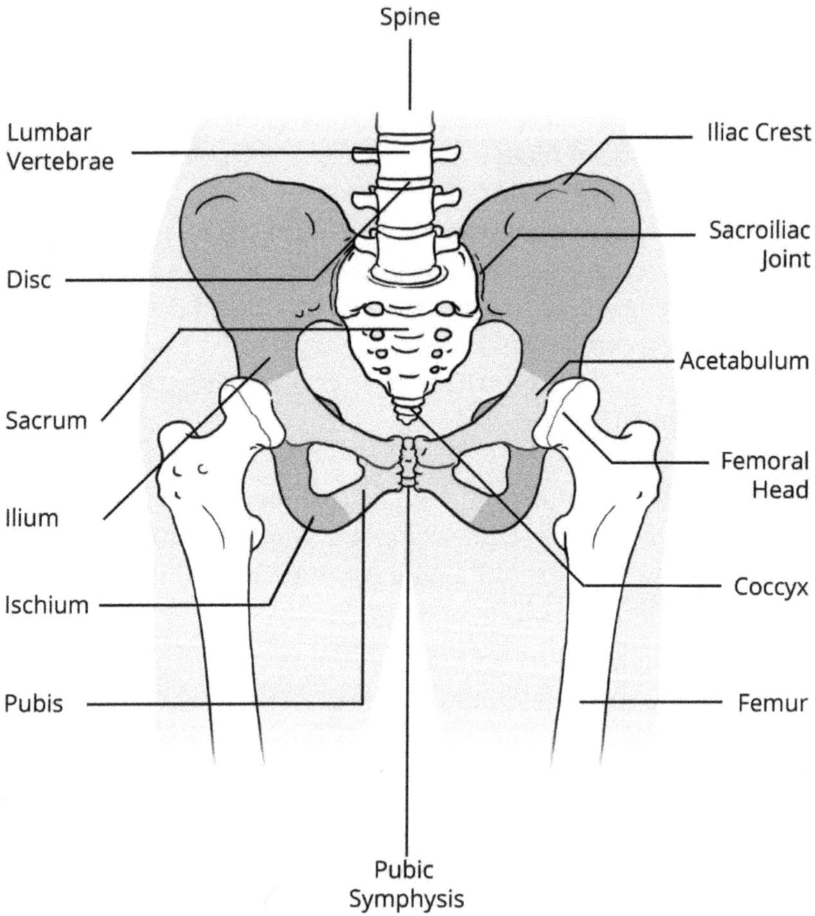

What are the signs and symptoms of a pelvic fracture?

Pelvic fractures typically present with localized pain, tenderness, and instability. Bruising or swelling in the lower abdomen, groin, perineum, or inner thighs may suggest underlying vascular injury. Blood at the urethral opening, difficulty urinating, or hematuria point to bladder or urethral damage, especially in anterior fractures. Rectal bleeding raises concern for open pelvic injury or colon perforation, particularly with high-energy or penetrating trauma.

A single gentle compression of the pelvic ring may reveal instability or pain. This should not be repeated, as it can worsen bleeding. Systemic signs of shock—pale skin, rapid heart rate, and low blood pressure—indicate severe internal bleeding and require immediate action.

In the field, management is limited to stabilization and preventing movement. Walking or repositioning a patient with a suspected pelvic fracture can worsen bleeding and accelerate shock. A pelvic binder is one of the few effective field interventions, helping to stabilize the ring and reduce venous bleeding.

In wilderness settings, early recognition and prompt evacuation are critical for presumed pelvic fractures.

How are pelvic fractures managed in the wilderness?

After airway and breathing, controlling hemorrhage is the next priority. Pelvic fractures can cause massive internal bleeding, most of it venous and concealed. The only effective intervention in the field is to reduce pelvic motion and compress the pelvic volume to slow the bleeding.

This is done with a pelvic binder placed firmly over the greater trochanters—the bony points at the top of the outer thighs, just below the hips. The binder works by stabilizing the bony pelvis and then by reducing the volume inside the pelvis, which limits the space for blood to collect and helps slow hemorrhage. Recent research has questioned whether binders improve perfusion or survival across all fracture types, but they continue to show benefit in pelvic ring injuries—fractures that can't be reliably identified in the field. For that reason, a binder—commercial or improvised—should still be applied when a pelvic fracture is suspected.

If a commercial binder isn't available, a folded sheet, blanket, or wide strap can be used. If no binder is available, tying the legs together at the knees and ankles can help limit movement and reduce further injury.

Additional field priorities include preventing hypothermia, avoiding unnecessary movement, and the judicious use of oral fluids to maintain volume.

All suspected pelvic fractures require immediate evacuation. These injuries are unstable by nature, and definitive care—surgery, blood products, and imaging—is not possible in the wilderness. Stabilization in the field buys time, but survival depends on evacuation.

Injuries to the Arms & Legs

What is the appendicular skeleton?

The appendicular skeleton includes the bones of the arms, legs, hands, feet, and the girdles—shoulder and pelvis—that connect them to the axial skeleton (skull, spine, ribs, and sternum). These structures provide mobility, support weight, and anchor muscles that enable movement. In wilderness settings, where mobility may be essential for self-rescue or evacuation, injuries to the appendicular skeleton can quickly become disabling.

These bones also protect major blood vessels and nerves. The femur, humerus, radius, and tibia are closely associated with critical neurovascular structures, making fractures in these areas a risk for severe bleeding or nerve injury. The femur is particularly vascular and can result in significant blood loss when fractured. The pelvic girdle, part of the appendicular skeleton, serves as a base for the spine and lower limbs while housing major vessels like the iliac arteries and veins.

In remote settings, rapid assessment and stabilization of these injuries is critical. Evaluation should include inspection for deformity, palpation for tenderness or abnormal movement, and neurovascular checks—circulation, sensation, and motor function—to determine if the injury threatens life or limb. Proper immobilization reduces pain, prevents further damage, and increases the chance of successful evacuation and recovery.

What are some general principles of fracture management?

Wilderness fracture management focuses on early recognition, stabilization, pain control, and evacuation decisions. Without imaging or surgery, outcomes depend on field assessment and care. The goal is to limit movement, prevent soft tissue damage, maintain circulation, and reduce complications.

Fractures are either open (bone exposed) or closed (beneath the skin). Open fractures carry a high risk of infection and require immediate irrigation, dressing, and antibiotics if available. Closed fractures can still threaten limbs if swelling compromises blood flow or if nearby vessels or nerves are damaged.

Signs of fracture include pain, swelling, bruising, deformity, and loss of function. Skin tenting, pallor, coolness, delayed capillary refill, or weak pulses signal vascular compromise and demand immediate action. In the wilderness setting, any obvious deformity should be reduced with *slow*, steady in-line traction—both to relieve pain and reduce bleeding. Realignment improves comfort, protects tissue, and makes splinting and evacuation far easier. Be patient. Gentle traction takes time, and pain often improves after reduction is complete.

That said, if evacuation and definitive care are imminent—and there's no evidence of circulatory compromise—a fracture can be splinted in the position found or in a position of comfort. But with prolonged evacuation times or any signs of poor perfusion, reduction is the move.

Once realigned, the limb must be immobilized. Splints should stabilize the joint above and below the fracture. Use rigid materials—sticks, trekking poles, rolled magazines, or anything available—and pad them well. Secure with cloth, tape, or bandages. Take your time when splinting—this is the moment to get it right. Always check capillary refill, as discussed earlier, especially after reduction or splint placement.

Evacuation is indicated for almost all fractures except those isolated to fingers or toes. Evacuation is mandatory for open fractures, vascular compromise, suspected femur fractures, or signs of compartment syndrome (see below). Even stable-appearing fractures can deteriorate with time.

Reassess frequently. Swelling, pain, and circulation can change. Manage pain with ibuprofen and acetaminophen. In the wilderness, early stabilization and timely evacuation are critical to preserving life and limb.

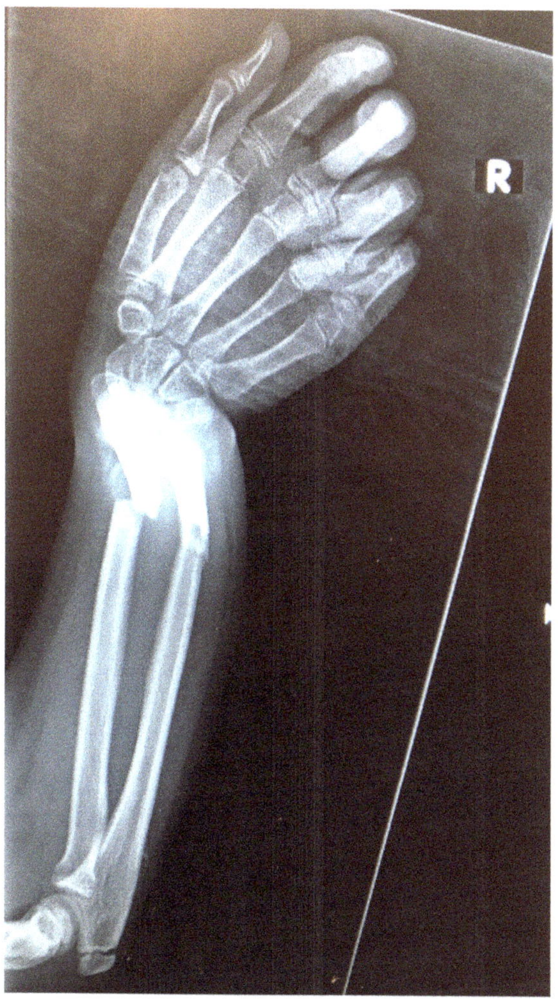

Fractures of the distal radius and ulna, sustained from a fall onto an outstretched hand (FOOSH). A common injury mechanism. Pre-reduction film. Image courtesy of the author.

What is a hematoma block?

A hematoma block is an underutilized but highly effective technique that should be in every guide's skill set. By injecting lidocaine or another anesthetic *directly into* the fracture site, significant pain relief can be achieved, making splinting and reduction far more tolerable. This procedure requires minimal training, carries a low risk, and can make the difference between a manageable evacuation and an unworkable situation. In remote settings, where advanced pain management options may be unavailable, a properly administered hematoma block is a game changer. This is one worth asking you favorite doc for some instruction on.

What is compartment syndrome?

Compartment syndrome is a limb-threatening condition that occurs when swelling causes increased pressure within a muscle compartment impairing circulation and oxygen delivery to tissues. It can result from fractures, penetrating trauma, crush injuries, burns, or prolonged compression (such as being pinned under heavy debris). As pressure rises inside the compartment, blood flow is restricted, leading to tissue ischemia, nerve compression, and, if untreated, irreversible muscle death and limb loss. Globally, delayed recognition of compartment syndrome remains a major cause of preventable amputations, particularly in wilderness settings where evacuation is prolonged and surgical intervention is unavailable.

The classic “five Ps” guide recognition of compartment syndrome:

- *Pain* - Severe, disproportionate pain that worsens with stretching is the most reliable early sign.
- *Paresthesia* - Tingling, numbness indicating nerve compression.
- *Pallor* - Pale or mottled skin, suggesting impaired circulation.
- *Pulselessness* - Diminished or absent distal pulses in advanced cases (though pulses may remain intact early on).
- *Paralysis* - Inability to move the affected limb, a late and ominous sign of severe tissue damage.

In a wilderness setting, the challenge is that compartment syndrome can develop gradually, with pain being the only reliable early symptom. Swelling, tightness, and increasing pain should raise suspicion before obvious vascular(pulse) changes appear.

How is compartment syndrome managed in the wilderness?

It's not—at least not definitively. Treatment requires fasciotomy, a surgical procedure to release pressure, which is not available in remote settings. The focus in the field is on preventing further harm and prioritizing evacuation.

Remove any external constriction, including tight splints, bandages, or clothing. This may relieve external pressure but will not stop internal compartment pressure from rising. The affected limb should be immobilized at heart level—not elevated—as elevation can reduce arterial inflow and worsen ischemia.

Pain management must be cautious. Overmedication may mask the progression of symptoms, delaying recognition. Once compartment syndrome develops, irreversible muscle and nerve damage can begin within hours. Delays beyond 6–8 hours significantly increase the risk of permanent disability or amputation.

Evacuation is urgent. Early recognition and rapid transport are the only actions that can preserve limb function in wilderness settings.

Why are femur fractures particularly dangerous?

Femur fractures are high-risk injuries in the wilderness due to massive blood loss into the thigh, and the risk of fat embolism syndrome. The femur is a highly vascular bone, and a closed fracture can bleed one to two liters into surrounding tissues. This blood loss is often hidden, and shock may develop before there are visible signs. Bone fragments can also damage nearby arteries and veins, compounding hemorrhage. Without access to transfusion, this internal bleeding can lead to hypovolemic shock.

Fat embolism syndrome (FES) is a potentially life-threatening complication of femur fractures. In FES, fat droplets from the exposed bone marrow enter the bloodstream and block vessels in the lungs, brain, or skin—triggering inflammation and organ dysfunction. Symptoms include sudden respiratory distress; confusion; and a rash across the chest, neck, or upper arms. It can appear hours to days after injury, even in patients who initially seem stable.

Stabilization and evacuation are mandatory. The femur must be realigned using slow, steady in-line traction. This reduces bleeding, relaxes muscle spasm, and improves circulation. Traction is effective even without anesthesia *if done gently and patiently*. Once realigned, apply a traction splint if available. If not, splint with rigid materials like trekking poles, tree branches, or foam pads, and secure with bandages or clothing. Securing the legs together may provide added stabilization during evacuation.

Evacuation is emergent. Even if the patient appears stable, the risks of continued bleeding, fat embolism, or sudden decompensation remain high. Early recognition, *careful* traction, and immediate evacuation are essential for successful recovery.

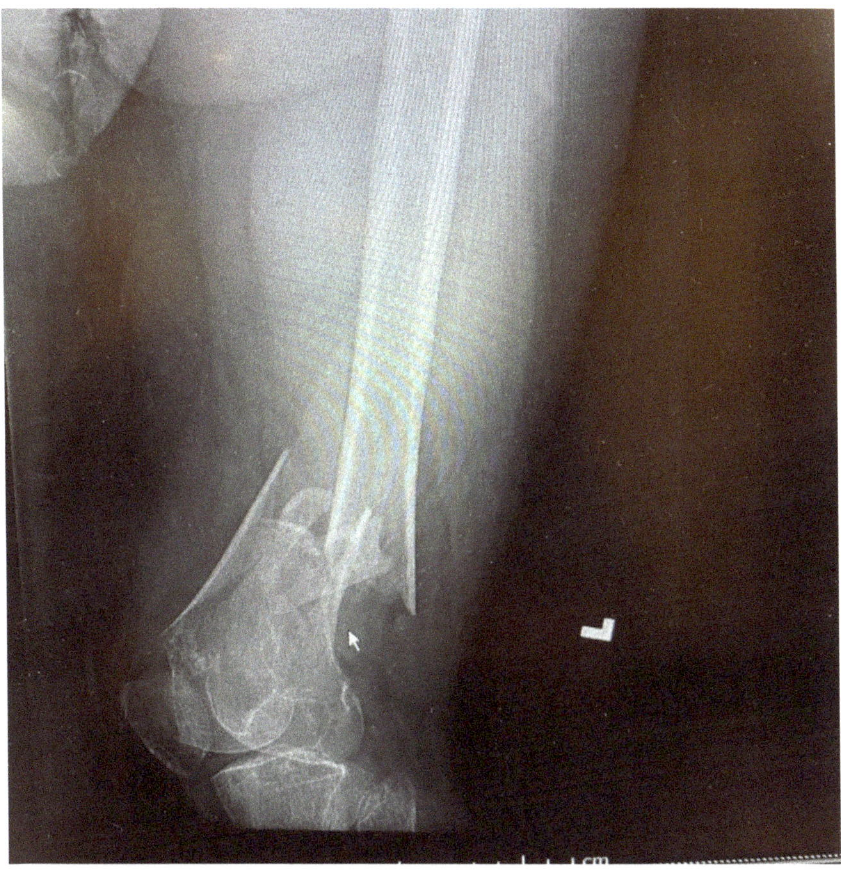

Comminuted distal femur fracture in a pediatric patient following a fall from a horse. After completing the primary trauma survey, the fracture was splinted in the field. The patient was then evacuated to the nearest landing zone for helicopter transport to definitive care. Image courtesy of the author.

What do guides need to know about clavicle fractures?

The clavicle, or collarbone, connects the sternum to the shoulder and serves as a strut to stabilize arm movement. Its exposed position and thin shape make it one of the most commonly fractured bones in the body.

Clavicle fractures are common in outdoor activities involving falls, direct shoulder impact, or high-force trauma—such as biking, skiing, or climbing. The clavicle (collarbone) connects the sternum to the scapula, forming a structural bridge between the axial and appendicular skeleton. It enables shoulder mobility, transmits force, and protects underlying neurovascular structures including the brachial plexus and subclavian vessels.

Fractures are categorized by location. Midshaft fractures are most common and often heal without surgery. Proximal fractures (near the sternum) carry higher risk due to their proximity to major vessels while distal fractures (near the shoulder) may destabilize the shoulder and limit arm use, complicating evacuation.

In the field, presentation includes pain, swelling, bruising, and deformity over the collarbone. The arm is typically held close to the chest. Tenting of the skin suggests displacement and increased risk for an open fracture. Initial management focuses on immobilization and pain control. Apply a sling and swathe to reduce motion and support the arm. A figure-of-eight bandage may help alignment but should not restrict breathing. Upright posture helps prevent shoulder hunching and malalignment—and helps with pain as well. Use ibuprofen *and* acetaminophen for pain, especially during long evacuations.

Evacuation is required for any fracture with skin tenting, neurovascular signs (cool, pulseless limb), severe shortening of the clavicle, or inability to perform essential tasks. Midshaft fractures without complications theoretically can be monitored in the field, but any sign of progressive swelling, suspected vascular injury, or respiratory compromise demands urgent transport. As always, early recognition and proper immobilization are key to recovery.

Hands & Feet

What is a subungual hematoma?

A subungual hematoma is blood trapped under a fingernail or toenail, usually from blunt trauma like crushing the fingertip or stubbing a toe. It results from bleeding beneath the nail and can cause throbbing pain due to pressure buildup. Small, painless hematomas typically resolve without treatment.

In the field, treatment focuses on relieving pressure and preventing infection. If the hematoma is painful, trephination—creating a small hole in the nail plate—can provide immediate relief. This can be done using a clean 18-gauge needle, the heated tip of a paper clip, or a small piece of wire. Gently melt or bore a hole through the nail to release the trapped blood. This is usually painless, as the nail has no nerve endings. After drainage, clean the area and apply a sterile dressing.

Avoid trephination if there's a nail bed laceration, underlying fracture, or signs of infection. If redness, swelling, or warmth appears, antibiotics and further medical care are needed.

Bony Anatomy of the Hand and Wrist

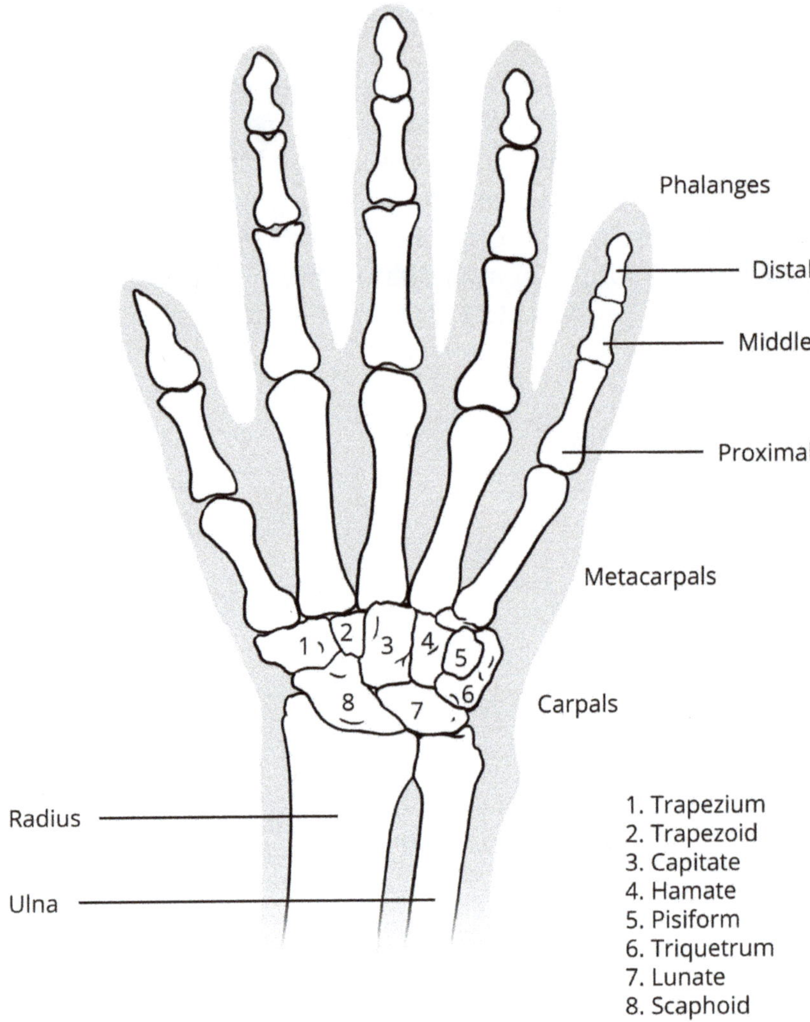

How are penetrating injuries to the hand or foot managed in the wilderness?

Penetrating injuries to the hand or foot are especially serious due to the density of tendons, nerves, blood vessels, and bones in a small space. Even minor-looking wounds can cause major complications—bleeding, infection, or long-term loss of function. In wilderness settings, delays in care increase the risk of permanent damage.

Initial management focuses on controlling bleeding, preventing infection, and preserving function. Apply direct pressure immediately—and if bleeding is uncontrolled, use a tourniquet—cautiously. Tourniquets prevent blood flow to the limb, and prolonged use increases the risk of nerve injury, tissue damage, or even amputation if evacuation is delayed.

Irrigate the wound thoroughly with clean water, initiate antibiotics if available, and lightly pack the wound with sterile gauze. Cover with a snug bandage and immobilize the hand or foot in a functional position using a splint or improvised support.

Do not remove small, impaled objects—they may be controlling the bleeding. Instead, stabilize them in place with padding or splints.

Evacuation is, required for uncontrolled bleeding (or tourniquet use), suspected arterial injury, visible deformity, loss of function, or signs of infection. Even seemingly minor wounds may need evacuation if structural damage, nerve involvement, or contamination is suspected.

Antibiotics should be given for all penetrating wounds, especially if there's exposure to dirt, organic material, or water. Signs of infection—redness, swelling, pus, or foul odor—require immediate evacuation for definitive care.

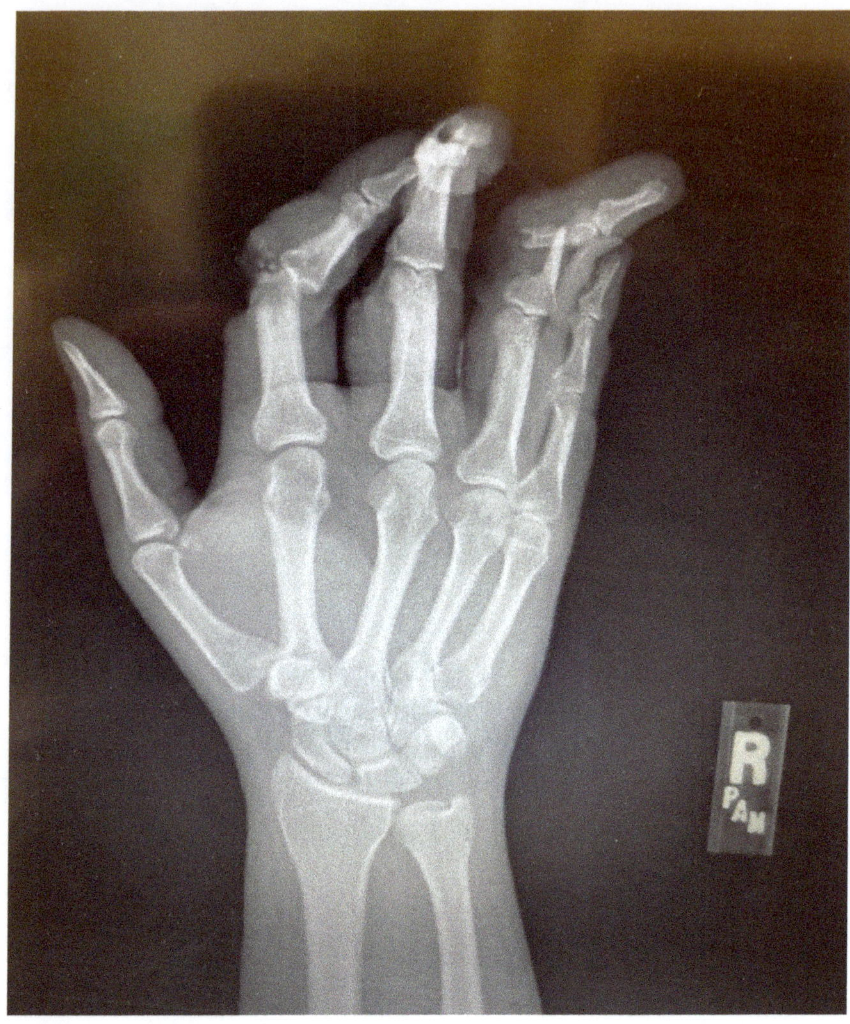

Open fracture-dislocations of the second and fourth fingers with visible deformity and joint misalignment following a crush injury between large boulders. Bone was exposed through the skin, classifying these as open fractures with high risk of infection. A thorough field washout was performed, antibiotics were initiated, the wounds were dressed, and the hand was splinted. Due to the instability and contamination, evacuation was required for surgical care. Image courtesy of the author.

What should guides know about finger and toe dislocations in the wilderness?

Dislocations occur when the bones of a joint are forced out of alignment—usually from falls, impact, or hyperextension.

Finger and toe joints are stabilized by ligaments, tendons, and a joint capsule, all of which can be stretched or torn. Each finger and toe has three bones (phalanges), except the thumb and big toe, which have two. The proximal interphalangeal (PIP) joint in the fingers is the most commonly dislocated. In the feet, big toe dislocations can significantly affect balance and mobility.

Dislocations present with pain, swelling, deformity, and loss of motion. Prompt reduction is important to restore alignment and prevent long-term damage. The proximal bone should be stabilized, and gentle, steady—in-line traction applied. While maintaining traction, the dislocated bone can be guided back into place by reversing the mechanism of injury. Slow and steady. A click or shift usually confirms reduction. If resistance is met, the attempt should be stopped and the patient evacuated.

After reduction, the joint should be immobilized. Buddy taping to an adjacent digit offers simple, effective support. The limb should be elevated, ice applied if available, and neurovascular status reassessed. Capillary refill, skin color, and sensation must be checked and monitored. Evacuation is required if reduction fails, circulation is compromised, or there is persistent numbness, visible deformity, or suspected fracture or tendon injury.

Bony Anatomy of the Foot

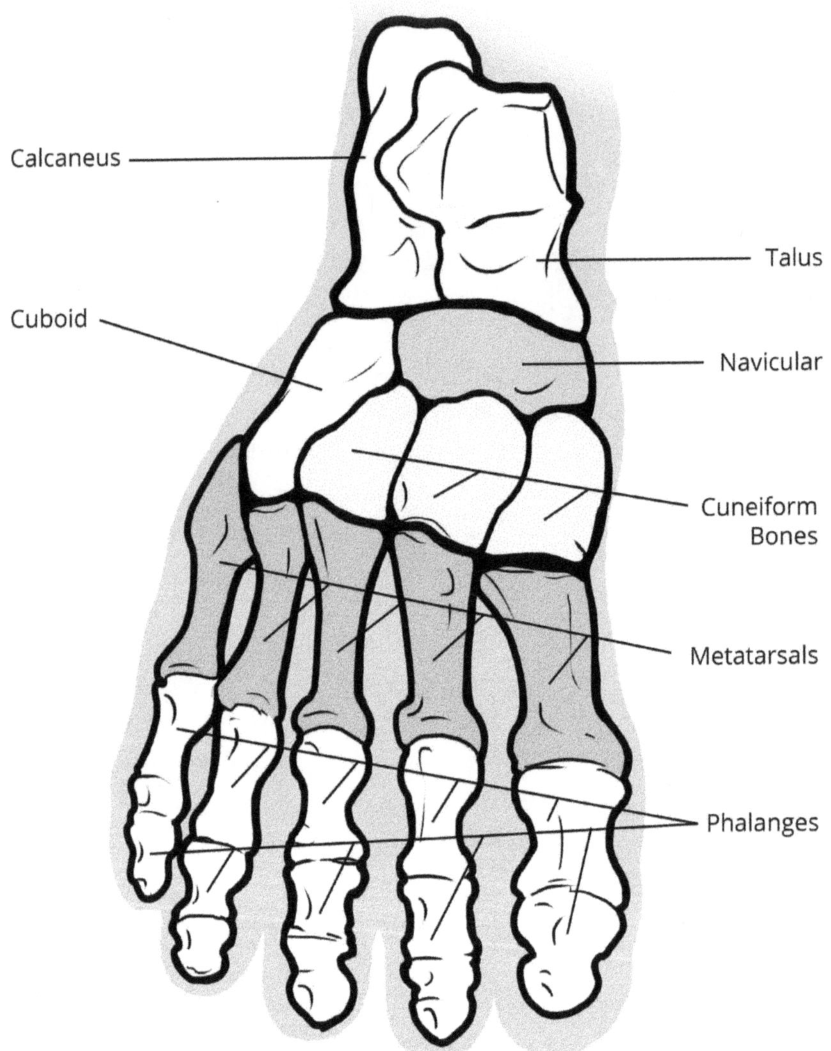

(Anterior View of Right Foot)

What is a field method for ring removal?

Rings, bracelets, or other accessories should be removed as soon as possible following injury, as swelling can turn them into tourniquets, restricting circulation and risking tissue loss. When cutting tools are unavailable, improvised methods can be quite effective.

A reliable technique involves using about two feet of dental floss, fishing line, or fine string. First, squeeze the string under the ring, leaving a short tail toward the palm. Then wrap the longer end snugly around the finger, starting at the ring and continuing past the first knuckle (proximal interphalangeal [PIP] joint). The goal is to compress the finger evenly, avoiding skin bulging between wraps. While maintaining gentle tension on the tail closest to the hand, slide and twist the ring over the compressed wraps. This helps guide the ring toward the narrower part of the finger for removal.

This method is simple, low-risk, and highly effective—widely used in emergency department and field settings when cutting is not an option.

Upper Extremity Dislocations

Shoulder Dislocation

What should guides know about shoulder dislocations?

Shoulder dislocations are among the most common joint dislocations encountered in remote settings. They typically result from falls, forceful arm movements, or direct impact—common in activities like climbing, biking, skiing, or paddling. The shoulder (glenohumeral joint) prioritizes mobility over stability, with the humeral head (ball) resting in a shallow glenoid fossa (socket), making it vulnerable to dislocation.

Most shoulder dislocations are anterior, with the humeral head displaced forward. The arm is often held slightly away from the body and internally rotated, with an inability to lift or externally rotate. Posterior dislocations are rare and usually associated with seizures, electrical injury, or high-force trauma.

Timely reduction is critical to restore alignment, relieve pain, and reduce the risk of nerve injury, vascular compromise, or chronic instability. In wilderness settings, where evacuation may be delayed, knowing how to assess and manage a shoulder dislocation is essential.

Before attempting reduction, guides should assess for obvious fractures, neurovascular deficits, or signs that reduction may be unsafe as severe pain, swelling, or abnormal limb positioning require caution. Numbness or tingling in the hand or arm may indicate nerve involvement, increasing the urgency and the need for careful, controlled intervention. If left unreduced, muscle spasms and swelling will worsen, making future reduction attempts significantly harder.

Immediate evacuation is required if reduction fails or if circulation, sensation, or motor function *remain* impaired. These findings may indicate a fracture, nerve, or vascular injury. Persistent numbness or absent pulses are red flags that demand urgent evacuation.

Evacuation is also recommended although not mandatory, after successful reduction in first-time dislocations due to the risk of ligament damage and likely future instability. Chronic dislocations with full motion and limited pain may not require immediate evacuation but should be monitored for recurrent instability or weakness.

A successful reduction provides relief, but it does not replace medical follow-up. Imaging and evaluation ensure joint stability, identify hidden injuries, and guide long-term management.

Bony Anatomy of the Shoulder

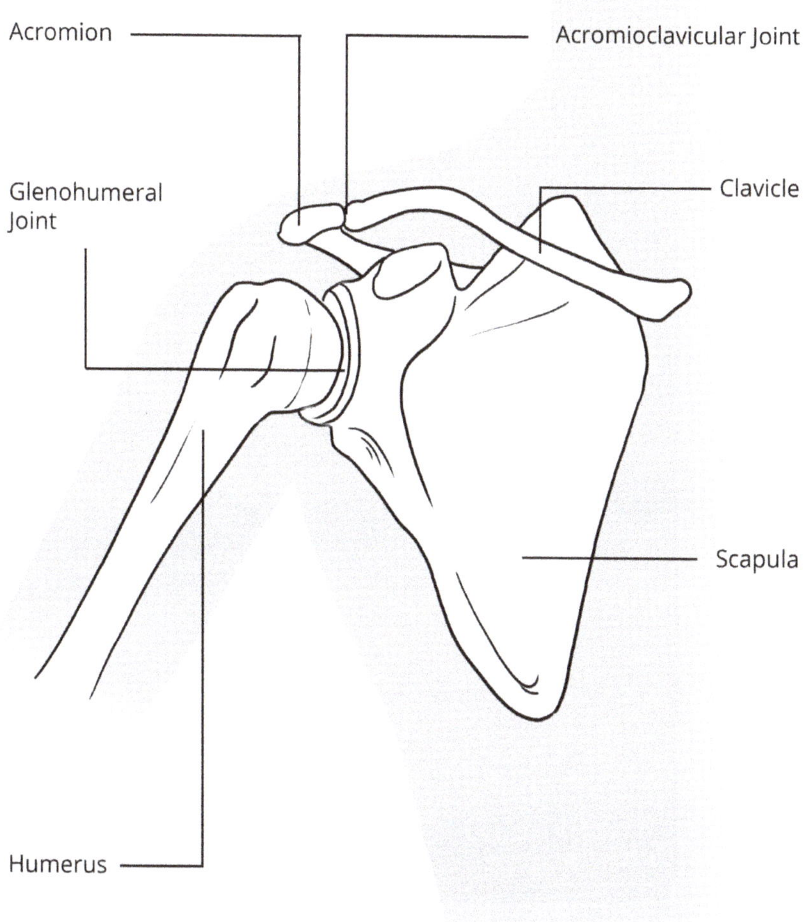

How does the Stimson Technique work?

The Stimson technique is a gravity-assisted method for reducing an anterior shoulder dislocation. It requires minimal equipment and no patient, effort, making it ideal in remote settings where mobility, pain, or fatigue may limit other approaches.

The patient lies face down on a stable surface with the injured arm hanging freely over the edge. Gravity alone may allow for reduction, but attaching a small weight—like a water bottle or sandbag—to the wrist provides gentle traction. A responder may also apply light manual traction by holding the wrist and pulling *steady* downward pressure.

The key is patience. Over several minutes, gravity will fatigue the muscles encouraging the humeral head to slide back into place. The patient must remain calm and relaxed, as muscle tension prevents reduction.

Once reduced, the arm should be immobilized with a sling and swathe. The patient should avoid using the arm until medically evaluated. Persistent weakness, numbness, or pain may indicate nerve or soft tissue injury and warrants further assessment.

The Stimson technique is low-risk and effective—often the difference between a tortured evacuation and a good story. If reduction fails or signs of vascular or neurological compromise are present, evacuation is mandatory.

The Stimson Technique

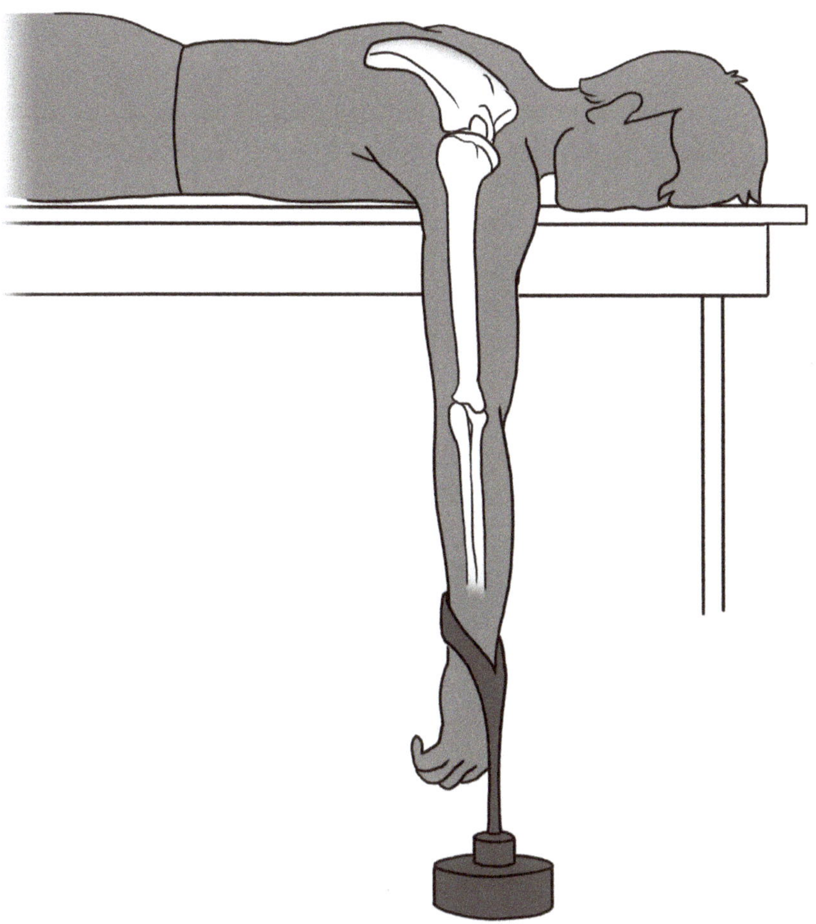

What is the Cunningham Technique?

The Cunningham technique is a muscle-relaxation method for reducing an anterior shoulder dislocation without force, sedation, or traction. Unlike the Stimson, method, which uses gravity, the Cunningham technique relies on patient cooperation and active relaxation—making it ideal when sedation isn't available, and the patient is calm and able to follow instructions.

The patient should sit upright with good posture (shoulders back). The rescuer faces the patient and supports the patient's bent elbow (at roughly 90°), resting the hand on the rescuer's forearm. This keeps the arm in neutral rotation and minimizes tension.

The patient is coached to roll the shoulders back and down while taking slow, deep breaths to relax the muscles. The rescuer gently massages the trapezius, deltoid, and biceps (in order) to reduce guarding. As tension eases, the patient may slowly "walk" their fingers up the rescuer's shoulder, while the responder is applying gently, steady downward pressure on the forearm—encouraging the natural reduction of the humeral head.

The key concept of the Cunningham Technique is that no force is used. Any pain, tension, or resistance should be respected, as forcing the joint will worsen spasms and make reduction more difficult.

Once the shoulder is reduced, check for joint stability, neurovascular status, and range of motion. Immobilize the arm in a sling and swathe. The patient should avoid movement until further evaluation is possible.

The Cunningham technique is low-risk, noninvasive, and field-friendly—especially valuable when patient is cooperative, and resources are limited.

The Cunningham Technique

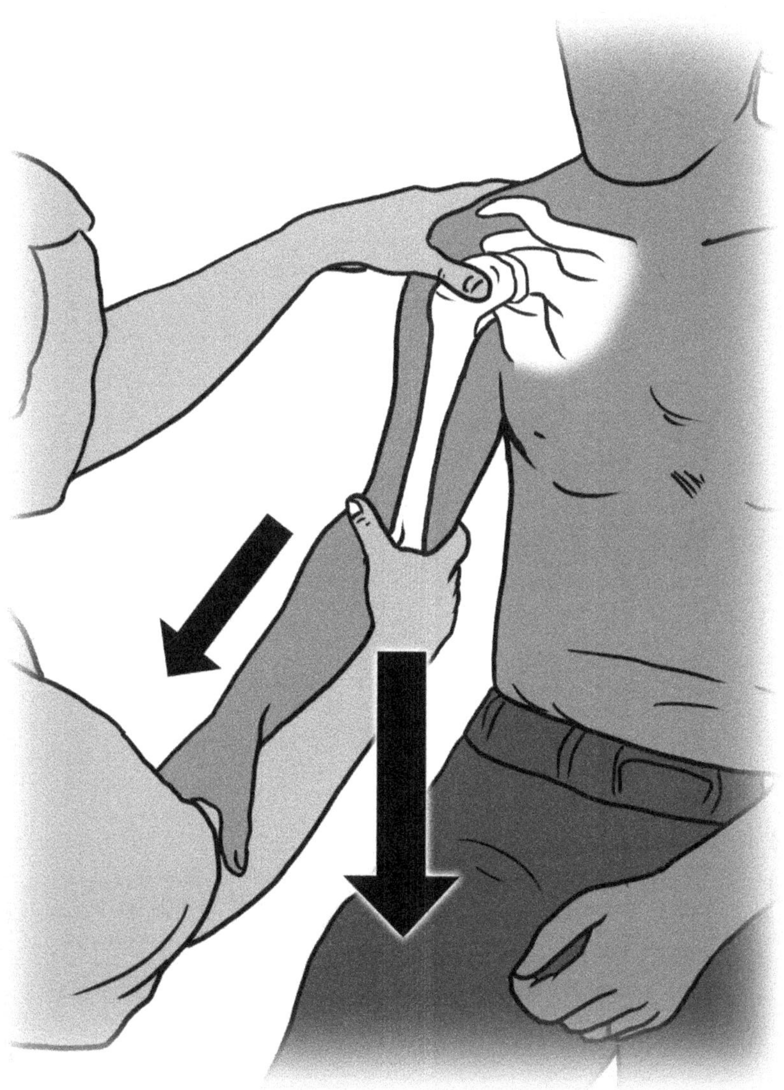

Elbow Dislocation

How are elbow dislocations reduced?

Elbow dislocations are one of the more dramatic joint injuries encountered in the field—painful, visibly deformed, and often functionally disabling. Posterior dislocations are by far the most common type and occur when the forearm is displaced *backward* relative to the humerus, typically from a fall onto an outstretched hand (FOOSH). These injuries can compromise circulation or nerve function below the elbow, and their appearance alone often prompts concern from both the patient and responders.

Early recognition and prompt intervention are critical, especially in wilderness settings where access to definitive care may be delayed.

The elbow joint is formed by three bones: the humerus (upper arm), the radius, and the ulna (forearm bones). The olecranon is the bony tip of the ulna that forms the point of the elbow. When the arm is extended, it fits into a notch on the back of the humerus called the olecranon fossa. This structure forms the point of the elbow and provides a mechanical stop at full extension. When a posterior dislocation occurs, the olecranon is displaced backward, out of alignment with the humerus.

Several major nerves and blood vessels run across the front of the elbow, including the brachial artery, median nerve, and radial nerve. Displacement of the joint can stretch, compress, or tear these structures—making neurovascular assessment before and after reduction critical.

In wilderness settings—where advanced care may be delayed—early reduction is critical. Prompt realignment reduces pain, facilitates evacuation, preserves limb function, and limits long-term damage.

Bony Anatomy of the Elbow

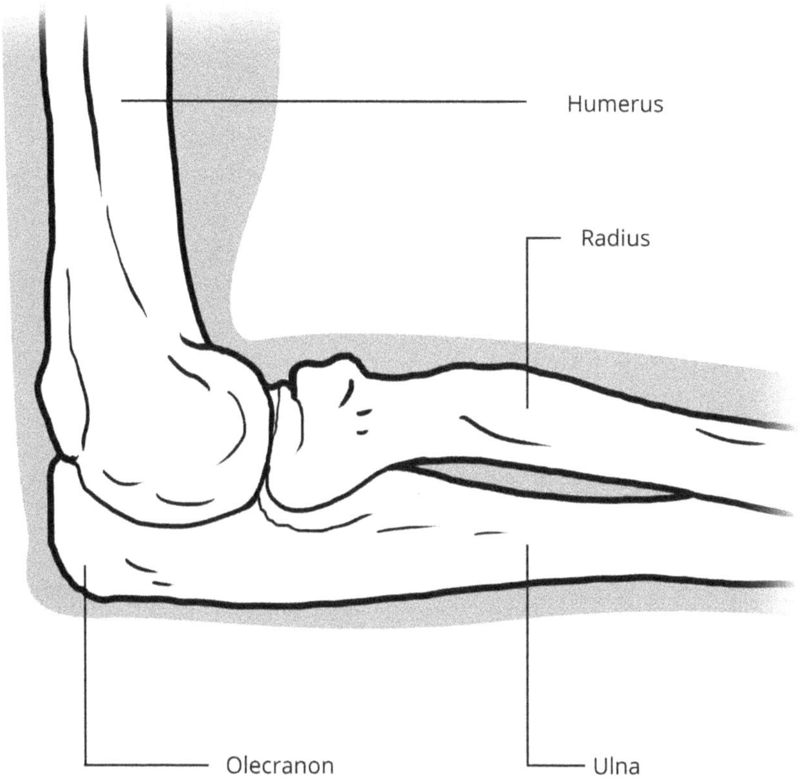

Traction-Countertraction Technique:

This is one of the more reliable methods for reducing a posterior elbow dislocation in the field. It requires two providers and should be performed carefully, step by step:

1. Position the Patient: Have the patient lie supine or sit upright with the injured arm supported, and the elbow slightly flexed, if tolerated.
2. Apply Countertraction: An assistant stabilizes the upper arm by grasping it firmly or using a sheet looped around the upper forearm just above the elbow. The sheet can be anchored around the assistant's back to provide steady countertraction.

3. Apply Traction: The primary provider holds the patient's wrist and applies slow, steady traction along the long axis of the forearm—in line with the bone, pulling away from the elbow.
4. Begin Elbow Flexion: While maintaining traction, gradually flex the elbow. This helps unlock the olecranon from its dislocated position behind the distal humerus.
5. Assist the Reduction: As the elbow flexes, gentle anterior pressure on the olecranon may help guide it forward into place.
6. Confirm Reduction: A palpable or audible "clunk," followed by improved alignment and relief of pain, usually signals a successful reduction.
7. Post-Reduction Care: Recheck pulses, sensation, and motor function. Immobilize the arm in a sling and swathe or a posterior splint and evacuate for definitive care.

Timely evacuation is mandatory for all elbow dislocations—even if successfully reduced—to rule out fractures, assess for ligament injury, and monitor for recurrent instability.

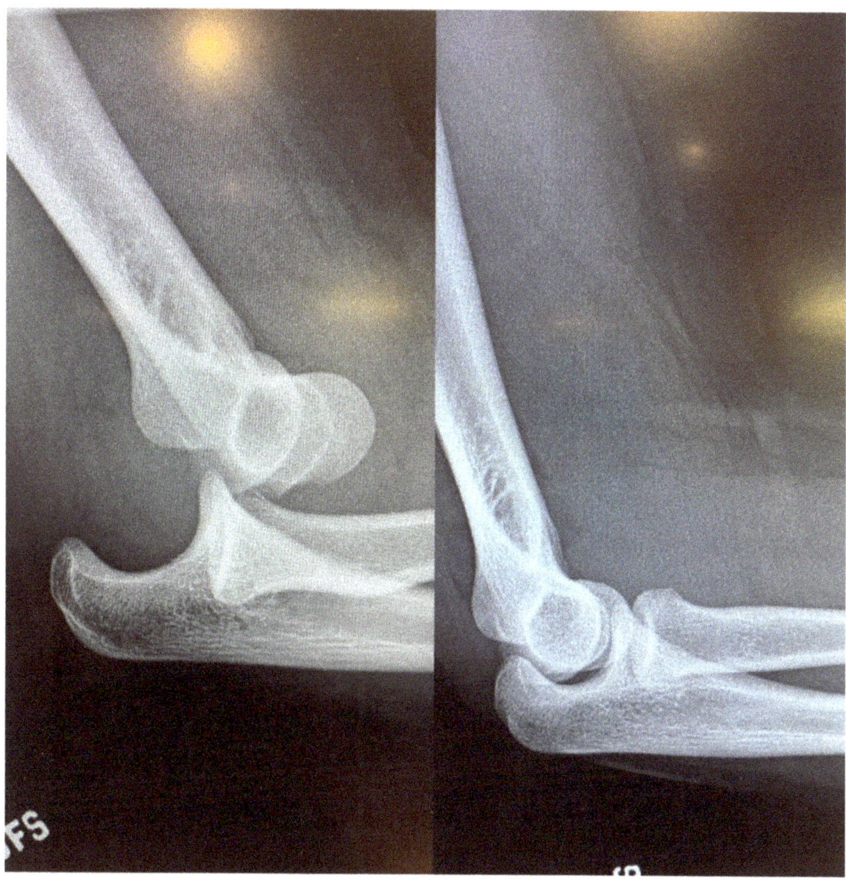

Posterior elbow dislocation, pre-and post-reduction. Initial film shows clear displacement of the ulna relative to the distal humerus. Post-reduction image confirms successful alignment following closed reduction. Both images courtesy of the author.

Lower Extremity Dislocations

Hip

What should I know about hip dislocations?

The hip joint is a ball-and-socket joint, where the femoral head (ball) fits into the acetabulum (socket) of the pelvis. It is deeply seated and highly stable, relying on strong ligaments, muscles, and the labrum (a cartilaginous rim around the socket) to maintain alignment. Because of this stability, for the hip to dislocate requires significant force, often resulting from falls, high-impact trauma, or severe twisting injuries.

Most hip dislocations are posterior dislocations, where the femoral head is forced backward out of the socket. This results in a shortened leg that is internally rotated and held in a fixed position. Anterior dislocations, where the femoral head is displaced forward, are much less common and present with an externally rotated and abducted leg. Both types disrupt the integrity of the joint and put critical structures at risk, including the sciatic nerve, which runs behind the hip, and the femoral artery and vein, which supply blood to the lower limb.

One of the most serious complications of hip dislocation is avascular necrosis (AVN), where the femoral head loses its blood supply due to compression or tearing of the surrounding blood vessels. If reduction is delayed, bone death and joint collapse can occur, leading to permanent disability. Because of this, hip dislocations are medical emergencies, requiring urgent reduction and immediate evacuation.

How do I reduce a hip dislocation in the wilderness?

In remote settings, the "Captain Morgan" technique is a controlled, field-appropriate method for reducing posterior hip dislocations. It uses mechanical leverage and slow, sustained pressure to safely reposition the joint without excessive force.

1. Position the patient: Lay the patient flat on their back on a stable surface. Flex the affected hip and knee to about 90°, or as tolerated. This helps relax the surrounding musculature.
2. Set up the fulcrum: The responder stands beside the patient and places their own knee *under* the patient's flexed knee. Their foot should be firmly planted behind the patient's buttock and on a solid object to brace.
3. Grip and control: One hand controls the ankle, while the other is placed firmly on the patient's thigh, just above the knee.

4. Apply pressure, slow and steady: Begin applying downward pressure on the ankle while slightly pulling the thigh out with the hand on the thigh. Let the mechanical advantage of your leg do the work. This is not a fast movement. Apply pressure to the ankle—and hold it. Don't jerk or use force. Be patient. Let the thigh muscles fatigue and the joint relax into reduction.
5. Feel for reduction: A successful reduction may produce a subtle shift or an audible "clunk." Once reduced, reassess circulation, motor function, and sensation immediately.

If significant resistance or pain persists, stop the attempt and initiate evacuation. Further attempts may worsen the injury.

What should I do after reduction?

Once the hip is reduced, it must be stabilized to prevent further injury. Position the leg in a neutral alignment and secure it using padding and splinting materials. If formal splints aren't available, tie the affected leg to the uninjured leg using soft materials to limit movement.

Evacuation is required for all hip dislocations, regardless of how well the reduction went. These injuries often involve ligament damage, acetabular fractures, or soft tissue trauma that can't be fully assessed without imaging. Check for neurovascular compromise—absent pulses, numbness, or weakness are red flags requiring urgent transport.

If evacuation requires ambulation, have the patient walk slowly and carefully. Avoid long strides and minimize movement over uneven ground. Support the limb, and use trekking poles, crutches, or improvised supports if available. The goal is to protect the joint while making safe progress toward definitive care.

Knee

What should I know about knee dislocations?

Knee dislocations are rare but high-risk injuries where the tibia (shin bone) is forcefully displaced from the femur (thigh bone), resulting in complete joint disruption. This is distinctly different from a patellar dislocation, which only involves the kneecap shifting out of place. True knee dislocations typically involve tearing of multiple ligaments and pose a serious threat to nearby blood vessels and nerves.

The popliteal artery, which runs directly behind the knee, is especially vulnerable—particularly in posterior dislocations, where the tibia moves backward. These injuries carry the highest risk of vascular compromise and can quickly lead to limb-threatening ischemia. Anterior dislocations, where the tibia shifts forward, are more common but still dangerous and can also compromise surrounding structures.

A deep indentation near the inner knee, known as the "pucker sign," may indicate a posterolateral dislocation. These are often locked in place and cannot be safely reduced in the field. Forced manipulation may cause further damage. Evacuation should be initiated immediately if this sign is present.

Every knee dislocation should be treated as a vascular emergency until proven otherwise. Assess for distal pulses, motor strength, and sensation. If pulses are absent—even if the joint appears realigned—evacuate without delay. Time-sensitive vascular injury can lead to permanent damage or limb loss.

How is a knee dislocation reduced in the wilderness?

Step-by-Step Procedure:

1. Position the patient flat on their back on a firm, stable surface. Keep the affected leg exposed and supported.

2. Assess Distally: Check foot pulses and capillary refill. Assess sensation and motor function, especially dorsiflexion and plantarflexion.
3. Set Hand Position: Place one hand firmly on the distal femur (just above the knee) for countertraction and control.
4. Grip the Tibia: With your other hand, grasp the distal tibia at the calf. Ensure a secure hold for steady traction.
5. Apply Traction—Slow and Straight: Pull gently but firmly along the long axis of the tibia. Avoid sudden jerks. The goal is to overcome muscle tension and create space between the bones, allowing the joint surfaces to disengage.
6. Maintain Traction—Be Patient: Keep steady pressure. As the tibia slides back beneath the femoral condyles, you may feel or hear a subtle "clunk." The leg will often visibly realign and partially extend.
7. Reassess Circulation and Alignment: Immediately recheck pulses, limb alignment, sensation, and motor function. If circulation improves, continue to monitor. If pulses remain absent, evacuate urgently—arterial repair may still be required.
8. Immobilize the Leg: Splint in a neutral, extended position using available materials—padding, trekking poles, sticks, etc. If gear is limited, tie the legs together for temporary support.
9. Evacuate Immediately: Even with a successful reduction and restored pulses, all knee dislocations require surgical evaluation. Ligament rupture, occult fracture, or vascular injury cannot be ruled out in the field.

What should I do after a reduction?

After reducing a knee dislocation, immediately reassess circulation, sensation, and movement in the affected leg. Check capillary refill by pressing on a toenail or toe pad—color should return within two seconds. If circulation is adequate, immobilize the leg in a straight, neutral position using available materials (splints, foam, trekking poles, etc.) and secure it to prevent motion. Elevate the leg, apply cold if available, and provide pain control with ibuprofen or acetaminophen. The patient should avoid bearing weight. Evacuate immediately—regardless of appearance, these injuries carry a high risk of vascular damage and ligament instability requiring surgical evaluation.

What should I know about kneecap dislocations?

Not a ton. The kneecap (patella) is a small, floating (sesamoid) bone that moves within a groove at the front of the thigh bone. It helps the quadriceps muscle extend the leg and provides stability to the knee joint. Normally, the patella stays in place as the knee bends and straightens, but if the stabilizing structures are weak or if enough force is applied, it can shift out of alignment, leading to a dislocation.

Most patellar dislocations happen when the kneecap shifts outward (laterally), often due to twisting movements, a direct blow, or landing awkwardly from a jump. People with naturally loose joints, weak supporting muscles, or a shallow groove in the thigh bone are at higher risk for dislocation. While this injury is not as severe as a full knee dislocation, it can still cause significant pain, swelling, and joint instability if not properly managed. Once a patella has dislocated, the risk of it happening again increases, especially if the surrounding muscles and ligaments do not fully recover.

How do I reduce a kneecap dislocation?

To restore normal alignment, position the patient on their back with the leg fully extended and supported. Keeping the leg straight relaxes the quadriceps, which otherwise contracts and prevents reduction. If needed, gently flexing the hip slightly can further reduce muscle tension. Apply gradual medial pressure to the lateral (outside) edge of the patella, guiding it back into the femoral groove. Reduction is often confirmed by a palpable or audible click, with immediate relief of tension. Forcing the patella back into place should be avoided, as aggressive pressure can worsen ligamentous injury or cause unnecessary pain.

What should I do after reduction?

After reduction, immediate stabilization is necessary to prevent recurrent dislocation and allow soft tissue healing. Immobilize the knee using a splint, knee brace, or padded rigid support secured with bandages or straps. Reassess circulation, capillary refill, and sensation in the lower leg, ensuring there is no neurovascular compromise. Applying cold packs and elevating the leg can help reduce swelling and discomfort. Pain management with ibuprofen and acetaminophen can improve comfort, especially in prolonged evacuation scenarios.

Evacuation may not be necessary for a first-time dislocation that reduces easily, with minimal pain, no instability, and the patient able to bear weight. However, evacuation should be considered if there are signs of ligament or cartilage damage, such as persistent pain, joint locking, or instability. Recurrent dislocations often indicate underlying structural weakness and should be evaluated for rehabilitation, bracing, or surgical intervention.

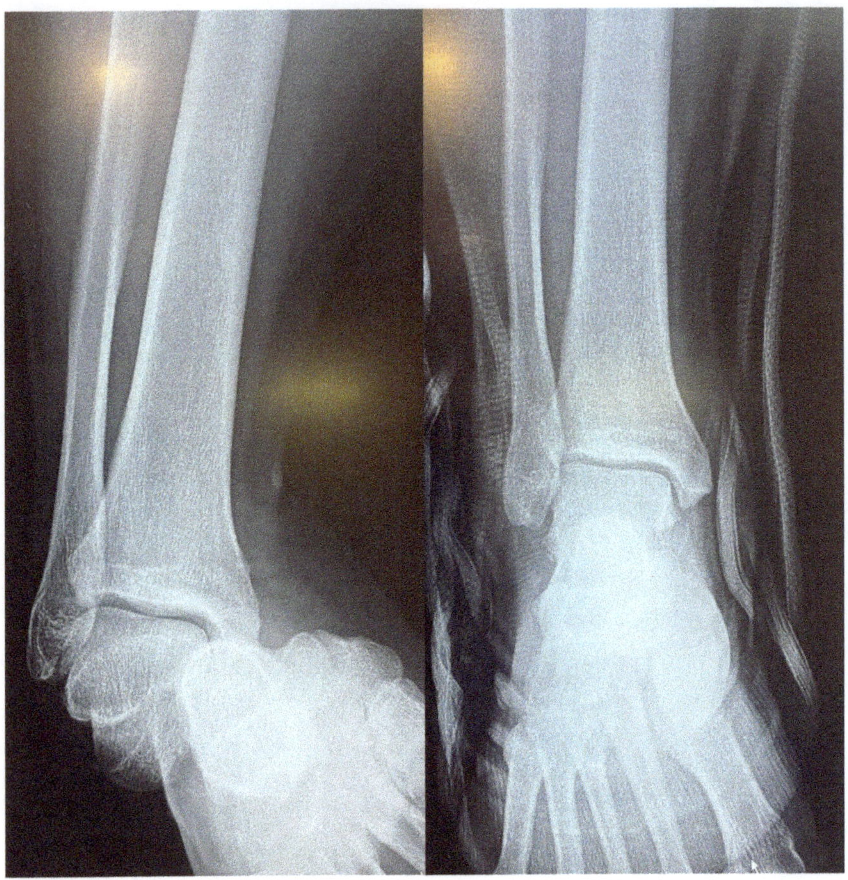

Pre-and post-reduction X-rays of an ankle fracture-dislocation in an 18-year—old male who jumped from a rock outcropping. The image on the left shows a dislocated joint with the talus pushed out of alignment beneath the tibia and fibula. The image on the right, taken after reduction, shows improved alignment of the bones and re-establishment of joint stability. Reduction helps restore circulation, relieve pressure on nerves and vessels, and prevent long-term damage. Image courtesy of the author.

Ankle

What should I know about ankle dislocations?

Ankle dislocations are severe injuries that typically also involve fractures due to the structural vulnerability of the joint. The ankle relies on bony congruency and ligament stability, making it highly susceptible to displacement under high-impact forces, such as falls, twisting injuries, or direct trauma. When the talus dislocates from the tibia and fibula, circulation and nerve function may be compromised, leading to severe swelling, impaired blood flow, and increasing tissue damage if not promptly addressed. Reduction is critical to restore joint alignment, relieve pressure on neurovascular structures, and prevent worsening soft tissue injury.

How do I reduce an ankle dislocation?

To perform a reduction, begin by positioning the patient on their back with the knee gently bent—this relaxes the calf muscles and reduces tension across the ankle joint. Expose the lower leg and support it securely to allow clear access to the foot.

1. Stabilize the ankle by grasping the heel firmly with one hand, while the other hand is positioned across the top of the foot. Apply gentle, steady traction in line with the leg, pulling the foot away slowly to slightly separate the joint surfaces. The goal is to create space and allow the dislocated bones to disengage.
2. Once you feel a release in tension or slight mobility, guide the foot back into its normal alignment using slow, controlled motion. Avoid any twisting or sudden movements. A successful reduction is usually indicated by improved alignment, decreased resistance, and visible relief in pain.
3. Afterward, reassess circulation using capillary refill along with checks for sensation and motor function. Press on a toenail—color should return within two seconds. If refill is delayed or there are signs of numbness, weakness, or impaired movement, assume a vascular injury.

Once the joint is reduced, immediate immobilization is necessary. Splint the ankle and lower leg using a rigid support that extends from just below the knee to the foot to prevent further movement during evacuation. Reassess circulation, capillary refill, and sensation in the toes to ensure proper blood flow and nerve function. Persistent numbness, a pulseless foot, or increasing swelling after reduction suggests ongoing vascular compromise, requiring immediate evacuation.

Even with a successful reduction, evacuation is mandatory. These injuries carry a high risk of fracture, ligament damage, and arterial injury—all requiring imaging, surgical evaluation, and close follow-up. In the wilderness, early recognition, reduction, stabilization, and timely evacuation are key to preserving limb function.

Red Flag Framework: Traumatic Emergencies

What's an easy way to remember what signs and symptoms warrant evacuation using the Red Flag Framework?

For Traumatic Emergencies: **FRACTURE**

- **F**: Fractures or Deformities – Visible signs of fractures, joint dislocations, or irreducible injuries. This can include deformities, abnormal bone positioning, or inability to move the affected area.
- **R**: Rigid Abdomen – Severe pain, distension, or guarding indicating possible internal injuries. Immediate evaluation for internal bleeding or organ damage is critical.
- **A**: Altered Mental Status – Confusion, unresponsiveness, or signs of traumatic brain injury (TBI) suggest serious damage, requiring urgent stabilization and transport.
- **C**: Cervical Spine Tenderness –Midline neck pain or deformity following trauma, suggesting a potential spinal injury. Immediate immobilization is necessary to prevent further damage.
- **T**: Thoracic Injuries – Difficulty breathing, severe chest pain, or suspected rib fractures (e.g., pneumothorax) should prompt immediate intervention. Protect the airway and prepare for rapid transport.

- **U**: Uncontrolled Bleeding – Persistent external bleeding or signs of internal hemorrhage require swift action to control and stabilize the injury, especially in cases of significant blood loss.
- **R**: Restricted Movement – Inability to move a limb, bear weight, or perform basic tasks indicates a severe injury, such as a fracture or dislocation that requires immobilization and stabilization.
- **E**: Entrance or Exit Wounds – Penetrating trauma to the chest, abdomen, or head demands immediate intervention. Apply pressure to control bleeding and stabilize the patient during transport.
- Any of these signs are a clear indication of a serious injury, requiring prompt attention and likely evacuation to prevent further harm.

Any of these signs indicate a potentially serious condition, requiring immediate evaluation and possible evacuation. When in doubt, follow the Red Flag Framework: FRACTURE = Evacuate.

Trauma at the Fenceline

The morning snowmobile run up to the fence line was oddly uneventful—no new slide paths, no snowdrifts blocking the road—quiet. Should've been my first clue. The stillness broke with a crackle on the radio: a call for help from fellow guides who had come across an injured snowmobiler.

I ran the sled down to the supply shack. Two snowmobiles were parked outside. Inside, the guides were tending to a middle-aged rider who'd hit a tree at high speed. The impact threw him forward, but not before his right leg clipped the handlebars—snapping his femur. It was obvious: angulated, with the bone tenting the skin but, thankfully, not open—at least not yet.

But before touching the injury, we ran a full primary trauma survey. That head-to-toe approach is standard and important for a reason—major mechanisms can hide lethal injuries.

He was in pain but alert. No respiratory issues. No chest wall tenderness with deep breathing. His head, neck, spine, and pelvis were all nontender. Aside from some superficial scalp abrasions, nothing else jumped out.

Once life threats were ruled out, it was time to stabilize and move. The helicopter was still 30 minutes out. Steady, manual traction was applied—slow and deliberate—with one hand on top of the foot, the other under the heel. At first, there was resistance: pain, muscle guarding. But within moments, the leg gave, the bone came back into rough alignment, and the skin tenting melted away. His toes were warm, with capillary refill under two seconds. Confident he had adequate perfusion, we immobilized the leg, bound both legs together, and secured him to a backboard.

From there, it was a toboggan ride to the LZ.

He made a full recovery. The case was a reminder: just because the injury is obvious doesn't mean it's the only one. The methodical, step-by-step trauma approach matters—especially out here.

Hope that cowboy's back out cutting powder somewhere.

Wound Management in the Wilderness

What are the initial priorities in wound management?

In wilderness settings, the priorities in wound management are controlling bleeding and preventing infection from further environmental contamination.

Ensuring safety for both the responder and the patient is the first priority, and using gloves or protective barriers minimizes exposure to infectious agents. Once safety is established, *thorough* wound cleaning is the most important step in preventing complications that could become life-threatening in remote environments.

Removing dirt, debris, and nonviable tissue is critical, as infection risk increases with delayed or inadequate cleaning. Animal bites require special attention due to their high bacterial load and deep puncture nature, which make infection almost inevitable without aggressive irrigation, antibiotics, and wound care.

How should wounds be cleaned in the wilderness?

Thoroughly. Effective wound cleaning depends on available resources, but the goal remains the same: reduce contamination and remove debris without harming healthy tissue.

Start by washing the skin around the wound with soap and potable water. This step helps prevent bacteria from the surrounding area from entering the wound during irrigation.

Use clean, drinkable water for irrigation. If a syringe or squeeze bottle is available, use it to create steady, moderate pressure to flush out dirt and bacteria. If none is available, pour water from a height to produce a similar flushing effect. The key is to remove visible debris while avoiding trauma to the tissue.

For wounds that are heavily contaminated, a diluted povidone-iodine solution (the color of weak tea) can help reduce bacterial load. Always rinse thoroughly with clean water afterward—povidone-iodine left in the wound can impair healing by damaging healthy cells.

After cleaning, inspect the wound for signs of deep tissue injury, retained foreign material, or the need for closure. Keep the wound moist and covered with a clean dressing to support healing and reduce infection risk.

Watch closely for signs of infection—redness, swelling, warmth, increased pain, or pus. If these occur, antibiotics and evacuation may be necessary.

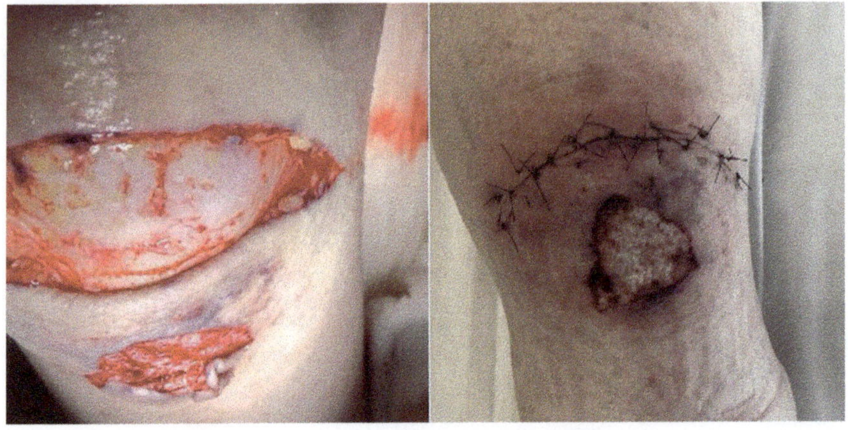

Full-thickness laceration over the anterior knee following a fall onto a rock. The wound was cleaned thoroughly in the field, antibiotics were initiated, and it was dressed to allow safe ambulation. Due to the remote setting, the patient was required to hike six miles out of the Grand Canyon to access definitive medical care. Image courtesy of the author.

When should I close a wound in the wilderness?

Closing a wound can help protect it, reduce discomfort, and promote faster healing—but only when the wound is clean, well-irrigated, and carries a low risk of infection. The best candidates for closure are shallow wounds in areas with minimal movement and good blood flow, where contamination is minimal, and drainage isn't needed.

Not all wounds should be closed. Heavily contaminated wounds, animal or human bites, and deep punctures should typically be left open to allow drainage. Closing these wounds too soon can trap harmful bacteria inside, increasing the risk of infection, abscess, or even systemic illness.

Timing matters. Wounds older than 8–12 hours, especially in dirty or high-risk environments, are more likely to become infected and are generally better left open. In some cases, delayed primary closure—where the wound is cleaned and monitored for a few days before being closed—may be the safer option.

Before closing any wound, perform thorough cleaning and irrigation. Remove all visible dirt and debris. If there's any doubt about whether the wound is fully clean, it's safer to leave it open and monitor closely.

In remote settings, ongoing observation is critical. Watch for signs of infection such as redness, swelling, warmth, drainage, or worsening pain. If any of these signs appear, antibiotics and evacuation may be necessary.

What are some options for wound closure techniques in the wilderness?

In a wilderness setting, wound closure depends on several factors: depth, contamination, location, bleeding control, responder experience, and available resources. Closure may be delayed, improvised, or avoided entirely if infection risk outweighs the benefit. When appropriate, here are the main options:

1. *Delayed Primary Closure*

   In contaminated or high-risk wounds, the best option may be to irrigate thoroughly, pack the wound open, and allow it to drain for 48–72 hours before closing. This lowers infection risk and gives the body time to control bacterial load. It's the safest approach when evacuation is delayed, and the wound is not immediately life-threatening.
2. *Steri-Strips or Medical Adhesive Strips*

   If available, adhesive strips work well on clean, superficial wounds with minimal tension. They're easy to apply and low-risk but require dry skin and some skin apposition. Reinforce with tape or improvised dressing to prevent peeling.
3. *Superglue (Cyanoacrylate)*

   Commercial or medical-grade cyanoacrylate can be used for superficial skin closure. Pinch the wound edges together and apply a thin layer over—not inside-the wound. Allow it to dry before releasing tension. It's fast, reasonably secure, and useful when Steri-strips or sutures aren't available. Do not use in deep or contaminated wounds.

4. *Hair Apposition (Scalp Wounds)*

   For scalp lacerations, twist small bundles of hair from each side of the wound and tie them together with a square knot or simple overhand tie. This method works well on small bleeding scalp wounds when suture is not available.
5. *Suturing*

   If you have sterile equipment and training, sutures provide the strongest closure. Only close wounds that are clean, less than 12 hours old (24 on the face), and not heavily contaminated. Always irrigate thoroughly. Avoid closing puncture wounds, animal bites, or wounds with devitalized tissue.
6. *Improvised Closure (Butterfly Tapes, Duct Tape)*

   If no medical supplies are available, narrow strips of tape, cloth, or even duct tape can approximate wound edges. This is a temporary solution meant to protect deeper tissue and minimize contamination, not to create a surgical-quality seal.

Always reassess perfusion and signs of infection. Any closure in the wilderness carries risk. If swelling, redness, pus, or worsening pain develops, *reopen the wound* and manage it as an open and contaminated wound. In questionable cases, it's safer to leave open, pack with gauze, and monitor than to seal in infection.

How can I tell if a skin infection needs antibiotics?

Recognizing when a skin infection needs antibiotics is critical in wilderness settings, where delays in treatment can lead to serious complications. Minor redness or irritation around a wound often resolves with proper cleaning and dressing. However, if the redness begins to spread beyond the wound edges, the area becomes increasingly swollen, warm, or painful, or if pus begins to drain from the site, the infection is likely progressing, and antibiotics are required. Red streaks moving up the limb (lymphangitis), fever, chills, body aches, or tender lymph nodes near the affected area are all signs that the infection is spreading beyond the skin. These symptoms indicate the need for systemic treatment and possible evacuation. Additionally, if the wound fails to improve within 48 to 72 hours despite proper care, antibiotics should be initiated. When in doubt, it's safer to treat early than to risk the infection progressing beyond control.

How are abscesses managed in the wilderness?

The principle for treating abscesses is well established: *Ubi pus, ibi evacua*—"Where there is pus, evacuate it." This Latin aphorism, widely attributed to the Dutch physician Herman Boerhaave (1688-1738), has been a cornerstone of medical practice for centuries. Regardless of the setting, an abscess will not resolve until the pus is drained, making this principle just as relevant in wilderness medicine as in any hospital.

The first step in managing an abscess is identifying the point of maximal fluctuance. Fluctuance refers to the sensation of trapped fluid beneath the skin, often with a subtle rebound when compressed. It indicates where the pus pocket is most superficial and is the ideal spot for the incision.

The incision should be made directly over this point and must be large enough to allow complete drainage. If the opening is too small, the wound will seal prematurely, trapping bacteria and pus inside, increasing the risk of recurrence. Once opened, the cavity should be gently probed to break up loculations—internal pockets where pus can remain trapped, preventing full resolution.

After drainage, irrigate the cavity thoroughly with clean water or a diluted antiseptic solution, such as a 50:50 mix of hydrogen peroxide and water. This helps clear debris and reduce bacterial load. Packing the cavity with sterile gauze keeps it open and promotes continued drainage, preventing early closure that could lead to reinfection. Packing should be changed at least twice daily, and the site monitored for worsening redness, swelling, or pain—signs that may indicate retained pus or spreading infection.

Antibiotics are not a substitute for drainage, but they are necessary if systemic symptoms are present, such as fever, chills, or expanding redness. Without proper evacuation of pus, antibiotics alone are unlikely to resolve an infection.

In wilderness settings, early intervention is critical. Large, deep, or high-risk abscesses—especially on the face, hands, or groin—or those that don't drain fully, should prompt evacuation. Effective wound care, continued monitoring, and ensuring full drainage are essential to prevent a localized infection from becoming a serious or even life-threatening condition.

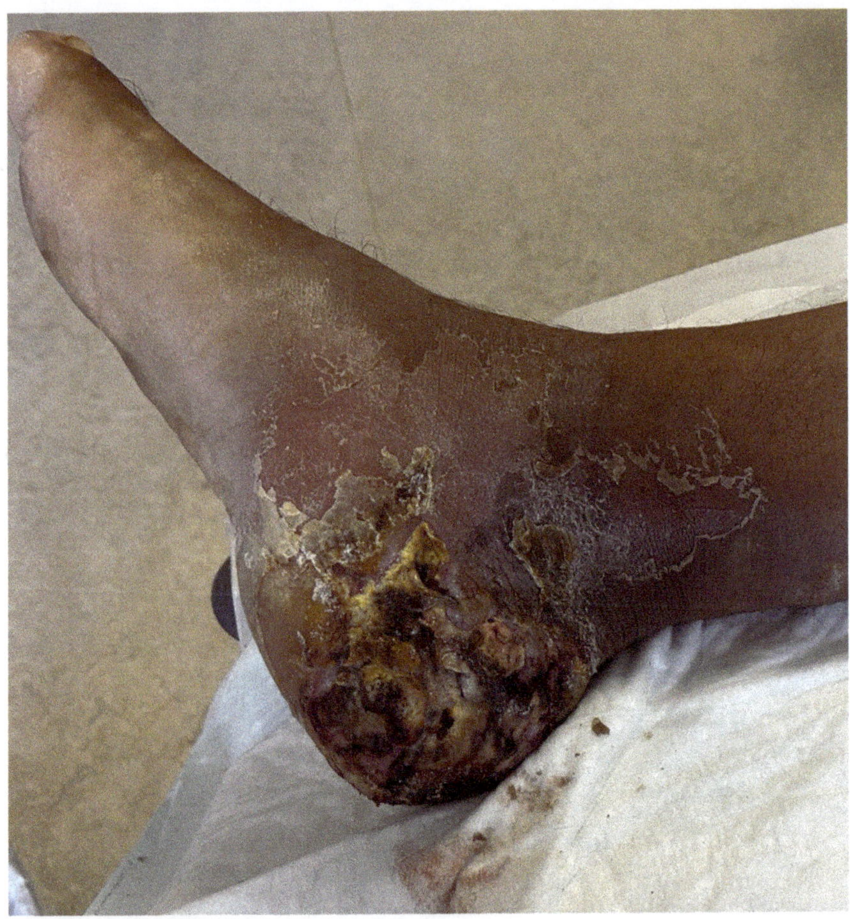

Infected heel wound in a 46-year-old diabetic male following a prolonged backcountry trip. Poor wound hygiene, extensive necrosis, and surrounding cellulitis led to deep tissue involvement. Delayed presentation significantly complicated care, and an amputation was ultimately required. Image courtesy of the author.

Why are wounds in diabetics especially concerning?

Diabetic wounds are concerning in any setting, but especially in the field, where limited hygiene and delayed care compound the risks. The underlying physiology of diabetes creates a perfect storm for delayed healing, unrecognized injury, and serious infection.

Chronically elevated blood sugar damages small blood vessels through a process called glycation, where excess glucose binds to proteins in vessel walls. Over time, this causes thickening and stiffening of small blood vessels, reducing their elasticity and impairing circulation. The result is poor perfusion—particularly in the feet and lower legs, where gravity and distance from the heart already challenge oxygen delivery and waste removal.

At the same time, hyperglycemia impairs immune function. White blood cells become less effective at killing bacteria and coordinating inflammation in high-sugar environments. Nerve damage (neuropathy) adds another layer of risk: that same vascular damage also affects peripheral nerves, leading to loss of sensation, typically starting in the toes and progressing upward. As a result, patients may not feel pressure, pain, or early injury—allowing small wounds to worsen without detection.

All of this translates into a higher risk of deep infection, poor healing, and serious complications—even from minor injuries. In wilderness settings, any wound on a diabetic patient, especially on the foot or lower leg, should be treated as high risk. Clean it thoroughly, start antibiotics if there's any sign of infection or tissue involvement, monitor closely, and maintain a low threshold for evacuation if the wound deteriorates or fails to improve.

Why are coral cuts particularly dangerous, and how should they be managed in the field?

Coral cuts are more than just surface abrasions—they carry a high risk of infection, delayed healing, and persistent inflammation. The jagged surface of coral creates irregular wounds that often trap tiny fragments deep in the tissue. These embedded particles can lead to ongoing pain, irritation, and firm nodules under the skin that may last for weeks if not properly cleaned. Many corals also contain toxins, stinging cells (nematocysts), and harbor marine bacteria like *Vibrio* species, which can cause rapidly worsening soft tissue infections.

Field management starts with immediate, aggressive cleaning. Rinse the wound thoroughly with clean water or sterile saline, then scrub it with soap and water to dislodge fine coral particles. Irrigation alone isn't enough—mechanical scrubbing is essential to prevent long-term irritation or infection. Avoid home remedies like lime juice, which can worsen tissue damage.

Coral cuts should be left open to air when possible. Avoid petroleum-based ointments, which trap moisture and create a low-oxygen environment where bacteria can thrive—just like underwater. Let the wound dry completely before applying a breathable, nonstick dressing.

These cases rarely require immediate evacuation. If the wound stays clean, stable, and improves with basic care, it can usually be managed in the field. However, if redness, swelling, worsening pain, or fever develop, start oral antibiotics such as doxycycline or ciprofloxacin, and arrange for evacuation. These infections can progress *quickly* and should not be taken lightly.

What's the deal with "staph" infections, and what is MRSA?

Staphylococcus aureus, often referred to as "staph," is a common bacterium found on the skin and in the nasal passages of many healthy individuals. It typically causes no harm, but when it enters the body through a break in the skin—like a cut, abrasion, or puncture—it can lead to infection. These infections range from minor issues like pimples, boils, or small abscesses to more serious conditions involving deeper soft tissue, joints, bones, or even the bloodstream. Staph is opportunistic—it takes advantage of breaches in the skin's natural barrier, particularly in settings where hygiene is limited, or wounds go untreated.

MRSA (Methicillin-resistant *Staphylococcus aureus*) is a particularly concerning strain because it has evolved resistance to several commonly used antibiotics, including methicillin, amoxicillin, and cephalexin. This makes it more difficult to treat. MRSA often presents as a painful, swollen, red lump that may resemble a spider bite or boil. It typically develops quickly, may feel warm to the touch, and often drains pus.

The concern with MRSA is twofold: antibiotic resistance, which limits treatment options, and its tendency to cause more aggressive and rapidly spreading infections. Left untreated or managed inadequately, MRSA can invade deeper tissue or spread into the bloodstream, leading to serious systemic illness. In wilderness or remote environments, this becomes a high-risk scenario due to delayed access to advanced care.

Early recognition is essential. If a wound becomes more swollen, painful, or begins draining pus—especially if accompanied by fever or red streaks moving up a limb—MRSA should be suspected. Start antibiotics effective against MRSA, such as doxycycline, clindamycin, or trimethoprim-sulfamethoxazole, if available and tolerated. Evacuation should be arranged as soon as possible, particularly if there is no improvement within 24 to 48 hours or if systemic symptoms develop. In remote medicine, a small staph infection that goes unrecognized can rapidly become a major medical problem.

Why don't healthcare professionals use the term "flesh-eating bacteria"?

Because it's inaccurate, dramatic, and clinically unhelpful. The term usually refers to necrotizing soft tissue infections, most often necrotizing fasciitis—a rapidly progressing infection that destroys skin, fascia, and muscle. Necrotizing simply means tissue death. These infections don't involve bacteria "eating" flesh—they involve toxins and inflammation that kill tissues.

There's no single "flesh-eating" organism. These infections can be caused by *Group A Streptococcus, Clostridium, Vibrio*, or mixed aerobic and anaerobic bacteria. The damage comes from bacterial toxins and the body's inflammatory response.

The phrase makes it sound rare or exotic, but necrotizing infections can occur anytime a serious wound, poor blood flow, or delayed care gives aggressive bacteria a foothold. What matters is early recognition: pain out of proportion, rapid swelling, systemic symptoms. The language doesn't help.

How about vodka or rubbing alcohol to clean wounds in the field?

How about it? No. Neither vodka nor rubbing alcohol should be used directly on open wounds. Vodka contains only about 40% alcohol—far below the 60% threshold needed to kill bacteria and viruses. It also contains impurities and sugars that can irritate tissue, promote infection, and delay healing. It's ineffective and potentially harmful.

Rubbing alcohol (usually 70% isopropyl) is a stronger disinfectant and works well on intact skin or for cleaning instruments. But pouring it into an open wound damages healthy tissue, delays healing, and causes unnecessary (and often significant) pain. No doubt it kills bacteria—but it also kills the cells trying to repair the wound. Keep the alcohol as a last consideration.

In the wilderness, your best option for wound care is clean water or sterile saline. These flush out debris and reduce bacterial load without harming tissue. If no other options are available, alcohol can be used to clean the skin around the wound or to disinfect instruments—not the wound itself.

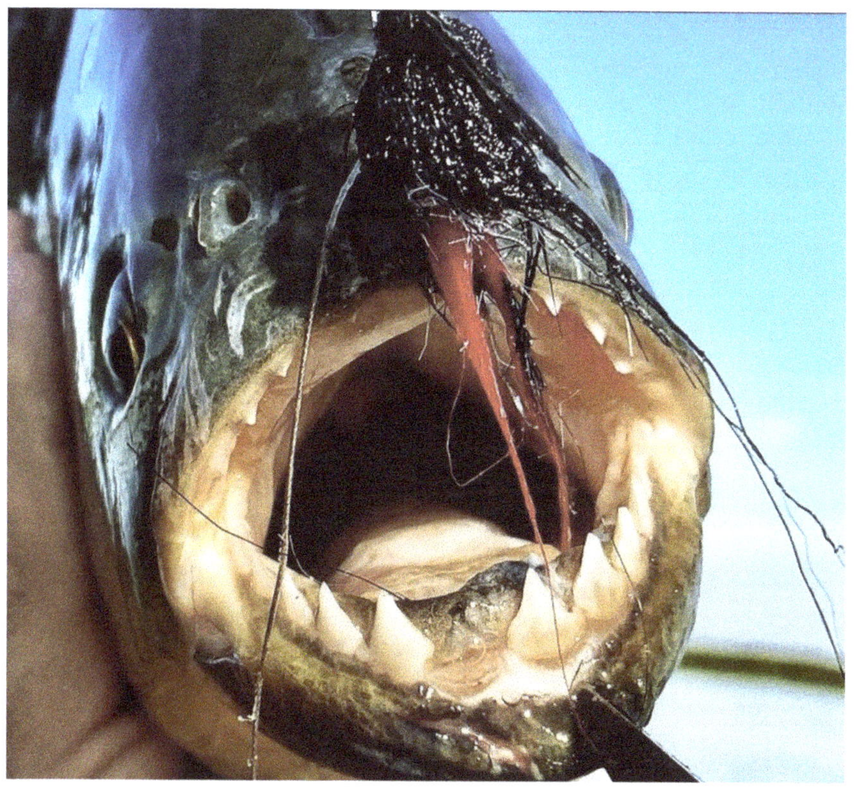

Dentition of a piraña, photographed in the Paraná system near the Iberá Marsh, Argentina. These sharp, triangular teeth are adapted for rapid shearing and can inflict serious lacerations. The mouth is heavily colonized with freshwater bacteria, including *Aeromonas* and *Pseudomonas* species, making even superficial wounds high risk for infection. Image courtesy of the author.

How do saltwater and freshwater wounds differ?

The type of water directly affects the bacterial risk. Freshwater wounds are typically contaminated with organisms like *Aeromonas* and *Pseudomonas*, which can cause cellulitis or soft tissue infections and usually respond well to antibiotics such as ciprofloxacin or trimethoprim-sulfamethoxazole if treated early.

Saltwater wounds, especially in warm or brackish environments, tend to be more dangerous. They carry a higher risk of infection from aggressive marine bacteria like *Vibrio vulnificus*, which can invade tissue rapidly and lead to necrotizing fasciitis or sepsis—especially in people with are immunocompromised. These infections progress quickly and can become life-threatening within hours.

All water-related wounds should be irrigated thoroughly with clean water or sterile saline to remove debris or organic matter completely. For saltwater injuries, especially puncture wounds or lacerations in warm coastal environments, empiric antibiotics targeting *Vibrio*—such as doxycycline or ciprofloxacin—should be considered. Any increasing redness, swelling, pain, or fever should prompt concern. Saltwater wounds require a lower threshold for antibiotics and evacuation due to the speed and severity of potential infection. You've been warned.

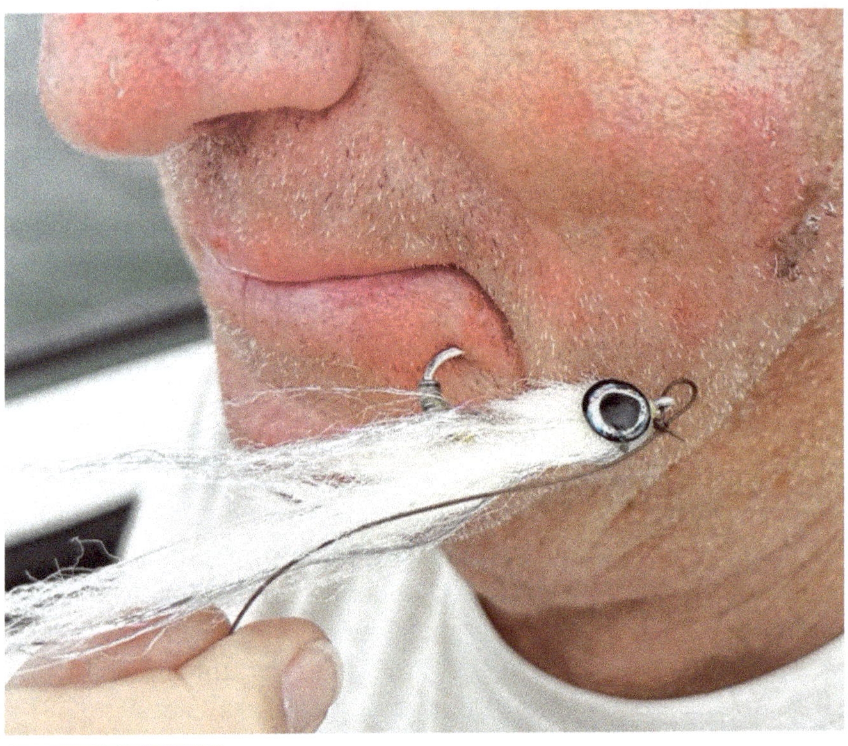

A common but painful mishap—barbed saltwater fly embedded in the lower lip of an angler. The hook was removed using the Quick Release Method with 30 lb. fluorocarbon fishing line, and the wound was thoroughly scrubbed in the field. No infectious complications developed. Facial hook injuries bleed heavily and carry a risk of infection, especially in warm, salt-water environments. Image courtesy of the author.

How do I remove a fishhook?

Removing a fishhook requires careful consideration of the hook's type, location, and depth to minimize tissue damage and prevent complications. In wilderness settings, where medical care may be delayed, proper technique reduces additional trauma and lowers infection risk.

Quick-Release Method:

This method is best for superficially embedded or barbless hooks where the barb has not deeply penetrated. It relies on momentum to extract the hook quickly with minimal tearing.

- Loop a strong string or fishing line around the midpoint of the hook's bend.
- While pressing firmly on the hook's shank (to the skin) to disengage the barb, pull the string sharply and forcefully along the entry path in a swift, controlled motion.
- Do not hesitate on the pull, as hesitation can cause additional tearing.

This technique is simple and effective, but improper execution can worsen injury. It should not be used for deeply embedded hooks or those near sensitive structures like tendons, eyes, or joints.

Push-and-Cut Technique:

This method is best for deeply embedded barbed hooks when backing the barb out is not feasible.

- Push the hook forward through the skin until the barb fully emerges.
- Once exposed, cut the barb off using wire cutters or pliers.
- Back the remaining portion of the hook out through the original entry point.

This technique avoids backward retraction of the barb, reducing soft tissue damage and unnecessary tearing.

However, it should be used with caution in areas with poor circulation, high infection risk, or when swelling makes manipulation difficult.

Surgical Removal:

This method is reserved for deeply embedded hooks or when less invasive techniques fail. It is more invasive but allows for precise removal with minimal additional tissue damage.

- Cut the hook's shank about 1cm above the skin to reduce unnecessary movement.
- If available, infiltrate the area with a local anesthetic to improve comfort.
- Using a sterile scalpel, make a small incision directly *over* and cut *down* to the embedded hook.
- Once the scalpel frees the hook from the surrounding tissue, lift it straight out to avoid unnecessary trauma.
- Irrigate the wound thoroughly with clean water or sterile saline to remove debris and bacteria.
- Apply a sterile dressing, monitor for infection, and consider antibiotics if the wound is contaminated or in a high-risk area, such as the hands, feet, or face.

Fish Hook Removal (Quick-Release Method)

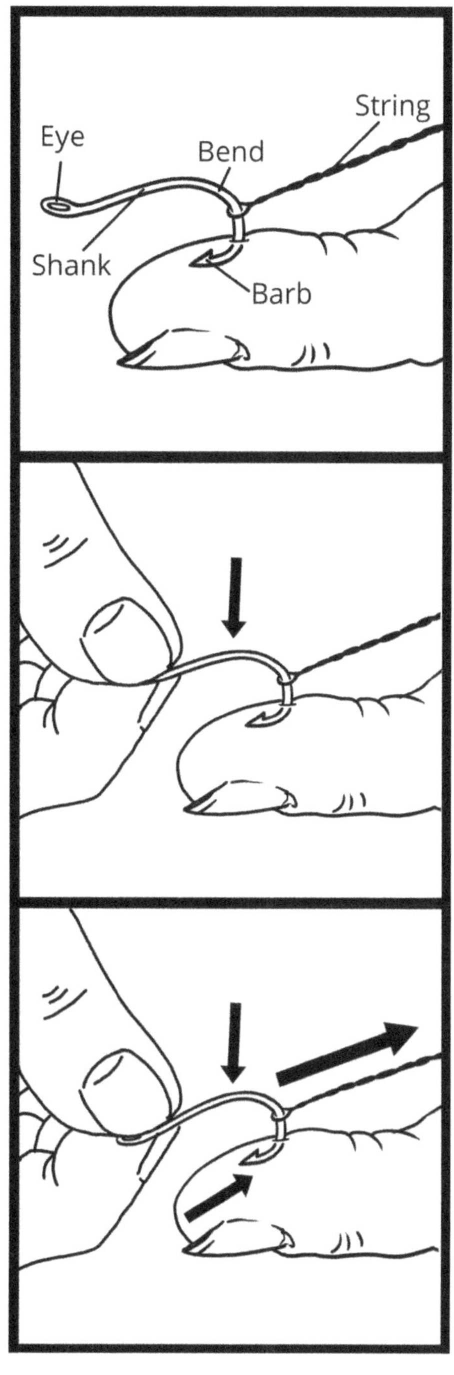

What should I do if a fishhook injures a joint or the eye?

Fishhook injuries involving a joint or the eye require extreme caution and should not be managed in the field beyond stabilization. These are medical emergencies that warrant immediate evacuation. If the hook is near or inside a joint, there's a high risk of septic arthritis, which can rapidly destroy cartilage and lead to permanent loss of function. Do not attempt removal if the hook is deeply embedded or if there's concern it has penetrated the joint capsule. Stabilize the limb to prevent movement and start antibiotics if available. Even if the injury appears minor, any hook in or near a joint should be treated as serious. If the hook is in or around the eye, do not touch it. Any movement-even slight-can cause permanent damage or vision loss. Shield the eye with a rigid covering (like a cup or taped gauze) to limit involuntary movement. Do not apply pressure. Evacuate urgently to an ophthalmologist or trauma center.

If the hook or lure is large and interferes with immobilization, you may carefully clip the shaft with wire cutters to reduce its size for transport. Stabilize the hook before cutting to prevent additional trauma. This step is only for cases where the size of the hook prevents safe evacuation—not for removing the embedded portion.

In both cases, the priority is stabilization, the field administration of antibiotics, and rapid evacuation—not field removal.

Okay, so what is septic arthritis?

Septic arthritis is a bacterial infection inside a joint space, most commonly caused by *Staphylococcus aureus*, including MRSA, but also sometimes by *Streptococcus* species or organisms such as *Pseudomonas*. It can occur when bacteria enter the joint through a penetrating injury, such as a fishhook or dirty puncture wound, or even through the bloodstream in cases of systemic infection. Once inside the joint, bacteria trigger an aggressive inflammatory response that begins breaking down cartilage within hours. Without early treatment, permanent joint destruction can occur in a matter of days. Clinically, septic arthritis presents with rapid-onset joint pain, swelling, warmth, and marked tenderness. The joint may appear red and will usually have a severely limited or painful range of motion. Systemic symptoms such as fever, chills, or malaise may follow if the infection spreads. The affected joint is typically held in a position of comfort, and the patient will resist movement due to pain. Treatment involves urgent joint drainage, intravenous antibiotics, and surgical consultation—none of which can be performed in the field. However, in remote settings, if evacuation is delayed, starting oral antibiotics may help slow the infection. Any suspected joint infection following a penetrating injury should be treated as septic arthritis until proven otherwise. Do not attempt to explore or manipulate the joint. Instead, immobilize the limb, start antibiotics, monitor for systemic signs, and arrange for timely evacuation to definitive care.

What is tetanus?

Tetanus is a life-threatening infection caused by *Clostridium tetani*, a bacterium found in soil, dust, and animal feces. It enters the body through wounds—particularly punctures or contaminated injuries—and produces a powerful neurotoxin that disrupts nerve signals. This results in severe muscle rigidity, painful spasms, and, in advanced cases, lockjaw, respiratory failure, and death. While tetanus is rare in individuals born in the U.S. who completed their childhood vaccination series, the risk isn't zero—especially if boosters are overdue, the wound is high-risk, or medical care is delayed. Wilderness injuries involving soil, wood, fishhooks, or animal-contaminated environments increase exposure risk, particularly when evacuation options are limited.

Prevention starts with thorough wound cleaning using soap and clean water to flush out contaminants. Puncture wounds, deep lacerations, and injuries involving organic material carry the highest risk. The CDC recommends a tetanus booster every ten years—or sooner if a high-risk wound occurs. In the field, knowing the tetanus vaccination status of guests is essential. Medical attention should be sought as soon as possible for a booster shot, or tetanus immune globulin (TIG) if the wound is high risk and immunization is uncertain or incomplete.

Symptoms typically begin about a week after exposure. In remote settings, once symptoms start, outcomes are often poor—even with evacuation. The best protection remains up-to-date vaccination and immediate, aggressive wound care.

Red Flag Framework: Skin & Soft Tissue Emergencies

What's an easy way to remember what signs and symptoms warrant evacuation using the Red Flag Framework?

For skin and soft tissue: **HARM**

- **H**ot, red, swollen wounds with spreading redness or warmth
- **A**bscess with purulent (pus-filled) drainage
- **R**apidly progressing tissue damage or blackening (e.g., necrotizing infection)
- **M**arked pain or tenderness that extends beyond the wound, indicating possible deep or spreading infection.

Any of these signs indicate a potentially serious condition, requiring immediate evaluation and possible evacuation. When in doubt, follow the Red Flag Framework: HARM = Evacuate.

Welcome to the Jungle

Fly fishing for giant tarpon in the Nicaraguan jungle is something every adventure angler should experience at least once. This isn't sight fishing on bright sand flats—it's deep, tannin-stained rivers where prehistoric fish lurk. The kind of place that makes you question whether a fly rod is even the right tool for the job. I mean, it took us a few trips before anything under 150 pounds was landed. The stories were good; the grins were the best.

That's when I noticed one of the guides, off to the side, cradling his elbow. Maybe a strain or bruise from guiding the boats and landing fish day after day. But as I got closer, I saw it was more than that. His elbow was red, taut, and seemingly radiating heat—classic signs of an infection. The skin over the joint had a pale, fluctuant pocket, something that immediately caught my attention.

The guide had already put himself on antibiotics for two days with little improvement. Worse, he'd tried draining the abscess himself with a needle—he'd managed to pull off a little pus, but the infection reset again once the skin closed. It was clear this wasn't going to resolve on its own.

A clean incision was made with a scalpel over the area of maximal fluctuance—I was immediately met with nearly a shot glass volume of pus. The guide had waved off anesthesia—not his favorite decision—but as soon as the pressure released, his relief was obvious. He exhaled, his elbow relaxed, and he flexed his arm, already moving better.

The cavity was flushed with nearly a liter of water, clearing out as much debris as possible. By the time the procedure was complete, the swelling had eased, and the redness nearly resolved. He was told to leave the wound open, irrigate it daily, and let it heal from the inside-out.

If an infection like this were left untreated, it could spread into the joint, causing septic arthritis—eroding the joint capsule—leading to permanent damage, or worse. Fortunately, the guide had full range of motion in his elbow and no tenderness or warmth in the joint itself, so the risk seemed low. Still, he was told to continue the antibiotics for a few more days, that if the pain worsened, swelling deepened, or if he felt ill, he needed to get to Managua immediately.

Some things can be managed in the jungle, but a worsening infection isn't one of them.

Burns

What is a burn?

Burns occur when tissues are damaged by heat, chemicals, electricity, or radiation. The skin, the body's largest organ, acts as a critical barrier against infection, regulates temperature, and prevents fluid loss. When damaged, these functions are compromised, leading to risks such as dehydration, hypothermia, and infection. The skin has three layers: the epidermis (outer protective layer), dermis (housing nerves, blood vessels, and glands), and hypodermis (fatty tissue providing insulation and shock absorption).

Globally, burns account for over 180,000 deaths annually, with the majority occurring in resource-limited settings. In wilderness environments, burns are often caused by campfires, cooking mishaps, sun exposure, or chemical spills. Understanding burn evaluation and management is critical for wilderness guides to prevent complications and improve patient outcomes.

How do I determine the severity of a burn?

The severity of a burn is assessed based on its depth and the total body surface area (TBSA) affected. Depth is categorized into three main types: Superficial burns, involve only the epidermis, causing redness, warmth, and pain without blistering (e.g., sunburn). Partial-thickness burns, extend into the dermis and present with significant pain; redness; blistering; and moist, weeping wounds. Full-thickness burns, destroy all skin layers, appearing white, leathery, or charred, often with little pain due to extensive nerve damage.

TBSA estimation uses the Palmar Method, where the *patient's* palm (including the fingers) approximates 1% of their body surface area. In the wilderness setting, partial-thickness burns involving more than 10% TBSA, and all full-thickness burns are considered major burns and carry a significant risk of systemic complications, including fluid loss, infection, and shock. Burns on critical areas such as the face, hands, feet, genitals, or over major joints also elevate the severity, as they can impair function or healing.

Accurate assessment of depth and extent allows for proper triage and prioritization of care. Superficial burns often require minimal intervention, while partial-and all full-thickness burns demand advanced care, particularly when large areas or vital structures are involved. Severe burns or those showing signs of systemic compromise should prompt immediate evacuation, as early medical intervention is critical to reduce complications and improve outcomes. That clock is definitely ticking.

How should minor burns be managed in the wilderness?

Burn management begins with immediate intervention. Remove the patient from harm and cool the burn with clean, cool water for 20 minutes. Carefully remove restrictive items like jewelry or tight clothing before swelling develops, but do *not* remove clothing stuck to the burn. For chemical burns, irrigate with copious clean water for at least 20 minutes, taking care not to spread the chemical to unaffected areas. Cover the burn with a clean, nonstick dressing or even food-grade cling film to protect the wound and reduce the risk of infection. Use antibiotic ointments like silver sulfadiazine if available, or resource-limited alternatives like honey, banana peels, or boiled potato skins, which provide antimicrobial benefits (albeit limited). Keep the wound moist and monitor for signs of infection, such as increasing redness, swelling, foul-smelling drainage, or fever. Pain management with ibuprofen, acetaminophen and even opioids are often needed for patient comfort.

How should severe burns be managed in the wilderness?

Severe burns are high-risk injuries in remote settings due to fluid loss, infection, and rapid systemic decline. Field management focuses on stabilization, preventing complications, and arranging immediate evacuation. Burns over joints should be splinted in an extended or functional position to reduce the risk of contractures and long-term disability. Circumferential burns—those encircling a finger, limb, or the torso—can act like a tourniquet as swelling progresses, restricting blood flow and potentially even causing compartment syndrome. When located on the chest or abdomen, this same effect can impair ventilation and lead to respiratory failure.

Facial burns, soot in the mouth or nose, hoarseness, or difficulty breathing suggest airway involvement. Swelling may be delayed but can progress rapidly and without warning. Once airway compromise begins, management in the field is extremely difficult. Any sign of inhalation injury warrants immediate evacuation.

Electrical burns always require evacuation, regardless of how minor they appear externally. These injuries can cause serious internal damage—cardiac arrhythmias, muscle necrosis, and delayed organ failure—that may not be immediately visible.

Burns involving more than 10% of total body surface area or those affecting the face, hands, feet, genitals, or major joints carry a high risk of shock and lasting morbidity. In wilderness settings, fluid replacement is often limited to oral intake, but maintaining hydration is critical to slow the onset of hypovolemia. Prophylactic antibiotics may be considered in large burns, given the high infection risk and delays in definitive care.

Monitor for red flags which are easy for burns—*any* worsening of the patient's condition, in any way, warrants urgent evacuation. I told you—the clock is ticking.

Drowning

How common is drowning?

Drowning is a major global health concern, accounting for an estimated 236,000 deaths annually, according to the World Health Organization. Nonfatal drownings are even more common and many result in long-term complications, including permanent neurological injury from prolonged hypoxia. In wilderness settings, the risk of drowning increases during activities such as swimming, rafting, kayaking, or river crossings, where strong currents, cold-water, unpredictable conditions, and delayed rescue responses significantly reduce survival chances. Limited access to advanced medical care further complicates outcomes, making immediate intervention essential. Delays in restoring oxygenation increase the risk of irreversible brain injury or death.

Are there different types of drowning?

Yes and no. Medically, drowning is defined as respiratory impairment resulting from submersion or immersion in liquid. Modern terminology recognizes only two outcomes: fatal drowning (resulting in death) and nonfatal drowning (survival, with or without long-term effects). Older terms like "near drowning," "dry drowning," and "secondary drowning" are now considered outdated and misleading.

Historically, labels like "dry drowning" implied that the presence or absence of water in the lungs determined the severity of injury. In reality, the key injury in any drowning event is hypoxia—oxygen deprivation—not the volume of water inhaled. This can result from airway obstruction, laryngospasm (vocal cord spasm), or actual water aspiration. Regardless of the mechanism, the outcome is the same: impaired oxygen delivery to vital organs, which can lead to organ failure or death if not treated promptly.

The idea of "delayed" or "secondary drowning"—where someone appears fine and then deteriorates days later—has been widely debunked. If no symptoms are present shortly after the incident, the likelihood of a serious medical problem directly related to the submersion is extremely low. However, this doesn't mean complications can't arise. What may follow is not a continuation of the drowning process, but secondary complications from water exposure or hypoxia. These can include aspiration pneumonitis, pulmonary edema, pneumonia, or neurologic injury, depending on the severity of the initial event.

That's why post-incident observation is important. If symptoms such as coughing, shortness of breath, fever, or confusion develop within hours, they should be taken seriously and evaluated. Still, these issues are best understood as complications of a nonfatal drowning, not a separate type of drowning. Framing drowning as a single process driven by hypoxia clarifies treatment priorities and avoids confusion caused by outdated terminology.

What should guides prioritize when managing a drowning incident?

The immediate goal in any drowning event is restoring oxygenation. Remove the patient from the water as quickly and safely as possible, avoiding unnecessary risk to rescuers. Once on land, assess for breathing and a pulse. If the patient is not breathing, begin rescue breathing immediately. If there is no pulse, initiate CPR.

Protecting the airway is essential, as vomiting is common during resuscitation. Turn the patient to their side to prevent aspiration of stomach contents. Hypothermia is also a concern, especially in cold-water drownings, so rewarming efforts should begin early. Even if the patient regains consciousness, close monitoring is necessary, as symptoms like persistent coughing, difficulty breathing, or confusion may indicate ongoing respiratory impairment or secondary complications requiring evacuation. In remote settings, early recognition and aggressive management can mean the difference between recovery and fatal deterioration.

What is the mammalian dive reflex?

The mammalian dive reflex is a physiological survival response triggered when the face is submerged in water—particularly cold-water. It slows the heart rate, reduces breathing effort, and constricts blood vessels in the extremities, prioritizing oxygen delivery to the brain and heart. By conserving oxygen, this reflex can extend survival time in low-oxygen environments, which is especially relevant in cold-water drownings.

Cold-water drowning differs significantly from warm-water drowning due to this reflex. In extremely cold-water, the body's oxygen demand decreases, slowing metabolism and delaying brain and heart damage. This has led to cases where victims have been successfully resuscitated after prolonged submersion in icy conditions. Generally speaking, the colder the water, the greater the potential benefit of this response, though factors such as the individual's health, and how quickly hypothermia sets in all influence survival. *Because of this effect, aggressive and prolonged resuscitation efforts are often warranted in cold-water drowning cases.*

Warm-water drowning, on the other hand, lacks this protective mechanism. Oxygen deprivation progresses much faster, leading to irreversible brain and organ damage in a shorter period. Regardless of water temperature, restoring breathing and oxygenation as quickly as possible remains the priority, as hypoxia is the primary cause of death in drowning victims.

The mammalian dive reflex was first described by English physician Edmund Goodwyn in 1786 and later expanded upon by French physiologist Paul Bert in the 1870s. Today, it is well established in diving medicine and survival physiology. For wilderness guides, understanding this reflex reinforces why prolonged resuscitation efforts may be successful after cold-water submersion. The concept of the dive reflex challenges traditional assumptions about time limits in drowning cases by showing how cold-water can slow metabolism and preserve brain function, even after extended periods without spontaneous breathing.

What are the evacuation considerations for submersion incidents in the wilderness?

Evacuation decisions depend on the severity of symptoms and the patient's vital signs. Any patient who has experienced submersion and presents with persistent symptoms—such as confusion, difficulty breathing, chest pain, or abnormal vital signs—rapid breathing or pulse rate, or low oxygen saturation—requires urgent evacuation to advanced medical care.

Even if a patient appears well immediately after a submersion event, they must be closely monitored for delayed complications such as pulmonary edema, which can develop hours later. New symptoms, including coughing, shortness of breath, or fatigue, indicate potential respiratory compromise and necessitate evacuation. Frequent reassessment of vital signs is essential, as subtle changes may signal deterioration. If there is any uncertainty about the patient's condition, evacuation is the safest course of action.

How should prolonged resuscitation be handled in the wilderness?

Prolonged resuscitation may be justified in wilderness settings, especially in cases of cold-water drowning. Hypothermia slows cellular metabolism, reducing oxygen demand and delaying irreversible brain injury. The medical adage "They're not dead until they're warm and dead" reflects the principle that CPR should ideally continue until the patient is fully rewarmed and assessed in a medical setting. Cold-water drowning victims have survived extended submersion with intact neurological function due to the combined effects of the mammalian dive reflex and hypothermia-induced metabolic suppression.

With all of that said—whether to continue resuscitation depends on several factors. If evacuation is feasible and the patient has a reasonable chance of reaching definitive care, prolonged CPR is appropriate. If rescue is imminent, resuscitation should continue without hesitation. In contrast, when evacuation is significantly delayed or physically impractical, the decision to continue must also consider rescuer fatigue and available resources.

Warm-water drowning follows a different trajectory. Without the protective effects of cold exposure, hypoxia causes irreversible brain damage within minutes. In these cases, while early CPR remains critical, prolonged efforts are unlikely to succeed unless advanced care is immediately accessible.

In all drowning cases, the priority is airway control, high-quality CPR, and oxygenation. When in doubt, continue resuscitation until the patient is assessed by medical personnel or until all reasonable efforts have been exhausted. Cold-water victims in particular warrant extended attempts, as their survival window is significantly longer.

Bleeding

How is bleeding controlled in the wilderness?

There are multiple ways to control bleeding in the wilderness—direct pressure, wound packing, tourniquets, and balloon tamponade—but all interventions should begin with focused, direct pressure. Nearly all external bleeding can be controlled with proper technique, and hemorrhage remains one of the few preventable causes of death in trauma. The key is to apply deliberate, targeted pressure directly over the bleeding vessel. Stacking gauze or applying broad hand pressure is rarely effective. Find the source, isolate the vessel, and compress it with precision—ideally using a gauze-covered fingertip. Maintain continuous pressure without releasing to check for continued bleeding as disrupting early clot formation resets the process.

Direct pressure works by mechanically compressing the vessel at the point of injury, collapsing the lumen of the blood vessel and stopping blood flow. This allows platelets to adhere and activate the local coagulation cascade, leading to fibrin clot formation. Broad or diffuse pressure fails to achieve this full occlusion. In the field—without blood products or surgical backup—this mechanical control is everything. Remember, bleeding must be *fully* controlled before moving on to anything else.

When and how are wounds "packed"?

If direct pressure is ineffective—especially in deep or irregular wounds—packing becomes the next move. Insert gauze, tampons, or even a clean shirt if needed into the wound cavity, layer by layer, while maintaining firm downward pressure as you fill. The goal is to build internal pressure directly against the bleeding vessels. Once the wound is fully packed, hold steady external pressure for several minutes. Commercially available hemostatic agents (kaolin or chitosan-based) accelerate local clotting, but technique matters more than products.

What is a tourniquet, and how do they work?

A tourniquet—from the French *tourner*, to turn—is a device used to apply *circumferential* pressure to a limb to stop blood flow and control life-threatening bleeding. Tourniquets stop bleeding by generating enough pressure to collapse the arterial wall and halt distal flow. To be effective, the applied pressure must *exceed* the systolic blood pressure, compressing the artery either against bone or by collapsing it within the surrounding soft tissue. This halts both arterial inflow *and* venous outflow, preventing further blood loss beyond the application point.

The compression must be circumferential and uniform. Narrow devices—like cords or wires—create localized pressure that can damage tissue *without* adequately occluding the vessel. A proper tourniquet uses a broad band—typically 2 to 3 inches wide—to distribute pressure across a larger surface area. This reduces tissue injury while providing the force needed to occlude arterial flow. Wider compression also reduces the risk of nerve damage and increases the chance of success without repeated tightening.

Apply the tourniquet high and tight, upstream to the injury, especially when the exact bleeding site is unclear. The goal is full occlusion—partial compression will worsen bleeding by obstructing venous return while leaving arterial inflow intact. Always reassess after application—the absence of distal pulses and cessation of visible bleeding confirms proper placement. If bleeding continues, tighten further or reposition.

Tourniquets are indicated for *severe* extremity hemorrhage that does not respond to direct pressure or packing. In remote settings, where surgical control may be hours to days away, early tourniquet use is critical. Concerns about limb ischemia are secondary to controlling hemorrhage. Tourniquet time can be managed later—what matters in the field is stopping the bleeding immediately and then figuring out the plan.

How do I improvise a tourniquet?

If a commercial tourniquet is unavailable, a wide, strong material such as a belt, cloth, or strap can be used. Wrap it around the limb above the wound, avoiding joints, and tie a firm overhand knot.

To tighten the tourniquet, place a rigid object such as a stick or tool on top of the knot, then tie a second overhand knot over it, securing the object in place. Twist the object until the bleeding stops, then secure it by tying it down with another piece of cloth, cordage, or tape. If a single tourniquet does not fully stop the bleeding, apply a second one adjacent to the first.

Avoid using narrow materials like shoelaces, paracord, or wire, as these can cause severe tissue damage without effectively stopping blood flow. A properly applied tourniquet must fully stop the bleeding, not just slow it down-if blood continues to flow, tighten the device, adjust its position, or apply a second tourniquet.

What is junctional bleeding?

Junctional areas like the groin, neck, and axilla (arm pit) are high-risk zones for fatal exsanguination. Tourniquets won't work here—you must pack deeply and apply *continuous* pressure. If bleeding persists, balloon tamponade is often your last viable option. A Foley catheter or any long, slender balloon, latex glove, or even condom can be inserted fully into the wound tract. Advance to the base of the wound, inflate slowly and fully, and monitor for bleeding control. The balloon must reach the base to be effective. Shallow inflation is unlikely to tamponade the actual source of bleeding. Inflate fully, ensure the bleeding has stopped, and secure the balloon (or whatever you used) in place for evacuation.

How do blood thinners affect bleeding?

Blood thinners—like warfarin (Coumadin), apixaban (Eliquis), rivaroxaban (Xarelto), and dabigatran (Pradaxa)—make it harder for the body to form clots. That means even small cuts can bleed more than expected, and serious injuries can lead to uncontrolled or delayed bleeding. These medications work by interfering with different parts of the body's clotting system, either by blocking clotting proteins or slowing down the process entirely.

In the backcountry, this becomes a real problem. In a city, hospitals can provide reversal drugs, blood transfusions, or surgery. In the wilderness, stopping the bleeding is much harder, and internal bleeding can go unnoticed until it's too late.

A guest on these medications might seem fine after a fall or cut, but without normal clotting, what looks minor can quickly become serious. Head injuries, belly trauma, or deep cuts are especially dangerous. Bleeding in the brain or abdomen can progress silently and become life-threatening before symptoms appear.

That's why it's critical to know what medications your guests are taking before the trip. If someone is on blood thinners, they should be treated as high risk for bleeding. If they get hurt—especially in the head, chest, or abdomen—don't wait for symptoms to appear. In the wilderness, delayed recognition of internal bleeding in an anticoagulated patient can be catastrophic.

What's the bottom line for wilderness hemorrhage control?

Control life-threatening bleeding first. Everything else can wait. Expose the wound, locate the vessel, and apply *targeted* pressure. Use gauze, pack deeply when needed, and escalate to balloon tamponade or tourniquet without waiting or debating. *Almost any improvised tools are acceptable if they meet the physiological goal—to stop the bleeding.*

Pain Control & Practical Pharmacology for Guides

Overview

Why does a guide need to understand pharmacology?

A basic understanding of pharmacology is essential for guides—not because they're expected to act as healthcare providers, but because medications are relevant to both preexisting conditions and acute care in the field. Clients often arrive with prescriptions for preexisting conditions, and in the field, factors like temperature, altitude, hydration, and exertion can alter how drugs are absorbed, metabolized, and tolerated. These environmental stressors can reduce a medication's effectiveness, increase side effects, or lead to unexpected interactions. Medications that behave predictably in clinical settings may act differently in the wilderness, and certain combinations can create complications that wouldn't surface under normal conditions.

Understanding how common medications function and interact in remote environments allows guides to make safer, more informed decisions when definitive care is hours or even days away. This chapter isn't meant to be a comprehensive pharmacology reference—it's a practical guide to using medications safely in the field. The goal is to recognize potential risks; adjust treatments when necessary; and ensure that when medications are used, they're administered as safely and effectively as the setting allows. Choosing a treatment isn't just about managing symptoms—it's about minimizing risk when medical backup isn't readily available. And in some remote areas, a basic pharmacy or rural clinic may be accessible. In those moments, the more you know, the more useful you become.

Pain Control

What is pain?

Pain is the body's built-in alarm system, signaling injury or illness through the nervous system. Nerve endings called nociceptors detect damage or irritation and send signals to the brain, triggering an inflammatory response and the release of stress hormones like cortisol. While pain serves a protective role, unmanaged pain in the wilderness can lead to increased anxiety, reduced mobility, and difficulty with evacuation. Effective pain control improves function, reduces suffering, and supports recovery, making it a critical component of wilderness medicine.

How should pain be managed in the wilderness?

Pain management in remote settings is about selecting the right drug for the right type of pain while considering risks, side effects, and potential Interactions.

- Acetaminophen acts in the brain to reduce pain and fever with less effect on inflammation or swelling. It's a safe first-line option for headaches, fevers, and general pain relief, but because it's processed by the liver, excessive doses or alcohol use can cause liver damage. International formulations include Tylenol, Panadol, and Calpol.
- NSAIDs (nonsteroidal anti-inflammatory drugs) block prostaglandins, the compounds responsible for pain, fever, and much of inflammation. This makes them ideal for musculoskeletal injuries, joint pain, and swelling. Ibuprofen (Advil, Motrin, Nurofen), naproxen (Aleve, Naprosyn), and ketorolac (Toradol) are widely available for short-term, severe pain relief. Of note, the

combination of acetaminophen and ibuprofen provides stronger pain relief than either drug alone and has been shown to be *as effective as opioids* for the short-term management of musculoskeletal injuries and fractures, making it the preferred first-line approach in remote settings.

- Aspirin (acetylsalicylic acid) functions as an NSAID but also irreversibly interferes with platelets required for clotting, increasing bleeding risk. Unlike ibuprofen or naproxen, its effects last for the lifespan of a platelet—about 7 to 10 days—until the body generates enough new platelets. While acknowledging aspirin has some use in cardiovascular protection and altitude sickness prevention, its bleeding risk often makes it a poor choice for pain management in injuries. Internationally, it is sold as Bayer, Ecotrin, and Aspro.

How do opioids work, and when should they be used?

Opioids bind to mu (μ), delta (δ), and kappa (κ) receptors in the brain and spinal cord, all of which contribute to pain modulation. While all three play a role in pain relief, activation of the mu receptor significantly reduces pain perception, slows breathing, and triggers dopamine release, leading to both euphoria and addiction potential. These effects make opioids highly effective for pain management while increasing the risk of significant respiratory depression especially when combined with other central nervous system depressants like muscle relaxants (benzodiazepines) or alcohol.

Common opioids include morphine, oxycodone, and hydrocodone, which are used clinically for severe pain such as fractures, burns, and major trauma. However, in the wilderness, the risks may outweigh the benefits. Opioids cause sedation, respiratory suppression, impaired judgment, and significant constipation—all of which could turn into a major problem in remote settings where close monitoring, hydration and mobility are already limited. Internationally, morphine is available as MS Contin and Sevredol, oxycodone as OxyContin and OxyNorm, and fentanyl as Durogesic and Sublimaze. Opioids should be a last resort in remote environments, with NSAIDs and acetaminophen prioritized whenever possible.

International travelers should exercise caution when carrying opioids across borders, as many countries have strict drug laws that classify these medications as controlled substances. Even with a prescription, possession of opioids can result in legal complications, detainment, or arrest in some regions.

Are there nonpharmacological techniques for managing pain?

For certain. Nonpharmacological methods play a critical role in pain management, particularly in remote environments where medication may be limited or unavailable. These techniques not only provide relief but also help stabilize the patient and improve overall outcomes.

- Controlled Breathing – Encouraging slow, deliberate breathing stimulates the parasympathetic nervous system (promoting rest, digestion, and energy conservation) and releases endorphins, which helps reduce anxiety and ease pain. Techniques like box breathing (inhale for 4 seconds, hold for 4 seconds, exhale for 4 seconds, and pause for 4 seconds) can be extremely effective, particularly for patients experiencing stress-induced pain responses.
- Distraction Techniques – Keeping the mind occupied can reduce the perception of pain. Engaging the patient in conversation, storytelling, or simple mental tasks shifts focus away from discomfort and can be particularly useful during prolonged evacuations.
- Positioning, Splinting, and Elevation – Properly positioning an injured limb, applying a well-fitted splint, and elevating swollen extremities above heart level help minimize inflammation and pain. Elevation is especially useful for managing fractures, sprains, and

soft tissue injuries, reducing swelling and preventing additional complications.

- Cold Therapy (Ice or Snow) – When available, applying cold to an injury can significantly reduce pain and swelling by slowing inflammation and numbing the area. In the absence of commercial ice packs, snow or chilled water bottles can be effective alternatives. Cold should be applied intermittently to prevent tissue damage, particularly in colder environments where frostbite is a concern.
- Reassurance and Communication – *A calm, confident guide sets the tone for the patient's response to pain.* Explaining what's happening in simple terms; setting clear expectations; and maintaining steady, controlled mannerisms can alleviate distress and improve the patient's ability to tolerate discomfort.

Pain management in the wilderness is often about more than medication; it's about practical interventions with an understanding of physiology, and sometimes even a bit of psychology. Simple measures, when applied correctly, can make a substantial difference in both comfort and even recovery.

Pharmacology for Guides

How do antihistamines work, and when should they be used?

Antihistamines block histamine receptors that control allergic reactions, inflammation, and stomach acid production. Histamine acts on two primary receptor types—H1 and H2—which each serve different functions. H1 antihistamines target skin, respiratory tract, and blood vessels. They are used for allergies, insect stings, and mild allergic reactions. First-generation H1 blockers like diphenhydramine (Benadryl, Dimedrol) cause sedation, while second generation options like loratadine (Claritin, Alavert, Clarityn) and cetirizine (Zyrtec, Reactine) are longer lasting and nonsedating. H2 antihistamines primarily reduce stomach acid production but also play a secondary role in vascular response and inflammation. Famotidine (Pepcid, Famocid, Gaster) and ranitidine (Zantac) are used for acid reflux, ulcers, and indigestion and can be combined with H1 blockers, providing greater histamine buffering to manage more severe allergic reactions.

How do blood pressure medications work, and why do they matter in remote settings?

Blood pressure medications help regulate circulation, but their effects can change significantly in wilderness environments. Dehydration, altitude, physical exertion, diarrhea, and alcohol use all influence how these drugs behave—sometimes dangerously. To understand blood pressure medication in the field, you have to understand that blood pressure is a system dependent on fluid volume. When the body loses fluids, blood volume drops—and so does pressure.

Diuretics like hydrochlorothiazide (Microzide, Esidrix) and furosemide (Lasix, Frumil, Furosed) reduce blood pressure by increasing urine output, directly reducing circulating fluid. In hot, humid conditions or when illness causes diarrhea or vomiting, these medications can amplify dehydration and cause lightheadedness, weakness, or fainting, especially when water intake is limited.

Beta-blockers such as metoprolol (Lopressor, Betaloc, Metolar) and propranolol (Inderal, Avlocardyl, Deralin) lower blood pressure by slowing the heart and reducing its force. While this helps in stable conditions, it can become a liability during exertion or at altitude, where the heart needs to beat faster to compensate for lower oxygen. These medications can blunt that response, leading to reduced exercise tolerance and poor acclimatization.

ACE inhibitors like lisinopril (Zestril, Prinivil, Hipril) and enalapril (Vasotec, Renitec, Enap), as well as ARBs like losartan (Cozaar, Presartan, Losium), lower blood pressure by relaxing blood vessels. In dehydrated individuals, especially in hot climates or after fluid loss from illness, these drugs can lead to dizziness, orthostatic hypotension, or fainting as the body struggles to maintain blood flow with less circulating volume.

Alcohol worsens all of this. It promotes fluid loss, impairs judgment, and exaggerates the blood pressure-lowering effects of diuretics and vasodilators—making volume depletion and low blood pressure even more likely.

In short, these medications work by influencing a fluid-driven system, and when fluids are lost—through sweat, illness, or heat—the effects of blood pressure meds can become unpredictable and dangerous. Guides and travelers taking these medications need to stay ahead of hydration, recognize early signs of low blood pressure like dizziness or fatigue, and adjust activity and fluid intake to stay safe in the field.

What should guides know about antibiotics?

Antibiotics can be life-saving in remote settings when evacuation is delayed, but they must be used appropriately. Not every infection requires antibiotics, and unnecessary use increases the risk of side effects, allergic reactions, and long-term resistance. Guides should understand which infections are likely to benefit from antibiotics—such as cellulitis, urinary tract infections, infected wounds, or gastrointestinal illness—and when their use is unwarranted—as in most sinus complaints.

Antibiotics are especially important when treating bites, puncture wounds, and penetrating injuries, where the risk of deep tissue infection is high. Selection depends on the likely organisms, the exposure source (e.g., water, soil, animal bite), and the patient's history—including known drug allergies. While many reported allergies—especially those from childhood—may not reflect a true immune-mediated reaction, guides should err on the side of caution. In remote settings where anaphylaxis cannot be easily managed, any stated allergy should be respected unless the individual is confident it was a side effect (e.g., nausea or mild rash) rather than a true allergy. When in doubt, choose an alternative class of antibiotic and avoid re-exposure.

The goal is to start antibiotics when there's a suspected bacterial source or when symptoms are *worsening*. In wilderness medicine, guides should carry a small, targeted supply of oral antibiotics, understand their appropriate field use, and document all administration for medical follow-up.

What should guides do if an infection worsens despite using antibiotics?

If an infection spreads or symptoms worsen while on antibiotics, it suggests progression beyond what oral treatment can manage. Signs like increasing pain, redness, swelling, fever, or systemic symptoms (fatigue, confusion, weakness) indicate that the infection may require surgical drainage or advanced medical care. Evacuation is mandatory in these cases.

Some infections—particularly abscesses—require drainage to resolve. If a fluctuant pocket is clearly present, responders may need to open, drain, and irrigate the site under clean technique. However, if the infection involves the face, hands, joints, or genitals, or if the patient is systemically ill, do not attempt drainage—evacuation is the priority.

In the field, worsening infection means the current plan is failing. Continuing the same treatment without reassessment risks further deterioration, and when in doubt, evacuate.

How do steroids work?

Steroids mimic cortisol, a naturally occurring, (endogenous) hormone produced by the adrenal glands that is essential for human life. Cortisol regulates inflammation, immune response, metabolism, blood pressure, and the body's ability to handle stress, making it a key component of normal physiological function. Steroid preparations are widely used to reduce tissue swelling, allergic reactions, and inflammatory responses. In remote settings, they can help manage severe allergic reactions (as an adjunct to epinephrine), asthma attacks, altitude illness, and many musculoskeletal injuries. Common oral steroids include prednisone (Deltasone, Rayos), prednisolone (Orapred, Panafcort), and dexamethasone (Decadron, DexPak, Ozurdex). Injectable forms such as methylprednisolone (Solu-Medrol, Depo-Medrol, Urbason) and hydrocortisone (Cortef, Solu-Cortef) are used in emergency situations for severe inflammation or adrenal crisis. Topical formulations like triamcinolone (Kenalog), betamethasone (Diprolene, Celestone), and hydrocortisone cream are effective for skin inflammation, insect bites, and allergic dermatitis. Of note, long-term or high-dose steroid use suppresses the body's natural cortisol production, leading to adrenal suppression.

The adrenal glands normally produce cortisol, a hormone essential for daily function and the body's stress response. With long-term steroid use, the body reduces its own cortisol production and becomes dependent on the medication. If steroids are stopped suddenly, the body may not be able to produce enough cortisol on its own—leading to fatigue, dizziness, low blood pressure, nausea, and, in severe cases, shock.

To prevent this, steroids must be tapered gradually over weeks to allow the adrenal glands time to slowly ramp up their natural cortisol production. In remote settings, the stakes are even higher. If someone on long-term steroids loses their medication, the body can't quickly resume adequate cortisol levels. Without access to replacement steroids, adrenal suppression can become life-threatening—especially during illness, injury, or other physical stress.

This makes it critical for anyone on chronic steroid therapy to carry extra doses, and for guides to ask about medications before departure.

How do benzodiazepines (benzos) work?

Benzodiazepines enhance the effects of GABA (gamma-aminobutyric acid), the brain's main inhibitory neurotransmitter. This increased GABA activity leads to sedation, reduced anxiety, muscle relaxation, and anticonvulsant effects. Commonly prescribed benzos include diazepam (Valium, Stesolid, Apaurin), lorazepam (Ativan, Temesta, Lorans), and alprazolam (Xanax, Helex, Alprox). They're often used for anxiety, seizures, muscle spasms, and alcohol withdrawal.

While effective, these medications depress the central nervous system, causing drowsiness, poor coordination, slowed breathing, and impaired judgment. In wilderness settings, this increases the risk of falls, hypothermia, and delayed reaction to environmental threats. When combined with alcohol or opioids, their effects are amplified, significantly raising the risk of respiratory failure. In remote environments, it's important to understand both their benefits and their dangers. Benzodiazepines may be necessary in some cases—but they can also compromise safety. Their use in the field should always be weighed carefully.

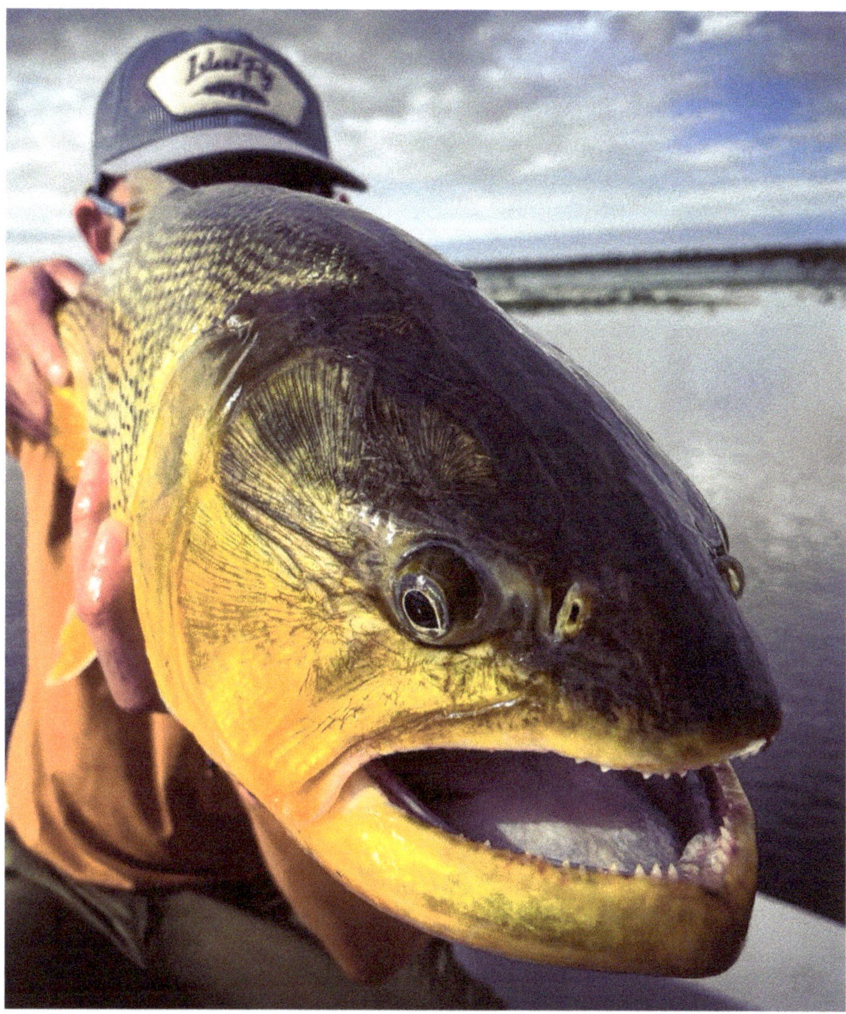

The Golden Dorado (Salminus brasiliensis)-an aggressive predator with powerful jaws and sharp teeth. Even minor bites or cuts from handling these fish carry a high risk of infection due to freshwater bacteria. Wounds should be irrigated thoroughly, dressed carefully, and followed with early antibiotics when deep or sustained in remote settings. Image courtesy of the author.

The Price of Gold

The golden dorado of Argentina's Paraná River are explosive predators that challenge every part of an angler's skill. They average 10 pounds but can blow past 30. These fish push the limits of freshwater fly fishing. Hosting trips here has been a true privilege—chasing these golden brutes while sharing Argentina's wild places, good wine, and great people.

Three days into a weeklong trip, after a banger of a day on the water, one of the guides came over with concern. A guest had been telling stories all afternoon of his battles with dorado. As things were winding down, the guide noticed his hand. At the base of the right thumb were clean tooth marks—red, swollen, and warm to the touch. No active bleeding, but definitely not nothing. The fish had twisted just enough while being unhooked to drag a row of teeth across the skin and leave a deep graze. It didn't look bad, but it hurt more than he expected.

A bite like that in warm freshwater carries real risk. Pseudomonas, Aeromonas—bacteria that thrive in these rivers—can turn a minor wound into a real problem fast. The site was scrubbed immediately with soap and water. That first scrub is critical and probably the most important step. "Scrub it till it bleeds" isn't about being rough—it's a reminder that you won't get a second chance to clean it right.

I started him on ciprofloxacin, which we always carry. It's known for treating traveler's diarrhea but also works well for some aquatic wound infections. By morning, the redness and swelling were already starting to ease. It still hurt, but the infection was in check.

By 48 hours, he was back on the water landing multiple dorado over 20 pounds.

That moment stuck with me. The core principles don't change—clean early and thoroughly, use the right antibiotics, and keep a close eye on it.

Improvisation matters, but preparation is what keeps things from unraveling. The goal is to keep the stories about the fish—not the infection.

Conclusion

So, what was the point of all this?

This book came out of two lives—one in medicine, one in the field. As a guide, former wilderness paramedic, ski patroller, and now emergency medicine provider, researcher, and educator, I've seen how fast things go sideways—and how quickly even the best-laid plans fall apart. Wilderness medicine is cold, hot, dirty, and full of variables you can't control. But the body still breaks. It still bleeds, shuts down, and fails the same way—whether you're in a hospital, the mountains, or waist-deep in mud.

You can't manage what you don't understand. What saves lives isn't a kit or a book. It's you—knowing what to look for, why it matters, and how to respond. If you know the why, you'll see the signs. Wilderness medicine is, by nature, improvisation—and real improvisation only works if you understand what's happening, especially when help is delayed or not coming at all.

Whether you're a guide, medic, or something else entirely—if you finish this book with a sharper sense of how to prioritize, adapt, and respond, then it did its job. If it leaves you more confident thinking through the chaos, that's enough.

Learn it. Use it. Pass it on.

Thanks for the read.

sjm

Appendix 1

Wilderness Antibiotic Reference Table

Ophthalmologic (Eye) Infections

Condition	Oral Antibiotic	Dose	Topical Antibiotic	Dose
Conjunctivitis (Bacterial)	Azithromycin	500 mg on Day 1, then 250 mg daily × 4d	Erythromycin ophthalmic ointment	Apply a thin ribbon 4× daily × 5–7 days
Corneal Abrasion (Infected, Contact Lens Wearer)	Ciprofloxacin	500 mg twice daily × 7 days	Ciprofloxacin ophthalmic drops	1–2 drops every 2h × 2d, then 4–6h × 5d
Orbital/ Periorbital Cellulitis	Amoxicillin–clavulanate	875 mg/125 mg twice daily × 7–10 days	Not applicable	Not applicable
(Alternate/ Penicillin Allergy)	Ciprofloxacin	500 mg twice daily x 3 days	Not applicable	Not applicable

Abdominal and Gastrointestinal Infections

Condition	Oral Antibiotic	Dose	Topical Antibiotic	Dose
Appendicitis (Delay in surgery)	Metronidazole + Ciprofloxacin	500 mg q8h + 500 mg twice daily	Not applicable	Not applicable
Infectious Diarrhea	Azithromycin	1 g orally once	Not applicable	Not applicable
(Alternative)	Ciprofloxacin	500 mg twice daily x 3 days	Not applicable	Not applicable
Abdominal Pain with Fever (Unspecified)	Ciprofloxacin + Metronidazole	500 mg twice daily + 500 mg every 8 hours × 5–7 days	Not applicable	Not applicable

Genitourinary Infections

Condition	Oral Antibiotic	Dose	Topical Antibiotic	Dose
Urinary Tract Infection (UTI)	Nitrofurantoin*	100 mg twice daily × 5 days	Not applicable	Not applicable
	*(Important Note)	Not for use in suspected pyelonephritis, flank pain, or in pregnant patients		
(Alternative)	Cephalexin	500 mg twice daily x 7 days	Not applicable	Not applicable
Pyelonephritis	Ciprofloxacin	500 mg twice daily × 7–14 days	Not applicable	Not applicable
Trichomoniasis	Metronidazole	2 g orally as a single dose	Not applicable	Not applicable
Bacterial Vaginosis	Metronidazole	500 mg twice daily × 7 days	Not applicable	Not applicable
Vulvovaginal Candidiasis (yeast infection)	Fluconazole	150mg orally, ONE TIME	Clotrimazole 1% cream	1 applicator vaginally for 7 nights
	*(Important Note)	Fluconazole not for use in pregnant patients		

Respiratory (Lung)Infections

Condition	Oral Antibiotic	Dose	Topical Antibiotic	Dose
Pneumonia (Community–Acquired)	Amoxicillin	1 g three times daily × 7–10 days	Not applicable	Not applicable
(Alternate/ Penicillin Allergy)	Azithromycin	500mg daily x 5 days	Not applicable	Not applicable

Skin and Soft Tissue Infections

Condition	Oral Antibiotic	Dose	Topical Antibiotic	Dose
Skin/Soft Tissue Infections	TMP–SMX (trimethoprim–sulfamethoxazole)	1–2 DS tablets twice daily × 7–10 days	Mupirocin ointment	Apply 3× daily up to 10 days
Cellulitis	Cephalexin	500 mg 4× daily × 7–10 days	Not applicable	Not applicable
Human/ Animal Bites	Amoxicillin–clavulanate	875 mg/125 mg twice daily × 5–7 days	Bacitracin/ Neomycin ointment	Apply 2–3× daily to superficial wounds
Open Fractures (Prophylaxis)	Cephalexin	500 mg 4× daily × 3–5 days	Not applicable	Not applicable
Saltwater Exposure	Doxycycline	100 mg twice daily x 10 days	Not applicable	Not applicable

Central Nervous System Infections (Meningitis/Skull Fracture)

Condition	Oral Antibiotic	Dose	Topical Antibiotic	Dose
Meningitis (Empiric, remote)	Ciprofloxacin	500 mg twice daily	Not applicable	Not applicable

Tooth and Gum Infections

Condition	Oral Antibiotic	Dose	Topical Antibiotic	Dose
Tooth/Mouth Infections	Amoxicillin–clavulanate	875 mg twice daily × 10 days	Chlorhexidine oral rinse	Rinse with 30 mL 2× daily × 7–10 days
(Alternate/ Penicillin Allergy)	Clindamycin	450 mg 3 x day x 10 days	Hydrogen Peroxide 3%; 1: 1 ratio with water	Rinse with 30 mL 2× daily × 7–10 days

Ear, Nose, and Throat Infections

Condition	Oral Antibiotic	Dose	Topical Antibiotic	Dose
Otitis Externa	Ciprofloxacin	500 mg twice daily × 7 days	Ciprofloxacin–dexamethasone otic drops	4 drops into ear 2× daily × 7 days
Otitis Media	Amoxicillin	500 mg 3× daily × 7–10 days	Not applicable	Not applicable
(Alternate)	Amoxicillin–clavulanate	875 mg twice daily × 10 days	Not applicable	Not applicable
Tonsillitis (Streptococcal)	Penicillin V	500 mg 2× daily × 10 days	Not applicable	Not applicable
(Alternate/ Penicillin Allergy)	Azithromycin	500mg daily x 5 days	Not applicable	Not applicable
Sinusitis	Amoxicillin–clavulanate	875 mg twice daily × 10 days		
(Alternate/ Penicillin Allergy)	Doxycycline	100 mg twice daily x 10 days		

Tapeworm Infections

Condition	Oral Antibiotic	Dose	Topical Antibiotic	Dose
Tapeworm	Praziquantel	5–10 mg/kg body weight, given as a single dose	Not applicable	Not applicable
(Alternate)	Niclosamide	2 gram as a single dose	Not applicable	Not applicable

Disclaimer:

This antibiotic reference table is provided for educational use only and is not a substitute for clinical judgment. Drug availability, resistance patterns, and treatment guidelines vary by region and may change over time. Readers are advised to consult current local protocols, professional guidelines, and a licensed medical provider before initiating any treatment. The author and publisher assume no liability for decisions made based on this material.

Appendix 2

Vaccination Recommendations for International Travelers

All Travelers (Routine Vaccinations)

- Measles-Mumps–Rubella (MMR)
- Diphtheria-Tetanus–Pertussis (DTaP)
- Varicella (Chickenpox)
- Meningococcal*
- Pneumococcal*
- Polio
- Influenza*
- COVID-19*
- Rabies*

North America and United States

- Hepatitis A
- Hepatitis B
- Influenza
- Measles-Mumps–Rubella (MMR)
- Tetanus-Diphtheria–Pertussis (Tdap)

South and Central America

- Hepatitis A
- Hepatitis B
- Yellow Fever
- Typhoid
- Malaria (as applicable)

- Measles-Mumps–Rubella (MMR)
- Tetanus-Diphtheria–Pertussis (Tdap)

Africa

- Hepatitis A
- Hepatitis B
- Yellow Fever
- Typhoid
- Cholera
- Malaria (as applicable)
- Measles-Mumps–Rubella (MMR)
- Tetanus-Diphtheria–Pertussis (Tdap)
- Meningococcal (ACWY)

Southeast Asia and Oceania

- Hepatitis A
- Hepatitis B
- Typhoid
- Malaria (as applicable)
- Japanese Encephalitis
- Measles-Mumps–Rubella (MMR)
- Tetanus-Diphtheria–Pertussis (Tdap)

Caribbean

- Hepatitis A
- Hepatitis B
- Typhoid
- Measles-Mumps–Rubella (MMR)
- Tetanus-Diphtheria–Pertussis (Tdap)

Indian Subcontinent

- Hepatitis A
- Hepatitis B
- Typhoid
- Cholera
- Measles-Mumps–Rubella (MMR)
- Tetanus-Diphtheria–Pertussis (Tdap)
- Japanese Encephalitis

Middle East

- Hepatitis A
- Hepatitis B
- Typhoid
- Measles-Mumps–Rubella (MMR)
- Tetanus-Diphtheria–Pertussis (Tdap)

Alaska and Northern Rivers

- Hepatitis A
- Hepatitis B
- Tetanus-Diphtheria–Pertussis (Tdap)

Tahiti and Pacific Islands

- Hepatitis A
- Hepatitis B
- Typhoid
- Measles-Mumps–Rubella (MMR)
- Tetanus-Diphtheria–Pertussis (Tdap)

*For travelers at increased risk due to underlying health conditions, age, or expected itinerary.

Disclaimer:

The vaccination recommendations provided here are intended for general educational purposes and do not replace individualized medical advice. Vaccine requirements and disease risks vary by country, region, and personal health status, and may change over time. Travelers should consult with a travel medicine specialist or licensed healthcare provider and refer to up-to-date resources such as the CDC or WHO prior to international travel.

Appendix 3

Wilderness Medicine Kit: Medications and Supplies

This guide covers recommended medications, and trauma supplies for a wilderness medical kit. Items requiring a prescription are noted. The focus of this list is on practicality, availability, and usability.

Medications

Pain Relief and Anti-Inflammatory

- Acetaminophen (Tylenol): For mild to moderate pain and fever reduction
- Ibuprofen (Advil, Motrin): NSAID for pain, inflammation, and fever
- Naproxen Sodium (Aleve): Long-acting NSAID for pain and inflammation
- Ketorolac (Toradol): Prescription NSAID for moderate to severe pain

Antihistamines and Allergy Relief

- Diphenhydramine (Benadryl): For allergic reactions and mild sedation
- Cetirizine (Zyrtec): Non-drowsy antihistamine for seasonal allergies
- Loratadine (Claritin): Non-drowsy antihistamine for allergies

- EpiPen (Epinephrine Auto-Injector): For anaphylaxis (prescription required)

Antibiotics

- Amoxicillin-Clavulanate (Augmentin): For respiratory, skin, and dental infections
- Doxycycline (Vibramycin): For tick-borne diseases, respiratory infections, and saltwater exposure
- Ciprofloxacin (Cipro): For gastrointestinal and urinary tract infections
- Azithromycin (Zithromax): For respiratory and gastrointestinal infections
- Cephalexin (Keflex): For skin and soft tissue infections
- Metronidazole (Flagyl): For gastrointestinal infections and bacterial vaginosis

Antiemetics and Antidiarrheals

- Ondansetron (Zofran): For nausea and vomiting (prescription required)
- Bismuth Subsalicylate (Pepto-Bismol): For diarrhea and upset stomach
- Loperamide (Imodium): For diarrhea control

Fungal and Yeast Infections

- Clotrimazole (Lotrimin): For topical fungal infections
- Fluconazole (Diflucan): For yeast infections (not for pregnant patients, prescription required)

Respiratory Medications

- Albuterol Inhaler (ProAir, Ventolin): For asthma or bronchospasm (prescription required)
- Prednisone: For severe allergic reactions, asthma, and inflammatory conditions (prescription required)

Wound Care and Local Anesthetics

- Povidone-Iodine (Betadine): Antiseptic for wound cleaning
- Bacitracin or Triple Antibiotic Ointment (Neosporin): For minor cuts and abrasions
- Lidocaine 1% (Xylocaine): Injectable anesthetic for local pain control (prescription required)
- Bupivacaine 0.25% (Marcaine): Longer-lasting injectable anesthetic (prescription required)
- Topical Lidocaine (Lidoderm Patch): For localized pain management (prescription required)
- Cyanoacrylate Glue (Super Glue): For minor wound closure and laceration repair

Emergency Medications

- Naloxone (Narcan): For opioid overdoses (prescription may not be required in some states)
- Glucose Tablets or Gel: For hypoglycemia
- Aspirin (81 mg and 325 mg): For suspected heart attack or clot prevention

Steroids

- Dexamethasone (Decadron): For altitude sickness, severe inflammation, or allergic reactions (prescription required)
- Methylprednisolone (Medrol): For severe allergic reactions and inflammation (prescription required)
- Triamcinolone Acetonide Cream: For inflammatory skin conditions and rashes

Other Essentials

- Water Purification Tablets (Potable Aqua): For emergency water treatment

- Electrolyte Replacement: Mix 1 liter of water with 1/2 teaspoon of salt and 6 teaspoons of sugar for oral rehydration
- Pregnancy Test Kit: For early detection of pregnancy
- Antimalarial Medications: Specific to travel destinations (e.g., Atovaquone-Proguanil [Malarone], prescription required)
- Preparation H (Hemorrhoid Cream): For swelling and localized irritation

Note: Ensure that all medications are stored appropriately and not expired. Include a copy of usage instructions and indications for each medication.

Trauma Supplies

Wound Care

- Sterile Gauze Pads (4x4): For cleaning and dressing wounds
- Adhesive Bandages (Assorted Sizes): For minor cuts and abrasions
- Non-Adherent Pads: For wounds requiring minimal sticking to dressing
- Roller Gauze (Kerlix): For securing dressings
- Medical Tape (Hypoallergenic): For securing dressings and bandages
- Elastic Bandages (ACE Wraps): For sprains and securing splints
- Wound Closure Strips (Steri-Strips): For small lacerations
- Skin Adhesive (Dermabond): For minor wound closure (prescription required)
- Tourniquet (CAT or SOF-T): For severe bleeding control
- Hemostatic Dressing (QuikClot): For controlling severe bleeding
- Irrigation Syringe (10-20 ml): For cleaning wounds

- Foley Catheter for junctional bleeding

Epistaxis (Nosebleed) Management

- Nasal Tampons: Traditional option for anterior nosebleeds
- Rhino Rocket® Nasal Packing: Made from PVA Expandacell® foam, these devices are designed for effective epistaxis management. They absorb moisture and expand to provide gentle, yet firm, mucosal compression

Chest Decompression Equipment

- Scalpel with #10 Blade: Essential
- 14-Gauge, 3.25-Inch Angiocatheter: Used for needle decompression in cases of tension pneumothorax

Fractures and Sprains

- SAM Splint: Moldable splint for immobilizing fractures
- Triangle Bandages: For slings or additional support
- Finger Splints: For minor digit injuries

Burn Care

- Burn Dressings (Water-Jel or Hydrogel): For minor burns
- Aloe Vera Gel: For soothing minor burns

Eye and Ear Care

- Eye Wash Solution: For flushing debris from eyes
- Ear Drops (Drying Solution): For swimmer's ear or minor irritation

General Trauma Supplies

- Trauma Shears: For cutting clothing and bandages
- Nitrile Gloves: For personal protection
- CPR Mask: For rescue breathing
- Thermal Blanket (Emergency Foil Blanket):For preventing hypothermia
- Cold Packs: For reducing swelling
- Splinter/Tick Remover: For removing debris or insects
- Digital Thermometer: For checking body temperature
- Tweezers: For removing splinters, ticks, or debris
- Notebook and Pen: For recording patient details

Note: Regularly review and update the trauma kit to ensure items are in good condition and not expired. Training on the proper use of supplies is highly recommended.

Glossary

A

Abduction: Movement of a limb away from the midline of the body, important in joint assessment.

Abrasion: A superficial wound caused by scraping the skin, often painful but not deep.

Abscess: A localized pocket of pus caused by infection; may need drainage in field conditions.

Acetaminophen: A pain reliever and fever reducer that is preferred in wilderness settings due to its low risk of bleeding.

Acidosis: A condition where blood pH drops below normal, often from shock, DKA, or poor perfusion.

Adduction: Movement of a limb toward the body's midline, tested in musculoskeletal exams.

Adrenaline: Another name for epinephrine; used in emergency care to stimulate the heart and open airways.

Agonal Breathing: Abnormal gasping breaths seen in cardiac arrest; ineffective for ventilation.

Air Embolism: Air bubbles in the bloodstream that can block circulation, often due to diving injuries.

Airway: The path air takes into the lungs; ensuring it remains open is the first priority in trauma care.

Altitude Illness: A group of disorders including AMS, HACE, and HAPE caused by rapid ascent to high elevation.

Analgesia: The relief of pain using medications or physical methods.

Anaphylaxis: A severe, rapid allergic reaction involving airway swelling and shock, requiring epinephrine.

Aneurysm: A weakened, bulging section of a blood vessel that can rupture and cause internal bleeding.

Anisocoria: Unequal pupil size, potentially indicating head injury or neurologic disorder.

Antibiotics: Drugs that kill or inhibit bacteria; often used in wound infections or contaminated injuries.

Antiemetic: A drug that helps control nausea and vomiting, important in dehydration and altitude illness.

Antihistamines: Medications that block histamine to reduce allergic symptoms like rash or swelling.

Antiseptic: A substance that inhibits the growth of microorganisms on living tissue, used for wound cleaning.

Anuria: The absence of urine output, often signaling kidney failure or severe dehydration.

Apical Pulse: The heartbeat heard at the chest's apex, often used in pediatric assessments.

Apnea: A temporary cessation of breathing can occur in head trauma or overdose.

Arrhythmia: An irregular heart rhythm that may impair cardiac output or cause palpitations.

Arterial Bleed: A high-pressure, spurting hemorrhage from an artery; requires immediate control.

Ascites: Fluid accumulation in the abdomen, often from liver disease or trauma.

Aspiration: Inhalation of food, fluid, or vomit into the lungs, leading to pneumonia or airway compromise.

Asystole: A flatline on the heart monitor; complete absence of electrical activity in the heart.

Ataxia: Lack of muscle coordination that can affect speech, eye movements, and walking.

Atopic: Describes a predisposition toward allergic hypersensitivity, often inherited.

Auscultation: Listening to internal body sounds, usually with a stethoscope, to assess lungs or bowel.

AVPU Scale: A quick way to assess consciousness; Alert, Verbal response, Pain response, Unresponsive.

Axillary Temperature: Temperature taken under the armpit; less accurate but non-invasive.

B

Bacteria: Single-celled organisms that can cause infections; often treated with antibiotics.

Barotrauma: Injury caused by pressure changes, often affecting ears, lungs, or sinuses during diving or flying.

Battle's Sign: Bruising behind the ears indicating possible skull fracture and brain trauma.

Bites: Wounds from insects or animals; may carry infection or venom depending on source.

Bivouac: A temporary camp used in wilderness settings, often without tents.

Blackwater Fever: A severe malaria complication with hemolysis and dark urine, seen in remote tropical regions.

Blister: A fluid-filled skin lesion from friction or burns; must be managed to prevent infection.

Body Substance Isolation: Precautions to prevent contact with fluids that may carry infectious diseases.

Boil: A skin infection involving a hair follicle and surrounding tissue, forming a painful pus-filled lump.

Bradycardia: An abnormally slow heart rate, which may occur in hypothermia or head injury.

Bronchospasm: Sudden tightening of the airway muscles, often seen in asthma or allergic reactions.

Brudzinski's Sign: Neck flexion causing involuntary hip/knee bending, suggestive of meningeal irritation.

Burn: Tissue injury from heat, chemicals, or electricity; classified by depth and size.

C

Cachexia: Severe muscle wasting from chronic illness or starvation.

Cairn: A pile of rocks used as a trail marker in remote or high-alpine environments.

Campylobacter: A bacterial cause of diarrhea from undercooked meat or contaminated water.

Capillary Leak: Fluid shifts from blood vessels to tissues due to inflammation, leading to swelling or shock.

Cardiac Arrest: The sudden cessation of heart function, requiring CPR and possibly defibrillation.

Cardiac Tamponade: Compression of the heart from fluid buildup in the pericardium, causing obstructive shock.

Cardiogenic Shock: Shock due to poor heart function, reducing blood flow despite adequate volume.

Catatonia: A state of immobility and unresponsiveness often associated with psychiatric emergencies.

Cellulitis: A skin infection that spreads through tissue layers, presenting with redness, swelling, and pain.

Cerebrospinal Fluid: Protective fluid surrounding the brain and spinal cord; leaks may indicate skull fracture.

Cervical Collar: A rigid device used to immobilize the neck in suspected spinal injuries.

Cheyne-Stokes Respiration: Abnormal breathing with periods of apnea, often seen in brain injuries or near-death states.

Chilblains: Painful inflammation of small blood vessels in skin exposed to cold, non-freezing temperatures.

Chin Lift: A manual airway maneuver that lifts the chin to open the airway in an unconscious patient without trauma.

Cholecystitis]: Inflammation of the gallbladder, typically caused by gallstones blocking the bile duct.

Cirrhosis: Chronic liver damage marked by scarring and impaired function, may lead to coagulopathy.

Clonus: Rhythmic, involuntary muscle contractions indicating upper motor neuron damage.

Coccyx: The tailbone at the base of the spine; injury can cause persistent sitting pain.

Coma: A deep state of unconsciousness where the patient cannot be awakened or respond.

Compartment Syndrome: Increased pressure within a muscle compartment that restricts blood flow and can cause permanent damage.

Concussion: A mild brain injury caused by impact, resulting in headache, nausea, and altered thinking.

Contusion: A bruise; bleeding under the skin without a break in the surface.

Crag: A steep or rugged cliff or rock face, relevant in wilderness rescues or climbing settings.

Crepitus: A crackling sound under the skin or in joints, often a sign of fractures or gas-producing infections.

Cyanosis: A bluish discoloration of skin or lips due to low oxygen levels.

D

Decerebrate Posturing: Extension of arms and legs due to severe brain injury, a grave neurologic sign.

Decorticate Posturing: Arm flexion and leg extension in response to brain injury, indicating upper brain damage.

Defibrillation: A procedure to reset the heart's electrical rhythm in cardiac arrest, using a shock.

Dehydration: Loss of body water and electrolytes, impairing circulation and temperature control.

Dermatitis: Skin inflammation from irritants, allergens, or prolonged moisture exposure.

Diabetic Ketoacidosis: A life-threatening complication of diabetes involving high blood sugar, ketones, and acidosis.

Dislocation: When a joint is forced out of position; requires reduction to restore function.

Distributive Shock: Shock from blood vessel dilation and poor distribution, common in sepsis and anaphylaxis.

Diverticulitis: Inflammation or infection of pouches in the colon wall, often causing lower abdominal pain and fever.

Dysphagia: Difficulty swallowing, seen in stroke or esophageal trauma.

Dysphoria: A profound state of unease or dissatisfaction, may indicate psychiatric crisis.

Dyspnea: Difficult or labored breathing, often associated with asthma, trauma, or altitude illness.

Dysrhythmia: A disturbance in heart rhythm, often used interchangeably with arrhythmia.

Dystonia: Abnormal muscle tone causing sustained, involuntary muscle contractions or postures.

E

Ecchymosis: Bruising due to blood leaking under the skin from injured vessels.

Eclampsia: Seizures in a pregnant patient with high blood pressure, a life-threatening emergency.

Ectopic Pregnancy: A pregnancy outside the uterus, usually in a fallopian tube, requiring urgent evacuation.

Electrolyte: Charged particles like sodium or potassium that are essential for nerve and muscle function.

Epinephrine: A drug that opens airways and raises blood pressure, used in severe allergic reactions.

Epistaxis: Nosebleed, which can result from trauma, dry air, or anticoagulant use.

Eustachian Tube: A canal that equalizes pressure between the middle ear and atmosphere; may cause discomfort in altitude changes.

Evacuation: The planned removal of a patient from a remote setting to a higher level of care.

Exertional Heat Illness: A spectrum of disorders caused by physical activity in hot environments, ranging from cramps to heat stroke.

Exposure: Part of trauma assessment—undress the patient to look for hidden injuries, then prevent heat loss.

F

Fainting: Temporary loss of consciousness from reduced brain perfusion, often due to dehydration or stress.

Fasciculations: Involuntary muscle twitches often seen in nerve injury or poisoning.

Febrile Seizure: Seizures triggered by fever in young children; typically, self-limited but concerning in the field.

Femoral Artery: A major artery in the thigh; critical to assess in leg trauma or tourniquet application.

Fibrillation: Disorganized heart muscle contractions; can be fatal if not corrected.

Field Amputation: The rare removal of a crushed or non-viable limb in extreme remote circumstances.

First-degree Burn: A superficial burn affecting only the outer skin, causing redness and pain.

Flail Chest: A condition where multiple broken ribs move independently, impairing breathing.

Flat Affect: Lack of emotional expression, can indicate head injury or psychiatric condition.

Fracture: A broken bone, which must be stabilized to reduce pain and prevent further injury.

Frostbite: Freezing of tissues from prolonged cold exposure, can lead to permanent damage.

G

Gangrene: Tissue death from infection or lack of blood supply, often requiring surgical removal.

Gastritis: Stomach lining inflammation, often from stress, alcohol, or infection, causing pain or nausea.

Gastroparesis: Delayed stomach emptying, common in diabetes and associated with nausea and bloating.

Glucagon: A hormone that raises blood sugar by prompting the liver to release stored glucose.

Greenstick Fracture: An incomplete fracture common in children where the bone bends and cracks.

H

Hallucination: A false sensory perception without an external stimulus, common in psychiatric and toxicological emergencies.

Heat Cramps: Muscle cramps from electrolyte loss during intense heat exposure or sweating.

Heat Stroke: A life-threatening condition where body temperature regulation fails; patient is hot and confused or unconscious.

Heimlich Maneuver: An abdominal thrust used to relieve airway obstruction in a choking conscious adult.

Hematoma: A localized collection of blood outside blood vessels, causing swelling and discoloration.

Hematuria: Blood in the urine, which may result from trauma, infection, or kidney stones.

Hemiparesis: Weakness on one side of the body, commonly seen in stroke.

Hemorrhage: Uncontrolled bleeding that can rapidly lead to shock if not stopped.

Hemostatic Dressing: A bandage treated to help blood clot faster in severe bleeding.

Hemothorax: Blood in the chest cavity, usually from trauma, that impairs lung expansion.

Hepatosplenomegaly: Enlargement of the liver and spleen, sometimes seen in infections like malaria.

Hives: Raised, itchy welts caused by an allergic reaction; may precede anaphylaxis.

Horner's Syndrome: A combination of drooping eyelid, constricted pupil, and decreased sweating on one side of the face due to disruption of the nerve pathway between the brain and the cervical spine most often caused by trauma, surgery, or tumor.

Hot Zone: An area with immediate danger, such as fire or hazardous materials.

Hypercapnia: Elevated carbon dioxide levels in the blood due to hypoventilation.

Hyperglycemia: High blood sugar that may be manageable in the field if not part of DKA.

Hypernatremia: High sodium levels in the blood, often from dehydration or saltwater ingestion.

Hypoglycemia: Low blood sugar that impairs brain function and can cause seizures or coma.

Hyponatremia: Low blood sodium from overhydration or prolonged exertion; can cause confusion or seizures.

Hypoperfusion: Inadequate blood flow to tissues, commonly referred to as shock.

Hypothermia: A drop in body temperature that worsens bleeding and mental status.

Hypoventilation: Inadequate breathing that results in elevated carbon dioxide levels.

I

Iliac Crest: The top of the hip bone, often used as a landmark for spinal procedures or trauma.

Immobilization: Restricting movement of an injured area to reduce pain and prevent further damage.

Infarction: Tissue death due to lack of blood supply, such as in a heart attack or stroke.

Insulin: A hormone that lowers blood sugar by helping cells absorb glucose.

Intracranial Pressure: The pressure inside the skull, which rises dangerously after a head injury.

Intubation: Insertion of a tube into the airway to support breathing or ventilation.

Irritant Contact Dermatitis: A skin rash caused by direct exposure to chemicals or allergens.

Ischemic Stroke: A brain injury caused by blocked blood flow, leading to sudden weakness or confusion.

J

Jaundice: Yellowing of the skin and eyes from bilirubin buildup, often due to liver dysfunction.

Jaw Thrust: A technique to open the airway while maintaining cervical spine precautions, used in trauma patients.

Jugular Vein: A large vein in the neck that carries blood from the head back to the heart; can be used as a visible sign of venous pressure.

Junctional Hemorrhage: Bleeding near the torso-limb junction that is difficult to control with a tourniquet.

K

Ketones: Acidic byproducts made when the body burns fat for fuel, often seen in DKA.

Kussmaul Breathing: Deep, labored breathing pattern seen in metabolic acidosis, and especially in DKA.

L

Lactic Acid: A byproduct of anaerobic metabolism that accumulates in shock and acidosis.

Laryngospasm: Sudden closure of the vocal cords, which can block airflow and cause panic.

Limp: An abnormal gait from pain, weakness, or joint injury; can indicate underlying trauma or infection.

Lingual Swelling: Swelling of the tongue, which can compromise the airway in allergic or angioedema reactions.

Lodgment: A foreign object becoming stuck in the body, such as a fishhook or piece of wood.

M

Maculopapular Rash: A flat and raised rash often seen in viral illnesses or drug reactions.

Mastoid Process: A bone behind the ear used as a landmark for head injury or infection.

Melena: Black, tarry stools indicating upper GI bleeding.

Meninges: The three layers of tissue that surround and protect the brain and spinal cord.

Metabolic Acidosis: A buildup of acid in the body due to illness, injury, or poor perfusion.

Miosis: Constricted pupils, often from opioid use or nerve agent exposure.

Monro-Kellie Doctrine: A premise stating that since the skull can't expand, swelling raises brain pressure dangerously.

Myalgia: Muscle pain, common after exertion or with viral infections.

Myocardial Infarction: Another term for a heart attack; caused by blocked blood flow to the heart muscle.

N

Necrosis: Irreversible tissue death from infection, trauma, or poor blood supply.

Needle Decompression: An emergency procedure to release trapped air from a tension pneumothorax.

Nephrolithiasis: Kidney stones, often presenting as severe flank pain and hematuria.

Neurogenic Shock: Shock caused by spinal cord injury disrupting autonomic control of blood pressure.

NSAIDs: Nonsteroidal anti-inflammatories like ibuprofen that reduce pain (but impair clotting).

O

Occlusive Dressing: A non-permeable dressing used to seal open chest wounds and prevent air entry.

Opioid Toxicity: A condition marked by pinpoint pupils, respiratory depression, and sedation; reversed with naloxone.

Oral Rehydration Solution: A mix of water, salt, and sugar used to treat dehydration and support absorption.

Oropharynx: The part of the throat behind the mouth; assessed during airway evaluation.

Orthostatic Hypotension: A drop in blood pressure when standing, often from dehydration or shock.

Overexertion: Physical strain beyond one's capacity, leading to heat illness, rhabdomyolysis, or collapse.

P

Palpation: Using hands to examine the body for tenderness, swelling, or deformity.

Paradoxical Movement: Opposite-direction chest motion during breathing, often from flail chest.

Parasite: An organism that lives in or on a host and derives nutrients at the host's expense.

Parasympathetic Nervous System: Part of the autonomic nervous system that promotes 'rest and digest' functions.

Parietal: Relating to the outer layer or wall of a body cavity or structure, like the parietal pleura or skull bone.

Pathogen: An organism that causes disease, including bacteria, viruses, parasites, and fungi.

Pericardial Tamponade: Fluid buildup in the sac around the heart that compresses and restricts pumping.

Peripheral Pulses: Pulses felt in the limbs; their presence helps assess circulation and perfusion.

Peritonitis: Inflammation of the abdominal lining, often from infection or ruptured organs.

Petechiae: Small red or purple spots from capillary bleeding, seen in infections or bleeding disorders.

Photophobia: Light sensitivity often seen with meningitis, migraine, or eye injury.

Piloerection: Goosebumps, caused by autonomic response to cold or fear.

Pneumomediastinum: Air in the central chest cavity from trauma or barotrauma, may cause chest pain or voice change.

Pneumothorax: A collapsed lung due to air in the chest cavity, causing breathing difficulty.

Polydipsia: Excessive thirst, commonly seen in diabetes and dehydration.

Precordial Thump: A rarely used forceful strike to the chest in witnessed cardiac arrest without defibrillator access.

Primary Survey: The initial trauma check for airway, breathing, circulation, disability, and exposure.

Protozoan: Single-celled parasitic organisms, often causing diarrheal or vector-borne diseases.

Ptosis: Drooping of the eyelid; can be a sign of nerve damage or stroke.

Q

Quarantine: The isolation of individuals exposed to infectious disease to prevent its spread, particularly important in remote group settings.

R

Rabies: A viral infection from animal bites, always fatal once symptoms appear without prior vaccination.

Raccoon Eyes: Bruising around both eyes, suggestive of a skull fracture.

Rebound Tenderness: Increased pain when pressure is released from the abdomen; may suggest peritonitis.

Rectal Hydration: A field method of giving fluids when oral intake isn't possible, using the colon.

Red Flag Framework: A memory aid to spot serious symptoms that demand evacuation developed by S. Jason Moore, PhD in 2024.

Rehydration: The process of restoring body fluids lost through sweating, vomiting, or diarrhea.

Respiratory Depression: Reduced drive to breathe, often due to opioids, head injury, or neurologic illness.

Rhabdomyolysis: Muscle breakdown releasing myoglobin into the bloodstream, can lead to kidney damage.

S

Scabies: A contagious skin infestation caused by mites, resulting in intense itching.

Scalp Laceration: A deep cut on the scalp that can bleed heavily and may indicate a skull fracture.

Scleral Icterus: Yellowing of the whites of the eyes, often the first visible sign of jaundice.

Scoop and Run: A trauma approach prioritizing rapid evacuation over on-site interventions—not appropriate in most wilderness environments.

Secondary Survey: A head-to-toe assessment after life threats are addressed to find other injuries.

Seizure: Sudden, uncontrolled electrical activity in the brain causing convulsions or altered awareness.

Sepsis: A life-threatening response to infection causing organ dysfunction and systemic inflammation.

Shock: A state of poor tissue perfusion and oxygen delivery, often caused by bleeding or infection.

Shock Index: Heart rate divided by systolic blood pressure; values >0.9 suggest possible shock.

Splenic Injury: Damage to the spleen, often from blunt trauma, leading to internal bleeding.

Splint: A device or improvised tool used to stabilize a broken or injured limb.

Stevens-Johnson Syndrome: A severe skin reaction often caused by medications, marked by mucosal involvement and skin detachment.

Strain: Muscle or tendon injury due to overstretching, often managed with rest and support.

Stroke: Loss of brain function from a blood clot or bleeding in the brain, requiring urgent care.

Subcutaneous Emphysema: Air trapped under the skin, often due to chest trauma or pneumothorax.

Suction: A method of clearing blood or vomit from the airway using negative pressure.

Sympathetic Nervous System: Part of the autonomic nervous system that triggers the 'fight or flight' response.

Syncope: Another term for fainting, typically caused by a drop in blood pressure or heart rate.

T

Tamponade: Compression of an organ or vessel by accumulated fluid or pressure.

Tension Pneumothorax: A life-threatening condition where air trapped in the chest compresses the lungs and heart.

Thoracostomy: Surgical creation of a chest opening to allow fluid or air to escape.

Thyroid Autonomy: A condition where parts of the thyroid function independently of regulation, possibly causing hyperthyroidism.

Tinnitus: Ringing or buzzing in the ears, sometimes from head trauma or barotrauma.

Tonic-Clonic Seizure: A seizure with muscle stiffening followed by rhythmic jerking; often results in postictal confusion.

Tooth Anatomy: Includes the crown, enamel, dentin, pulp, and root; damage or infection may require field management.

Torsion: Twisting of an organ such as the testicle or ovary, cutting off blood flow and causing acute pain.

Tourniquet: A tight band used to stop severe limb bleeding when pressure fails.

Toxic Epidermal Necrolysis: A life-threatening skin condition with widespread blistering and peeling, usually drug-induced.

Trauma: Physical injury from external forces like falls, weapons, or vehicle crashes.

Triage: The process of prioritizing patients based on injury severity and available resources.

Trismus: Inability to open the jaw fully, often due to infection, trauma, or tetanus.

Tympanic Membrane: The eardrum; injury can occur from pressure changes or trauma.

U

Ultrasound: A diagnostic tool that uses sound waves to visualize internal structures; portable versions are increasingly used in wilderness medicine.

Urosepsis: A systemic infection originating from the urinary tract, requiring antibiotics and evacuation.

Urticaria: Another name for hives; often part of an allergic response.

V

Vasoconstriction: Narrowing of blood vessels, which raises blood pressure and redirects blood flow.

Vasodilation: Widening of blood vessels, reducing blood pressure and increasing blood flow.

Vasovagal Syncope: Fainting caused by sudden drop in heart rate and blood pressure, often from stress or pain.

Vector: An organism that transmits disease, such as mosquitoes or ticks.

Venom: Toxic substance delivered by bites or stings, may cause systemic effects.

Ventilation: The process of moving air into and out of the lungs, essential for oxygenation and carbon dioxide removal.

Vertigo: A sensation of spinning or dizziness may be inner ear or neurologic in origin.

Virus: Microscopic infectious agents that replicate within host cells, causing various diseases.

Visceral: Relating to the organs within body cavities, such as visceral peritoneum covering abdominal organs.

W

Wheezing: High-pitched whistling sound during breathing, usually due to narrowed airways.

Wilderness First Responder: An advanced wilderness medical provider trained in field care and evacuation.

Wound Irrigation: The process of flushing a wound with clean fluid to remove debris and reduce infection risk.

X

Xerosis: Abnormal dryness of the skin, common in cold, dry environments and can lead to cracking or infection.

Xiphoid Process: The lower tip of the sternum, a key landmark in CPR and chest trauma.

Y

Yellow Fever: A mosquito-borne viral disease with fever, jaundice, and bleeding risk; preventable by vaccination.

Z

Zika Virus: A mosquito-borne infection that may cause fever, rash, or birth defects.

Zipper Injury: Soft tissue trauma caused by clothing fasteners; may involve genitals or skin folds.

Zoonosis: A disease that can be transmitted from animals to humans, including rabies and leptospirosis.

References

Things to Know

1. World Health Organization. *Drinking-water.* Updated June 14, 2023. Accessed April 12, 2025. https://www.who.int/news-room/fact-sheets/detail/drinking-water.
2. U.S. Food and Drug Administration. *Antibacterial Soap? You Can Skip It—Use Plain Soap and Water.* Last modified September 2, 2020. https://www.fda.gov/consumers/consumer-updates/antibacterial-soap-you-can-skip-it-use-plain-soap-and-water.
3. U.S. Food and Drug Administration. *FDA Issues Final Rule on Safety and Effectiveness of Antibacterial Soaps.* Last modified September 2, 2016. https://www.fda.gov/news-events/press-announcements/fda-issues-final-rule-safety-and-effectiveness-antibacterial-soaps.
4. Centers for Disease Control and Prevention. *Show Me the Science—How to Wash Your Hands.* Last modified November 15, 2022. https://www.cdc.gov/handwashing/show-me-the-science-handwashing.html.

Environmental Emergencies

1. National Safety Council. *Injury Facts.* https://injuryfacts.nsc.org.
2. Centers for Disease Control and Prevention. *Heat-Related Illness and Death.* https://www.cdc.gov/mmwr.
3. Zhao Q, Guo Y, Ye T, et al. Global, regional, and national burden of mortality associated with non-optimal

ambient temperatures: a systematic analysis. *Lancet Planet Health.* 2021;5(7):e415–e425.

4. Holle RL. Lightning: understanding and mitigation. In: Auerbach PS, ed. *Wilderness Medicine.* 7th ed. Elsevier; 2017.
5. National Weather Service. *Lightning Fatalities.* https://www.weather.gov/safety/lightning-fatalities.
6. Cherington M. Neurologic manifestations of lightning strikes. *Neurology.* 2003;60(2):182–185.
7. Hackett PH, Roach RC. High-altitude illness. *N Engl J Med.* 2001;345(2):107–114.
8. Basnyat B, Murdoch DR. High-altitude illness. *Lancet.* 2003;361(9373):1967–1974.
9. Isbister GK, Fan HW. Spider bite. *Lancet.* 2011;378(9808):2039–2047.
10. Vetter RS, Isbister GK. Medical aspects of spider bites. *Annu Rev Entomol.* 2003;53:409–429.
11. White J. Clinical toxicology of spider bites. In: Meier J, White J, eds. *Handbook of Clinical Toxicology of Animal Venoms and Poisons.* CRC Press; 1995:491–522.
12. Bush SP, King BO, Norris RL, Stockwell SA. Bites of the brown recluse spider and suspected necrotic arachnidism. *N Engl J Med.* 1995;332(9):523–527.
13. Bucaretchi F, Deus Reinaldo CR, Hyslop S, et al. A clinico-epidemiological study of bites by spiders of the genus *Phoneutria. Rev Inst Med Trop Sao Paulo.* 2000;42(1):17–21.
14. Diaz JH. The global epidemiology, syndromic classification, management, and prevention of spider bites. *Am J Trop Med Hyg.* 2004;71(2):239–250.
15. Maretić Z. *Loxosceles* and *Latrodectus* envenomations in Europe: a review. *Toxicon.* 1987;25(4):461–471.
16. Binford GJ. An analysis of venom gland transcriptomes from six-eyed sand spiders reveals toxin diversity and clues to evolutionary relationships. *Toxicon.* 2001;39(7):949–957.
17. Rash LD, Hodgson WC. Pharmacology and biochemistry of spider venoms. *Toxicon.* 2002;40(3):225–254.

18. Isbister GK, Seymour JE, Gray MR, Raven RJ. Bites by spiders of the family Theraphosidae in humans and canines. *Toxicon.* 2003;41(4):519–524.
19. Sutherland SK. *Australian Animal Toxins: The Creatures, Their Toxins and Care of the Poisoned Patient.* Oxford University Press; 1983.
20. Graudins A, Padula M, Broady K, Nicholson GM. Red-back spider (*Latrodectus hasselti*) antivenom prevents the toxicity of widow spider venoms. *Ann Emerg Med.* 2001;37(2):154–160.
21. Julian AF, King CM. Katipo spider bite in New Zealand: a review. *N Z Med J.* 1997;110(1052):48–50.
22. Bauer D, Varadi L, Budai P. False widow spider (*Steatoda grossa*) envenomation: case report and literature review. *Clin Toxicol.* 2020;5(5):456–460.
23. World Health Organization. *Snakebite Envenoming: A Strategy for Prevention and Control.* Accessed June 17, 2025. https://www.who.int/publications/i/item/9789241515641.
24. Kasturiratne A, Wickremasinghe AR, de Silva N, et al. The global burden of snakebite: a literature analysis and modelling based on regional estimates of envenoming and deaths. *PLoS Med.* 2008;5(11):e218. doi:10.1371/journal.pmed.0050218.
25. Smith TS, Herrero S, DeBruyn TD, Wilder JM. Efficacy of bear deterrent spray in Alaska. *J Wildl Manage.* 2008;72(3):640–645.
26. Clarke J. Does bear spray work on mountain lions? *Adventure.com.* Last modified June 26, 2024. https://adventure.com/.
27. U.S. Fish & Wildlife Service: Interagency Grizzly Bear Committee. *Bear Spray Safety Program.* Accessed June 17, 2025. https://www.wikipedia.org/.
28. Geng XY, Wang MK, Chen JH, Xiao L, Yang JS. Marine biological injuries and their medical management: a narrative review. *World J Biol Chem.* 2023;14(1):1–12. doi:10.4331/wjbc.v14.i1.1.

29. Moulin R, Joubert C, Chabanet P, et al. Clinical features of 27 shark attack cases on La Réunion Island. *J Trauma Acute Care Surg.* 2017;5(1). doi:10.1097/TA.0000000000001399.

Infectious & Travel-Related Diseases

1. World Health Organization. Yellow fever vaccine. *Wkly Epidemiol Rec.* 2013;88(27):269–284. https://www.who.int/publications/i/item/WER8827.
2. Centers for Disease Control and Prevention. *Hepatitis A Questions and Answers for Health Professionals.* https://www.cdc.gov/hepatitis/hav/havfaq.htm.
3. World Health Organization. Typhoid vaccines. *Wkly Epidemiol Rec.* 2018;93(13):153–172. https://www.who.int/publications/i/item/WER9313.
4. Centers for Disease Control and Prevention. *Rabies Pre-exposure Prophylaxis.* https://www.cdc.gov/rabies/medical_care/pre-exposure.html.
5. Centers for Disease Control and Prevention. *Japanese Encephalitis Vaccination.* https://www.cdc.gov/japaneseencephalitis/vaccine/index.html.
6. World Health Organization. Cholera vaccines. *Wkly Epidemiol Rec.* 2017;92(34):477–498. https://www.who.int/publications/i/item/WER9234.
7. Centers for Disease Control and Prevention. *Meningococcal ACWY Vaccination.* https://www.cdc.gov/vaccines/vpd/mening/public/index.html.
8. Centers for Disease Control and Prevention. *Polio Vaccination: What Everyone Should Know.* https://www.cdc.gov/vaccines/vpd/polio/public/index.html.
9. Centers for Disease Control and Prevention. Vaccine effectiveness: how well do the flu vaccines work? https://www.cdc.gov/flu/vaccines-work/vaccineeffect.htm.
10. Centers for Disease Control and Prevention. *COVID-19 Vaccine Effectiveness.* https://www.cdc.gov/coronavirus/2019-ncov/vaccines/effectiveness/index.html.

11. Centers for Disease Control and Prevention. *Measles, Mumps, and Rubella (MMR) Vaccination: What Everyone Should Know.* https://www.cdc.gov/vaccines/vpd/mmr/public/index.html.
12. Centers for Disease Control and Prevention. *Tetanus Vaccination.* https://www.cdc.gov/vaccines/vpd/tetanus/public/index.html.
13. Centers for Disease Control and Prevention. *Malaria: Prophylaxis.* https://www.cdc.gov/malaria/travelers/drugs.html.
14. Centers for Disease Control and Prevention. *Pneumococcal Vaccination: What Everyone Should Know.* https://www.cdc.gov/vaccines/vpd/pneumo/public/index.html.
15. Centers for Disease Control and Prevention. *Shingles Vaccination: What Everyone Should Know.* https://www.cdc.gov/vaccines/vpd/shingles/public/index.html.
16. Shattock AJ, Johnson HC, Sim SY, et al. Contribution of vaccination to improved survival and health: modelling 50 years of the Expanded Programme on Immunization. *Lancet.* 2024;403(10383):917-926. doi:10.1016/S0140-6736(23)02198-7.
17. Global Polio Eradication Initiative. *Polio Eradication Progress Report.*
18. World Health Organization. *The Global Eradication of Smallpox: Final Report.* Geneva: WHO.
19. Souayah N, Yacoub HA, Khan HM, et al. Guillain-Barré syndrome after vaccination in United States: a report from the CDC/FDA Vaccine Adverse Event Reporting System. *Vaccine.* 2009;27(52):7150-7154. doi:10.1016/j.vaccine.2009.09.026.
20. McNeil MM, Weintraub ES, Duffy J, et al. Risk of anaphylaxis after vaccination in children and adults. *J Allergy Clin Immunol.* 2016;137(3):868-878. doi:10.1016/j.jaci.2015.07.048.

21. National Safety Council. *Odds of Dying.* https://injuryfacts.nsc.org/all-injuries/preventable-death-overview/odds-of-dying/.
22. Li G, Warner M, Lang BH, et al. Epidemiology of anesthesia-related mortality in the United States, 1999–2005. *Anesthesiology.* 2009;110(4):759–765. doi:10.1097/ALN.0b013e31819b5a7d.
23. Steffen R, Amitirigala I, Mutsch M. Health risks among travelers—need for regular updates. *J Travel Med.* 2008;15(3):145–146.
24. Connor BA. Travelers' diarrhea. In: *CDC Yellow Book 2024.* https://wwwnc.cdc.gov/travel/yellowbook/2024/posttravel-evaluation/general-approach-to-the-returned-traveler.
25. Centers for Disease Control and Prevention. *Global Rabies: What You Should Know.* Accessed April 21, 2025. https://www.cdc.gov/rabies/around-world/index.html.
26. World Health Organization. *Global Tuberculosis Report 2023.* Geneva: WHO; 2023. https://www.who.int/publications/i/item/9789240079722.
27. World Health Organization. *Middle East Respiratory Syndrome Coronavirus (MERS-CoV).* Accessed April 21, 2025. https://www.who.int/health-topics/middle-east-respiratory-syndrome-coronavirus-mers.
28. Khidir RJY, Ibrahim BAY, Adam MHM, et al. Prevalence and outcomes of hyponatremia among COVID-19 patients: a systematic review and meta-analysis. *Int J Health Sci (Qassim).* 2022;16(5):69–84. PMID:36101848; PMCID:PMC9441642.
29. World Health Organization. *World Malaria Report 2023.* Geneva: WHO; 2023.
30. Centers for Disease Control and Prevention. Malaria's impact worldwide. Last modified November 6, 2023. https://www.cdc.gov/malaria/php/impact/index.html.
31. Bhatt S, Gething PW, Brady OJ, et al. The global distribution and burden of dengue. *Nature.* 2013;496(7446):504–507.

32. World Health Organization. Disease outbreak news: dengue situation update. Last modified April 2024. https://www.who.int/emergencies/disease-outbreak-news/item/2024-DON518.
33. Ivers LC. Cholera in Haiti: the equity agenda and the future of tropical medicine. *Am J Trop Med Hyg.* 2017;97(3):501–503. doi:10.4269/ajtmh.16-0781.
34. World Health Organization. *Cholera.* Accessed April 21, 2025. https://www.who.int/news-room/fact-sheets/detail/cholera.
35. Snow J. *On the Mode of Communication of Cholera.* London: John Churchill; 1849.
36. Centers for Disease Control and Prevention. *Guinea Worm Disease (Dracunculiasis).* Accessed April 21, 2025. https://www.cdc.gov/parasites/guineaworm.
37. Centers for Disease Control and Prevention. *Naegleria fowleri – Primary Amebic Meningoencephalitis (PAM).* Accessed April 21, 2025. https://www.cdc.gov/parasites/naegleria.
38. Olival KJ, Anthony SJ, Allen T, et al. *A Global Perspective on Emerging Zoonotic Diseases.* Springer; 2021.

Medical Emergencies

1. Troeger C, Blacker BF, Khalil IA, et al. Estimates of the global, regional, and national morbidity, mortality, and aetiologies of diarrhoea in 195 countries: a systematic analysis for the Global Burden of Disease Study 2016. *Lancet Infect Dis.* 2018;18(11):1211–1228. doi:10.1016/S1473-3099(18)30362-1.
2. Hristova M, Angelova M. International miscarriage rates: a comprehensive overview of prevalence and causes. *J IMAB.* 2024;30(3):5703–5709.

Traumatic Injuries in Wilderness Settings

1. McIntosh SE, Campbell AD, Dow J, Grissom CK. Wilderness Medical Society practice guidelines for

the prevention and treatment of acute injuries and illnesses in backcountry environments. *Wilderness Environ Med.* 2019;30(4S):S33–S70. doi:10.1016/j.wem.2019.05.005.

2. Smith WR, Hill RR, Berona K, Zafren K. Patterns of injury and illness during wilderness travel. *Wilderness Environ Med.* 2018;29(2):151–160. doi:10.1016/j.wem.2017.10.004.
3. Johnson DE, Rock PB, Bärtsch P. Environmental physiology of mountaineering: altitude illness and cold injury. *Clin Sports Med.* 2020;3(4):693–708. doi:10.1016/j.csm.2020.06.004.
4. Holmes JF, Akkinepalli R. Computed tomography versus plain radiography to screen for cervical spine injury: a meta-analysis. *J Trauma.* 2005;58(5):902–905.
5. Campbell JE, Li F, Martin DJ, et al. Prehospital pelvic binders and survival in pelvic fractures: a retrospective cohort study. *Injury.* 2024;55(1):35–41. doi:10.1016/j.injury.2023.11.015.
6. Faculty of Pre-Hospital Care, Royal College of Surgeons of Edinburgh. *The Pre-Hospital Management of Pelvic Fractures: Consensus Statement.* 2019. Accessed May 24, 2025. https://fphc.rcsed.ac.uk/media/1765/the-pre-hospital-management-of-pelvic-fractures.pdf.
7. World Health Organization. *Burns.* Last modified March 6, 2018. https://www.who.int/news-room/fact-sheets/detail/burns.
8. World Health Organization. *Drowning.* Last modified July 25, 2023. https://www.who.int/news-room/fact-sheets/detail/drowning.

Pain Control & Practical Pharmacology for Guides

1. Chang AK, Bijur PE, Esses D, Barnaby DP, Baer J. Effect of a single dose of oral opioid and nonopioid analgesics on acute extremity pain in the emergency department: a randomized clinical trial. *JAMA.* 2017;318(17):1661–1667. doi:10.1001/jama.2017.16190.

About the Author

Jason Moore is a wilderness medicine expert, guide, and educator whose nearly three-decade career blends exploration, teaching, and a commitment to safety in remote environments. His extensive experience—as both a medical provider and expedition leader—has shaped a practical understanding of the challenges faced in the field.

He has worked and traveled in some of the world's most remote places, from first-descent river expeditions in Tibet and Costa Rica to atolls in the Pacific and Indian Oceans, as well as the Amazon, Africa, and Australia. These experiences sharpened his approach to medical preparedness and deepened his respect for the unpredictability of the natural world.

An accomplished educator, author, and adventure angler, Jason is the founder of Island Fly, a premier fly-fishing outfitter, and an international host who shares his expertise through guide training, guest lectures, educational and media platforms.

As a clinician-scholar, Dr. Moore brings extensive experience in general and trauma surgery, critical care, and emergency medicine, with a PhD in epidemiology and public health complementing his clinical practice. Through peer-reviewed research, medical texts, field publications, and education, his work reflects a consistent commitment to advancing medical knowledge and practice.

His rare blend of field experience, clinical skill, and academic insight makes him a valued resource for those seeking both adventure and confidence in remote environments.

www.ingramcontent.com/pod-product-compliance
Lightning Source LLC
Chambersburg PA
CBHW042313210326
41599CB00038B/7111
9798892854382